PHARMACY REVIEW

ARCO MEDICAL REVIEW SERIES

PHARMACY REVIEW

SECOND EDITION

Walter Singer, Ph.D.
Dean and Professor of Pharmacy

Gary D. Hall, M.S.
Associate Professor of Pharmacy

Thomas E. Platek, Pharm.D.
Associate Clinical Professor of Pharmacy

Barry S. Reiss, Ph.D.
Associate Professor of Pharmacy

Albany College of Pharmacy
Union University
Albany, N.Y.

ARCO PUBLISHING, INC.
NEW YORK

Second Edition, First Printing, 1980

Published by Arco Publishing, Inc.
219 Park Avenue South, New York, N.Y. 10003

Library of Congress Cataloging in Publication Data

Main entry under title:

Pharmacy review.

(Arco medical review series)
Bibliography: p. *xiii*
1. Pharmacy—Examinations, questions, etc.
I. Singer, Walter.
RS98.P54 1980 615'.1'076 79-22434
ISBN 0-668-04878-6

Printed in the United States of America

Contents

Preface		*vii*
Professional Competency in Pharmacy		*ix*
Helpful Hints		*xi*
References		*xiii*
Chapter 1	PRETEST	1
	Answers	6
Chapter 2	PHARMACEUTICAL CHEMISTRY	8
	Answers and Commentary	25
Chapter 3	PHARMACOLOGY	39
	Answers and Commentary	52
Chapter 4	PHARMACEUTICAL CALCULATIONS	62
	Answers and Commentary	68
Chapter 5	PHARMACY	76
	Answers and Commentary	101
Chapter 6	BIOPHARMACEUTICS AND PHARMACOKINETICS	123
	Answers and Commentary	131
Chapter 7	CLINICAL PHARMACY	138
	Answers and Commentary	162
Chapter 8	POST-TEST	182
	Answers and Commentary	188

Preface

Pharmacy licensing examinations are designed to determine whether the applicant has the requisite ability to carry out the responsibilities of the profession. A candidate preparing for a licensing examination is faced with establishing competency in several fields, any one of which may be the subject for intensive questioning or which, alternatively in some years in some examinations, may hardly be touched upon at all.

This book is designed for self-testing to identify areas of weakness, for subject review, and for self-teaching. A pretest and post-test are provided for separate evaluations at the start and finish of the study period. Within the chapters, some questions have been ordered into groups on the basis of similar chemistry or pharmacology or use. Many questions have intentionally not been ordered so that there can be periodic reinforcement of prior learning of topic areas by return to them in later questions. Some comments are quite extensive and represent miniature reviews. Others are limited to brief specifics. The test items and comments relate to professional and scientific topics and not to legal or commercial considerations.

Passing the licensing examination does not guarantee continued competence. Practicing pharmacists must retain much of the knowledge and skill that they gain early in their professional education and careers and, in addition, they must somehow keep current with contemporary modes of practice over a long professional life. What is written above about the utility of this book for preparing for a licensing examination applies equally well to its other goal of providing a means for self-assessment of competency to practice and for stimulation of purposeful guided review. There are those who advocate mandatory periodic re-examination for relicensure. Voluntary self re-examination and subsequent study of areas of lesser competency is a more palatable avenue to achieving the desired goal.

A statement of professional competency in pharmacy that is distributed by the California State Board of Pharmacy is reproduced herewith. Test items in this book relate to those competencies in this statement that we have been able to fit into the selected format.

Professional Competency in Pharmacy

A competent pharmacist is capable of conferring with a physician concerning the care and treatment of his patient. He should appreciate the essentials of the clinical diagnosis and comprehend the medical management of the patient. He should have a knowledge of the drugs that may be used in the treatment of the patient's disease state, their mechanism of action, their commercial drug combinations and dosage forms, the fate and disposition of the drugs (if known), the factors which may influence the physiological availability and biological activity of the drugs from their dosage forms; how the age, sex, or secondary disease states might influence the course of treatment; and how other administered drugs, foods, and diagnostic procedures may interact to modify the activity of the drug.

A competent pharmacist is one whose overall functions result in optimum drug therapy. He should know the appropriate use and dosage regimen for the drug therapy being undertaken and the contraindications and potential untoward reactions which may result during therapy. He should be informed as to what proprietary products might interact adversely with such therapy or may be useful adjuncts to improve the convenience of administration or the overall patient care.

A competent pharmacist must know the proposed therapeutic actions of proprietary medications, their composition, and any uniqueness or potential limitations of their dosage forms. He should be capable of an objective appraisal of the advertising claims for the product. When requested by the patient, he should be capable of ascertaining the probable therapeutic usefulness of available proprietary medication in relation to the patient's complaints.

A competent pharmacist should be able to review a scientific publication and be able to summarize the practical implications of the findings as they may relate to the clinical use of drugs. He should be able to analyze a literature report of a clinical trial as to the appropriateness of the design of the study and of the statistical analysis made of the data. He should be able to prepare an objective summary of the significance of the data and the author's conclusions.

A competent pharmacist is a specialist on the stability characteristics and storage requirements of drugs and drug products, on the factors that influence the release of drugs from dosage forms, how the site of administration or environment within its location in the body may influence the absorption of a specific drug from the administered dosage form, and most importantly, how these may interact to influence the onset, intensity, or duration of therapeutic action.

A competent pharmacist should be precisely informed of the legal limitations on procurement, storage, distribution, and sale of drugs. He should be informed of the approved use of a drug as specified by federal authorities and acceptable medical practice and his legal responsibilities to the patient in the use of drugs in experimental therapeutic procedures.

A competent pharmacist should be capable, with the availability of appropriate source material, of recommending which drug product and/or dosage form may be potentially most useful for a particular therapeutic need, and he should be able to support objectively his choice. He should also be capable, within a reasonable time, of identifying a drug product on the basis of its described color and shape, and possibly its proposed use, using appropriate source material.

A competent pharmacist, on the basis of the symptoms described in an interview with the patient, should be aware of what additional information he should attempt to gain from the patient concerning his condition. Based on this information, he should be able to refer the patient to the proper medical practitioner, specialist, or agency which may be of most help to him in his case.

A competent pharmacist should have a knowledge of the toxic manifestations of drugs and the necessary measures which are the best available means of treatment of these toxic symptoms.

A competent pharmacist should be able to communicate effectively with a patient on the instructions for proper administration of prescription and proprietary drugs. He should know the limitations which should be placed on food intake, other medication, and physical activity.

A competent pharmacist should be able to communicate with other health professionals or to laymen on appropriate drug subjects. He should be able to make the recipient understand the contents of the message being communicated.

A competent pharmacist should be capable of compounding appropriate drugs or combinations in acceptable dosage forms.

Finally, a competent pharmacist is a person who undertakes appropriate measures to maintain his level of competency in each of the above areas.

Helpful Hints

There are several ways to maximize learning from this review book. For example, the reader could answer a short series of questions before looking for the answers at the end of the chapter. Keeping score will make these become miniature tests. If not sure of an answer, rather than guessing, look it up in the referenced book or a related one before checking the answer section. If your answer then does not agree with the one given herein, check it out again, perhaps in another source. Keep digging; learning cannot be passive. Recognize that a question which says "which of these does *not*" or "all of these *except*" gives you four statements or phrases which *do* apply positively and these should be considered a part of the commentary. Use the built-in internal review feature; if a question or commentary seems familiar to you, look back for the other one to affirm the relationship.

References

A numbered list of references is provided below. With the intention of encouraging the user of this book to enlarge his or her personal library, we have deliberately chosen to use multiple sources to support the answers and commentaries. Most are books, but other types (journals, drug information sources, etc.) are cited to stimulate awareness of sources of more frequently updated information. The reader should have available at least a general pharmaceutical science book (e.g., 1, 15, 20b, or 22 from the list), a pharmacology text or review handbook (e.g., 6, 7, 17, 32), a book with a clinical pharmacy orientation (e.g., 30, 31, 33b, 42, 44), a manual or book oriented toward therapy and treatment (e.g., 4, 5, 9, 16, 37), and a pharmaceutical chemistry text (e.g., 38 or 39). Individual interests and needs should dictate any requirement to obtain the specialized books in the areas of physical pharmacy, biopharmaceutics, pharmacokinetics, pharmacy calculations, parenteral medications, drug interactions, nonprescription drugs, etc.

On the last line of each test item there appears a number combination that identifies the reference source and the page or pages where information pertaining to the question and answer may be found. The first number refers to the source, the second to the pages. For example (1:117–19; 38:463) means pages 117 to 119 in the first source on the list and page 463 in the thirty-eighth. For the convenience of the reader, these identification numbers have also been included in the commentary sections of each chapter.

1. Osol, A. *Remington's Pharmaceutical Sciences,* Fifteenth Edition, Mack Publishing Co., Easton, PA: 1975.
2a. Penna, R.P. *Handbook of Non-Prescription Drugs,* Fifth Edition, American Pharmaceutical Association, Washington: 1977.
2b. Penna, R.P. *Handbook of Non-Prescription Drugs,* Sixth Edition, American Pharmaceutical Association, Washington: 1979.
3. Kastrup, E.K. *Facts and Comparisons,* Facts and Comparisons, Inc., St. Louis: 1979.
4. AMA Department of Drugs, *AMA Drug Evaluations,* Third Edition, Publishing Sciences Group, Inc., Acton, MA: 1977.
5. Osol, A. and Pratt, R. *The United States Dispensatory,* Twenty-seventh Edition, J.B. Lippincott Co., Philadelphia: 1973.
6. Goodman, L.S. and Gilman, A. *The Pharmacological Basis of Therapeutics,* Fifth Edition, Macmillan Publishing Co., Inc., New York: 1975.
7. Avery, G.S. *Drug Treatment,* Publishing Sciences Group, Inc., Acton, MA: 1976.
8. Hansten, P.D. *Drug Interactions,* Fourth Edition, Lea & Febiger, Philadelphia: 1979.
9. Costrini, N.V. and Tomson, W.M. *Manual of Medical Therapeutics,* Twenty-second Edition, Little, Brown and Co., Boston: 1977.
10. Product Literature—the drug inserts current in 1978 and 1979.
11. *Dorland's Illustrated Medical Dictionary,* Twenty-fifth Edition, W.B. Saunders Co., Philadelphia: 1974.
12. Martin, A.N., Swarbrick, J., and Cammarata, A. *Physical Pharmacy,* Second Edition, Lea & Febiger, Philadelphia: 1969.
13. Turco, S. and King, R.E. *Sterile Dosage Forms,* Second Edition, Lea & Febiger, Philadelphia: 1979.
14. Parrott, E.L. *Pharmaceutical Technology,* Burgess Publishing Co., Minneapolis: 1970.

15. Sprowls, J.B. *Prescription Pharmacy,* Second Edition, J.B. Lippincott Co., Philadelphia: 1970.

16. Thorn, G.W., et al. *Harrison's Principles of Internal Medicine,* Eighth Edition, McGraw-Hill Book Company, New York: 1977.

17. Meyers, F.H., Jawetz, E., and Goldfein, A. *Review of Medical Pharmacology,* Sixth Edition, Lange Medical Publications, Los Altos, CA: 1978.

18. United States Pharmacopeial Convention, Inc. *The United States Pharmacopeia,* Nineteenth Revision with current supplements, Mack Publishing Co., Easton, PA: 1975.

19. National Formulary Board. *The National Formulary,* Fourteenth Edition, American Pharmaceutical Association, Washington: 1975.

20a. Martin, E.W. *Dispensing of Medication,* Seventh Edition, Mack Publishing Co., Easton, PA: 1971.

20b. Hoover, J.E. *Dispensing of Medication,* Eighth Edition, Mack Publishing Co., Easton, PA: 1976.

21. Trissel, L.A. *Handbook of Injectable Drugs,* American Society of Hospital Pharmacists, Washington: 1977.

22. Dittert, L.W. *Sprowl's American Pharmacy,* Seventh Edition, J.B. Lippincott Co., Philadelphia: 1974.

23. Stoklosa, M.J. *Pharmaceutical Calculations,* Sixth Edition, Lea & Febiger, Philadelphia: 1974.

24. Ansel, H.C. *Introduction to Pharmaceutical Dosage Forms,* Second Edition, Lea & Febiger, Philadelphia: 1976.

25. *Physician's Desk Reference,* Thirty-third Edition, Medical Economics Co., Oradell, N.J.: 1979.

26. Block, J.H., et al. *Inorganic Medicinal and Pharmaceutical Chemistry,* Lea & Febiger: 1974.

27. Wade, A. *Martindale The Extra Pharmacopoeia,* Twenty-seventh Edition, The Pharmaceutical Press, London: 1978.

28. Cadwaller, D.E. *Biopharmaceutics and Drug Interactions,* Roche Laboratories, Nutley, N.J.: 1971.

29. Gibaldi, M. *Biopharmaceutics and Clinical Pharmacokinetics,* Second Edition, Lea & Febiger, Philadelphia: 1977.

30. Francke, D.E. and Whitney, H.A.K., Jr. *Perspectives in Clinical Pharmacy,* Drug Intelligence Publications, Hamilton, IL: 1972.

31. Blissett, C.W., Webb, O.L., and Stanaszek, W.F. *Clinical Pharmacy Practice,* Lea & Febiger, Philadelphia: 1972.

32. Goth, A. *Medical Pharmacology,* Ninth Edition, C.V. Mosby Co., St. Louis: 1978.

33a. Melmon, L.K. and Morrelli, H.F. *Clinical Pharmacology,* Macmillan Publishing Co., Inc., New York: 1972.

33b. Melmon, L.K. and Morrelli, H.F. *Clinical Pharmacology,* Second Edition, Macmillan Publishing Co., Inc., New York: 1978.

34. Notari, R.E. *Biopharmaceutics and Pharmacokinetics,* Second Edition, Marcel Dekker, Inc., New York: 1975.

35. Alexander, S.F., Farage, D.J., and Hassan, W.E., Jr. *Martin's Hazards of Medication,* J.B. Lippincott Co., Philadelphia: 1971.

36. Guyton, A.C. *Function of the Human Body,* Third Edition, W.B. Saunders Co., Philadelphia: 1969.

37. Krupp, M.A. and Chatton, M.J. *Current Medical Diagnosis and Treatment 1979,* Lange Medical Publications, Los Altos, CA: 1979.

38. Wilson, C.O., Gisvold, O., and Doerge, R.F. *Textbook of Organic Medicinal and Pharmaceutical Chemistry,* Seventh Edition, J.B. Lippincott Co., Philadelphia: 1977.

39. Foye, W.O. *Principles of Medicinal Chemistry,* Lea & Febiger, Philadelphia: 1974.

40. *Diabetes Mellitus,* Seventh Edition, Lilly Research Laboratories, Indianapolis: 1973.

41. Morris, W. *The American Heritage Dictionary of the English Language,* American Heritage Publishing Co., New York: 1969.

42. Koda-Kimble, M.A., et al. *Applied Therapeutics for Clinical Pharmacists,* Second Edition, Applied Therapeutics Inc., San Francisco: 1978.

43. Dittert, L.W. and DiSanto, A.R. "The Bioavailability of Drug Products," *J Am Pharm Assoc,* Vol. NS 13, pp. 421–32, 1973.

44. Herfindal, E.T. and Herschman, J.L. *Clinical Pharmacy and Therapeutics,* Williams & Wilkins Co., Baltimore: 1975.

45. Agent, S.K. "Hyperalimentation and Electrolytes," *J Am Pharm Assoc,* Vol. NS 15, pp. 402-05, 1975.

46. Riley, T.N. "Report on New Drugs 1978," *U.S. Pharmacist,* Vol. 4, pp. 50-64, Feb. 1979.

47. Riley, T.N. "Report on New Drugs 1978—Part 2," *U.S. Pharmacist,* Vol. 4, pp. 34-48, Mar. 1979.

48. Madan, P.L., et al. "Total Parenteral Nutrition," *Drug Intell and Clin Pharm,* Vol. 10, pp. 684-96, 1976.

49. Niazi, S. *Textbook of Biopharmaceutics and Clinical Pharmacokinetics,* Appleton-Century-Crofts, New York: 1979.

PHARMACY REVIEW

CHAPTER 1

Pretest

This is a series of 50 representative questions. Correct answers are given without commentaries at the back of the chapter. Each answer is referred to a similar question (with commentary) in one of the chapters. This is explained in the introduction to the answer section, but don't look now. The 50-question post-test at the end of the book is similarly constructed.

The following procedure is suggested. (1) Answer all the pretest questions. (2) Check your answers against those supplied. If you answered 40 or more correctly you demonstrate good competency in our judgment. (3) Then only for the ones you *missed,* try to answer the similar questions in the chapters. If you miss again, you have probably even at this early stage identified areas that you need to study in the cited reference books and journals.

After completing the pretest (and perhaps some reading suggested by this preliminary self-assessment), try the questions in the subsequent chapters. Finally, your performance on the post-test should confirm learning and identify areas still to be reviewed.

Directions: Each of the questions or incomplete statements below is followed by five suggested answers or completions. Select the BEST answer in each case.

1. Terbutaline is used therapeutically as a/an
   A. bronchodilator
   B. nasal decongestant
   C. antiarrthythmic agent
   D. anti-inflammatory agent
   E. miotic

2. Based upon relative sensitivity requirements, the Class A prescription balance is how many times more sensitive than the Class B balance?
   A. two
   B. five
   C. 10
   D. 20
   E. 100

3. A pharmacist adds 30 mL of 6% Diluted Acetic Acid USP to a 1-liter bottle of Sodium Chloride Irrigation USP. What is the percent W/V concentration of acetic acid in the final dilution?
   A. 0.15%
   B. 0.175%
   C. 0.18%
   D. 0.19%
   E. 0.52%

4. Two oral formulations of equal doses of drug A will have equal bioavailability only if
   A. they produce the same blood level a half hour after administration
   B. the same total amount of drug A is absorbed into the systemic circulation from each formulation
   C. they disintegrate in the GI tract at the same rate
   D. they are excreted in the urine at the same rate
   E. they are bound to plasma proteins to the same degree

5. A pharmacist can best prepare 100 ml of Diluted Alcohol USP (49% V/V ethanol) by adding ____ ml of Alcohol USP to ____ ml of purified water.
   A. 47 and 47
   B. 47 and 53
   C. 49 and 51
   D. 50 and 50
   E. 52 and 52

6. Primidone is most similar in chemical structure to
   A. phenytoin
   B. imipramine
   C. primaquine
   D. procainamide
   E. phenobarbital

7. Diazoxide (Hyperstat®), when used parenterally, is indicated for the treatment of
   - A. diabetes
   - B. severe pain
   - C. hypertensive crisis
   - D. manic-depressive psychoses
   - E. shock

8. How much Keri Lotion® must be mixed with 45 g of triamcinolone cream (0.1% W/W) to obtain a final triamcinolone concentration of 0.015%?
   - A. 38.3 g
   - B. 45 g
   - C. 210 g
   - D. 255 g
   - E. 300 g

9. Which of the following antineoplastic agents is metabolized by xanthine oxidase?
   - A. 6-mercaptopurine (Purinethol®)
   - B. vincristine (Oncovin®)
   - C. procarbazine (Matulane®)
   - D. chlorambucil (Leukeran®)
   - E. 6-thioguanine

10. Which of the following is formed in the body as part of the usual action of methenamine mandelate (Mandelamine®)?
    - A. hexylresorcinol
    - B. ethanol
    - C. undecylenic acid
    - D. formaldehyde
    - E. benzocaine

11. How many ml of 17% Zephiran® Chloride Concentrate are needed to prepare 2 quarts of a 1:1000 solution?
    - A. 11.2
    - B. 17.0
    - C. 22.4
    - D. 44.8
    - E. none of the above

12. If a drug has a very small volume of distribution (V_d), it is likely that this drug
    - A. does not accumulate in various tissues and organs
    - B. has a short biological half-life
    - C. is not bioavailable
    - D. will not be effective
    - E. is widely distributed in the body

13. The chemical reaction shown below is an example of

$$C_3H_5\,(C_{16}H_{31}O_2)_3 + 3KOH \rightarrow 3K\,C_{16}H_{31}O_2 + C_3H_5\,(OH)_3$$

    - A. esterification
    - B. neutralization
    - C. hydrolysis
    - D. saponification
    - E. polymerization

14. The cardiac glycoside most irregularly absorbed from the gastrointestinal tract is
    - A. lanatoside C (Cedilanid®)
    - B. ouabain
    - C. digitoxin
    - D. digoxin (Lanoxin®)
    - E. gitalin (Gitaligin®)

15. What is the minimum volume that should be measured in a 100 ml conical graduate that is calibrated in 5-ml intervals from 5 to 100 ml?
    - A. 5 ml
    - B. 10 ml
    - C. 15 ml
    - D. 20 ml
    - E. 30 ml

16. Thrombophlebitis is most likely to occur when a drug is administered by
    - A. intravenous infusion (continuous)
    - B. intravenous push (bolus)
    - C. the intramuscular route
    - D. the subcutaneous route
    - E. the intradermal route

17. How many mg of sodium chloride should be present in the following formula to obtain an isotonic solution? (E value for cocaine hydrochloride is 0.16.)

Cocaine HCl	2.0%
Sodium Chloride	q.s.
Purified Water q.s.	30.0 ml

    - A. 48 mg
    - B. 96 mg
    - C. 174 mg
    - D. 222 mg
    - E. none of these

18. The levo isomer of propoxyphene is indicated for use as a/an
    - A. antitussive
    - B. urinary antiseptic
    - C. analgesic
    - D. anti-inflammatory agent
    - E. nasal decongestant

19. Blood flow through a capillary can best be described by which equation?
   A. Hildebrand
   B. Langmuir
   C. Noyes Whitney
   D. Poiseuille
   E. Stokes

20. Esters of high-molecular-weight alcohols and acids are
   A. stearins
   B. mineral oils
   C. glycols
   D. tweens
   E. waxes

21. Acetylcysteine (Mucomyst®) exerts its mucolytic effect by
   A. complexing with mucus protein
   B. altering the normal synthesis order of DNA
   C. altering the cellular synthesis of RNA
   D. breaking disulfide bonds of mucoproteins
   E. increasing the secretion of low viscosity fluids from the walls of the respiratory tract

22. Which of the following depends on the reduction of cupric ion to cuprous for a positive test?
   A. Benedict's solution
   B. Acetest® Tablets
   C. Tes-Tape®
   D. Ketostix®
   E. Clinistix®

23. Diluted Acetic Acid contains how much pure acetic acid?
   A. 6% W/V
   B. 6% W/W
   C. 10% W/V
   D. 10% W/W
   E. 36% W/W

24. Cholestyramine resin (Cuemid®, Questran®) is primarily used as a
   A. topical protectant
   B. keratolytic
   C. bile acid binder
   D. tyramine antagonist
   E. gallstone solubilizer

25. Determine the number of grains of silver nitrate needed to prepare three fluid ounces of a 0.5% silver nitrate solution.
   A. 2.9 gr
   B. 6.8 gr
   C. 7.2 gr
   D. 22.5 gr
   E. 45 gr

26. Two oral formulations of a drug that have radically different serum concentration–time curves but equal areas under these curves
   A. are bioequivalent
   B. will be equally effective
   C. release the drug from the dosage form at approximately the same rate
   D. release approximately the same total amount of drug
   E. will produce similar peak plasma levels at approximately the same time

27. How many grams of 2% aluminum paste must be mixed with a 10% aluminum paste to prepare exactly 120 g of 5% strength?
   A. 6 g
   B. 24 g
   C. 45 g
   D. 48 g
   E. 75 g

28. Which of the following symptoms is associated with drug-induced Parkinsonism?
   A. dry mouth
   B. constipation
   C. muscular rigidity
   D. convulsions
   E. drowsiness

29. The antihypertensive agent that acts directly to dilate arterioles is
   A. methyldopa (Aldomet®)
   B. hydralazine (Apresoline®)
   C. reserpine (Serpasil®)
   D. mecamylamine (Inversine®)
   E. veratrum alkaloids

30. The following structure is ____ hydroxybenzoic acid.

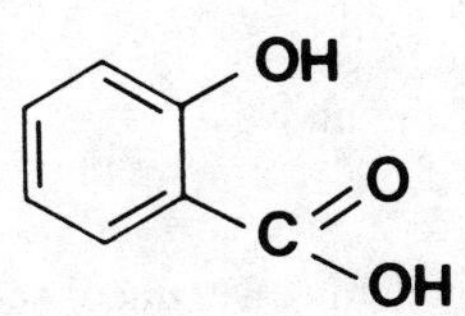

   A. meta-
   B. para-
   C. levo-
   D. ortho-
   E. pseudo-

31. A hospital pharmacy needs 1 gallon of Dilute Hydrochloric Acid USP (10% W/V). How many ml of Hydrochloric Acid USP (36% W/W; specific gravity = 1.18) will be needed?
    A. 320
    B. 378
    C. 891
    D. 1051
    E. 1240

32. Colchicine is usually administered orally in a dose of
    A. 5 mg
    B. 50 μg
    C. 50 mg
    D. 500 μg
    E. 5 μg

33. Doubling the blood concentration of a drug that follows first-order kinetics will
    A. not affect the half-life
    B. double the half-life
    C. increase the half-life by an unpredictable amount
    D. decrease the half-life by half
    E. decrease the half-life by an unpredictable amount

34. One picogram is equivalent to how many nanograms?
    A. 1×10^{-6} ng
    B. 1×10^{-3} ng
    C. 1×10^{-2} ng
    D. 1×10^{3} ng
    E. 1×10^{6} ng

35. Retinoic acid is structurally related to
    A. vitamin D
    B. riboflavin
    C. ascorbic acid
    D. thiamine
    E. none of the above

36. Acute hypoglycemia in an unconscious patient is usually treated with
    A. orange juice or a candy bar
    B. intramuscular cortisone
    C. intravenous glucagon
    D. subcutaneous epinephrine
    E. intravenous glucose

37. How many ml of Zephiran® Chloride Concentrate 17% are needed for the following prescription?

    Rx Zephiran Chloride Conc. q.s.
    Purified Water ad 180 ml
    M & Ft Sol
    Sig: f℥ i dil to f℥ iv = 1:10,000

    A. 0.071
    B. 0.127
    C. 2.03
    D. 2.54
    E. 30.6

38. Which of the following is *not* a pharmacologic effect of epinephrine?
    A. increases heart rate
    B. miosis
    C. increases blood pressure
    D. increases blood glucose levels
    E. bronchodilation

39. The compound formed by reacting theophylline with ethylenediamine is
    A. caffeine
    B. xanthine
    C. theobromine
    D. citrated caffeine
    E. aminophylline

40. Polymyxin B acts as an antibiotic by
    A. interfering with the synthesis of bacterial RNA
    B. promoting the formation of bacterial cell mutants
    C. interfering with the synthesis of bacterial DNA
    D. disrupting the bacterial cytoplasmic membrane
    E. none of the above mechanisms

41. Which of the following is *not* a category of surfactant?
    A. cationic
    B. amphoteric
    C. nonionic
    D. lympholytic
    E. anionic

42. The injection form of calcium gluconate, $Ca(C_7H_{13}O_8)_2$, contains 1 g of drug in 10 ml of solution. How many milliequivalents of calcium are present? (atomic wt. Ca = 40; mol. wt. calcium gluconate = 430)
    A. 0.78
    B. 2.3
    C. 4.7

D. 50
E. none of the above

43. Cyproheptadine (Periactin®) can best be classified pharmacologically as an
A. antihypertensive agent
B. antipsychotic
C. antidepressant
D. anti-inflammatory agent
E. antihistamine

44. If a fixed dose of a drug that is eliminated by first-order kinetics is administered at regular intervals, we would expect
A. the drug to keep accumulating in the blood indefinitely (as long as the drug is being administered)
B. no drug accumulation, because the rate of elimination will always increase sufficiently to prevent it
C. no drug accumulation, because the half-life of the drug is constant
D. the drug to accumulate until the rate of elimination equals the rate of administration
E. none of the above

45. Which of the following terms does *not* relate to the phenomenon of isomerism?
A. isosterism
B. cis-trans
C. conformational
D. equatorial
E. optical enantiomorphs

46. The term pK_a is used to express
A. acid strength
B. potassium ion concentration
C. buffer system potential
D. positive kalium association
E. gas pressure

47. Wilson's disease has been successfully treated by the administration of
A. gentamicin
B. propantheline
C. calcium lactate
D. thyroglobulin
E. penicillamine

48. The structure pictured below is characteristic of

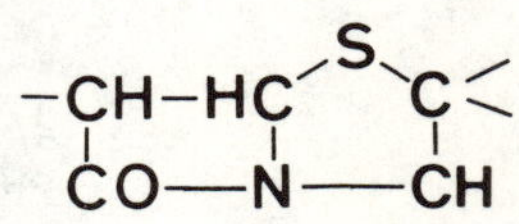

A. cephalosporins
B. thiazides
C. thiobarbiturates
D. penicillins
E. thioguanines

49. The hematocrit is useful for evaluating erythrocytes. It is a percentage expression reflecting the
A. amount of iron present in red blood cells
B. colorimetric red color of red blood cells
C. ratio of neutrophils to basophils
D. ratio of packed red cells to total blood volume
E. ratio of red blood cells to white blood cells

50. Which one of the following products for total parenteral nutrition does *not* contain a supply of nitrogen?
A. Amigen®
B. Aminosol®
C. CPH®
D. Intralipid®
E. all are sources of nitrogen

Pretest Answers

In the answer to question 1, the "A. (Pcol:21)" means A is the correct answer and a related question with an explanatory comment will be number 21 in the Pharmacology chapter (Chapter 3). The abbreviations used for the chapters are shown below.

Chapter Abbreviations

Abbreviations	*Chapter*
Ph Chem	Pharmaceutical Chemistry
Pcol	Pharmacology
Ph Calc	Pharmaceutical Calculations
Pharm	Pharmacy
Biopharm	Biopharmaceutics and Pharmacokinetics
Clin Pharm	Clinical Pharmacy

1. **A.** (Pcol:21)
2. **B.** (Pharm:13)
3. **C.** (Ph Calc: 41)
4. **B.** (Biopharm:1)
5. **E.** (Pharm:35)
6. **E.** (Pcol:28)
7. **C.** (Pcol:101)
8. **D.** (Ph Calc:50)
9. **A.** (Clin Pharm:184, 185)
10. **D.** (Pcol:109)
11. **A.** (Ph Calc:7)
12. **A.** (Biopharm:25)
13. **D.** (Ph Chem:96, 164)
14. **B.** (Pcol:64)
15. **D.** (Pharm:15)
16. **A.** (Clin Pharm:89)
17. **C.** (Ph Calc:47)
18. **A.** (Pcol:87)
19. **D.** (Pharm:37)
20. **E.** (Ph Chem:78)
21. **D.** (Pcol:10)
22. **A.** (Ph Chem:13, 14)
23. **A.** (Pharm:115)
24. **C.** (Pcol:13)
25. **B.** (Ph Calc:15)
26. **D.** (Biopharm:48)
27. **E.** (Ph Calc:14)
28. **C.** (Clin Pharm:10)
29. **B.** (Pcol:121)
30. **D.** (Ph Chem:147, 154)
31. **C.** (Ph Calc:26)
32. **D.** (Pcol:70)
33. **A.** (Biopharm:58)
34. **B.** (Ph Calc:2)
35. **E.** (Pcol:18)
36. **E.** (Clin Pharm:182)
37. **D.** (Ph Calc:40)
38. **B.** (Clin Pharm:132)

39. **E.** (Ph Chem:6)
40. **D.** (Pcol:38)
41. **D.** (Ph Chem:176–79)
42. **C.** (Ph Calc:19)
43. **E.** (Pcol:111)
44. **D.** (Biopharm:57)
45. **A.** (Ph Chem:21)
46. **A.** (Ph Chem:27)
47. **E.** (Pcol:37)
48. **D.** (Ph Chem:37)
49. **D.** (Pharm:80)
50. **D.** (Clin Pharm:226)

CHAPTER 2

Pharmaceutical Chemistry

Pharmaceutical chemistry has advanced from its early emphasis on synthesis and chemical structure and reactions to encompass many elements of pharmacology, biochemistry, and molecular biology. The test items in this chapter reflect this, although a considerable effort has been made to focus on the chemical aspects. Some quite elementary chemistry is also touched upon.

Directions: Each of the questions or incomplete statements below is followed by five suggested answers or completions. Select the BEST answer in each case.

1. Which of the following antihypertensive agents is most similar in chemical structure to hydrochlorothiazide?
   - A. hydralazine
   - B. methyldopa
   - C. guanethidine
   - D. diazoxide
   - E. reserpine (1:783; 33b:198)

2. Which of the following oral hypoglycemic agents is *not* a sulfonylurea?
   - A. Tolinase®
   - B. Diabinese®
   - C. Dymelor®
   - D. Orinase®
   - E. DBI® (37:764–65)

3. Benzalkonium chloride is a germicidal surfactant which is rendered inactive in the presence of
   - A. organic acids
   - B. gram-negative organisms
   - C. cationic surfactants
   - D. soaps
   - E. inorganic salts (6:1001–02)

4. Diphenoxylate (Lomotil®) is an agent useful in the treatment of diarrhea. It is structurally similar to
   - A. kaolin
   - B. meperidine
   - C. phenytoin
   - D. pectin
   - E. oxalic acid (38:681, 698)

5. Which of the following anesthetics is *not* a volatile liquid at normal room temperature and atmospheric pressure?
   - A. cyclopropane
   - B. halothane
   - C. ether
   - D. ethyl chloride
   - E. trichloroethylene (38:349–52)

6. Upon exposure to air, aminophylline solutions may develop
   - A. crystals of theophylline
   - B. a gas
   - C. a precipitate of aminophylline
   - D. a precipitate of ethylenediamine
   - E. a straw color (1:1067–68; 18:25–26)

7. Which of the following is an aminoquinoline antimalarial?
   - A. chloroquin phosphate (Aralen®)
   - B. quinacrine hydrochloride (Atabrine®)
   - C. proguanil hydrochloride (Guanatol®)
   - D. quinine bisulfate
   - E. pyrimethamine (Daraprim®) (38:255–58)

8. Quinine sulfate
   - A. may be dissolved in water by addition of a small amount of sulfuric acid to convert it to the more soluble bisulfate
   - B. has a sweet, pleasant taste
   - C. is official in the USP as the heptahydrate
   - D. is poorly absorbed from the GI tract
   - E. is not affected by exposure to light (1:1158; 38:255)

9. Quinine is
   A. prepared synthetically
   B. an optical isomer of quinidine
   C. legally available only on prescription
   D. an aminoquinoline
   E. weakly acidic (38:252, 254)

10. Paraldehyde solutions that are exposed to air rapidly become strongly acidic because paraldehyde is easily oxidized to
   A. acetaldehyde
   B. formaldehyde
   C. carbonic acid
   D. formic acid
   E. acetic acid (18:358; 38:370)

11. Petrolatum USP is *not* soluble in
   A. chloroform
   B. ethyl alcohol
   C. ether
   D. benzene
   E. petroleum ether (38:961)

12. Chloroform should be stored in airtight, light-resistant containers at a temperature not above 30°F. In the presence of air, sunlight, or open flames, chloroform is
   A. oxidized to phosgene
   B. unchanged
   C. converted to carbon tetrachloride
   D. hydrolyzed to hydrochloric acid
   E. reduced to methane (38:962)

13. Reagent strips impregnated with glucose oxidase, peroxidase, and orthotolidine are dipped into urine or blood as a test for the presence of glucose. The reaction(s) that occur are
   A. glucose is oxidized to CO_2, which forms carbonic acid, which turns the orthotolidine a blue color
   B. glucose oxidase is reduced to glucose reductase, which converts glucose to a blue color in the presence of orthotolidine and peroxidase
   C. glucose is oxidized to gluconic acid and hydrogen peroxide; then hydrogen peroxide in the presence of peroxidase converts the orthotolidine to a blue substance
   D. sucrose is oxidized by glucose oxidase to glucose, which is oxidized to glucuronic acid by peroxidase and orthotolidine to form a dye
   E. glucose oxidase and atmospheric oxygen oxidize glucose to aldehyde, which undergoes a Schiff test reaction with orthotolidine and peroxidase to yield colored compounds (1:588, 601; 8:450–52)

14. Which of the following is *specific* for the measurement of glucose?
   A. Benedict's solution
   B. Acetest® tablets
   C. Clinitest® tablets
   D. Tes-Tape®
   E. Ketostix®
   (3:1670–71; 8:450–52, 462; 44:283–84)

15. Acetazolamide (Diamox®) is rarely the drug of choice for diuretic therapy because it
   A. is too potent
   B. causes systemic acidosis and alkaline urine
   C. is habit forming
   D. does not exhibit tachyphylaxis
   E. induces enzymes, especially carbonic anhydrases (39:423, 425)

16. Lactic acid is
   A. ethandioic acid
   B. dihydroxysuccinic acid
   C. 2-hydroxypropionic acid
   D. ethanoic acid
   E. cis-butenedioic acid
   (1:1223; 38:83, 966, 967, 972)

17. Which is *not* true for Mineral Oil USP?
   A. an antioxidant may be added to prevent peroxide formation
   B. a mixture of liquid hydrocarbons obtained from petroleum
   C. immiscible with castor oil
   D. miscible with alcohol
   E. specific gravity is less than 1.0
   (1:744; 38:952)

18. A chelate must always contain a/an
   A. multivalent metal
   B. amine group
   C. triple bond
   D. ethylenediamine group
   E. polyoxyethylene chain (38:50, 239)

19. The most common and most stable chelate rings are _____ membered.
   A. three-
   B. four-
   C. six-
   D. eight-
   E. 10- (38:50)

20. Conformation of organic molecules is most commonly determined by which of the following analytical methods?
    A. nuclear magnetic resonance (NMR)
    B. optical rotation
    C. pK determinations
    D. biological assay
    E. mass spectrophotometry
    (1:647–49; 39:87–88)

21. Conformational isomerism is described as
    A. a form of optical isomerism
    B. cis-trans isomerism
    C. possession of a plane of symmetry so that the (+) and (–) rotation around two asymmetric centers is equal and opposite with a resultant cancellation of optical rotatory properties
    D. the nonidentical spatial arrangement of atoms in a molecule, resulting from rotation about one or more simple bonds
    E. the concept that the similarities in physicochemical properties of atoms, groups, radicals, and molecules arise from similar electronic structures
    (38:26; 39:77, 82–84)

22. In the chair conformation of cyclohexane, six hydrogens extend radially outward from an axis passing through the center of the molecules. These hydrogens are termed
    A. axial
    B. asymmetric
    C. bonded
    D. equatorial
    E. peripheral (38:26; 39:85)

23. Oleic acid exists in the cis form. This means
    A. there also exists an optical isomer of oleic acid
    B. two groups of atoms are spatially fixed around a double bond so that they are both on the same side of the molecule
    C. a mirror image of the oleic acid molecule exists
    D. there is asymmetry in the molecule
    E. two groups of atoms are spatially fixed around a double bond so that they are on opposite sides of the molecule (38:27)

24. The two compounds whose formulas follow are best described as

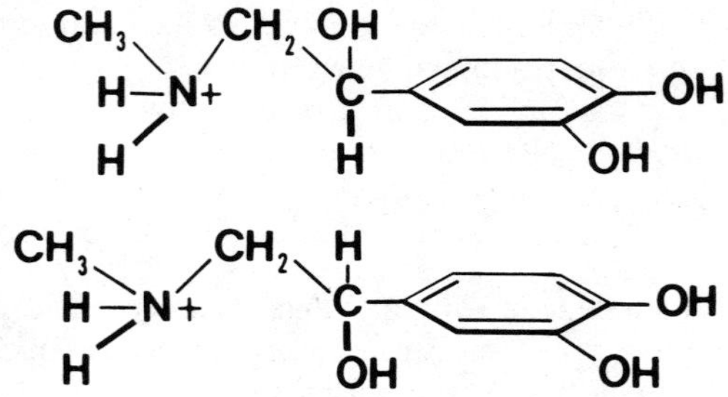

    A. isosteres
    B. diastereoisomers
    C. optical enantiomorphs
    D. conformational isomers
    E. cis-trans isomers (1:179; 38:31–33)

25. The prostaglandins are a group of related
    A. alcohols
    B. aldehydes
    C. alkaloids
    D. fatty acids
    E. amines (6:641; 33b:667–70; 39:30)

26. Which of the following actions is common to clofibrate (Atromid-S®), nicotinic acid, cholestyramine (Cuemid®), sodium dextrothyroxine (Choloxin®), and probucol (Lorelco®)?
    A. antilipemic
    B. hypoglycemic
    C. anticoagulant
    D. antihypertensive
    E. neuroleptic (3:502–13; 6:746–51)

27. The degree of dissociation of acids is often expressed in terms of pK_a. pK_a is
    A. directly measured by titration of the acid with sodium hydroxide
    B. calculated by determining the acid's buffer capacity
    C. directly determined by conductivity measurements
    D. the natural log of the acid's dissociation constant
    E. the reciprocal log of the dissociation constant (12:192)

Answer questions 28 to 30 by referring to the following table as necessary.

Table of pK_a values for acids

Acid	pK_a
acetic	4.76
acetylsalicylic	3.49
boric	9.24
lactic	3.86
salicylic	2.97

28. Which one of the following acids would have the greatest degree of ionization in water?
   A. acetic
   B. boric
   C. hydrochloric
   D. lactic
   E. salicylic (12:208)

29. Which one of the following acids would be considered the weakest (least amount of ionization) in water?
   A. acetic
   B. acetylsalicylic
   C. boric
   D. lactic
   E. salicylic (12:208)

30. To prepare a buffer system with the greatest buffer capacity at a pH of 4.0, one would utilize which one of the following acids?
   A. acetic
   B. acetylsalicylic
   C. boric
   D. lactic
   E. salicylic (12:249)

31. Ibuprofen has a pK_a of 5.5 If the pH of the patient's urine is 7.5, what would the ratio of dissociated to undissociated drug be?
   A. 2:1
   B. 100:1
   C. 20:1
   D. 1:2
   E. 1:100 (1:269)

32. The antipsychotic drug loxapine succinate (Loxitane®) is a ____ compound.
   A. phenothiazine
   B. benzodiazepine
   C. dibenzoxazepine
   D. thioxanthene
   E. butyrophenone (38:400)

33. Which of the following is *not* an androgenic or anabolic substance?
   A. calusterone (Methosarb®)
   B. dydrogesterone (Duphaston®, Gynorest®)
   C. stanozolol (Winstrol®)
   D. norethandrolone (Nilevar®)
   E. nandrolone phenpropionate (Durabolin®) (23:1113–14; 37:753–54, 756)

34. Which of the following antineoplastics is a plant alkaloid?
   A. cytarabine (Cytosar®)
   B. 6-mercaptopurine (Purinethol®)
   C. busulfan (Myleran®)
   D. chlorambucil (Leukeran®)
   E. vincristine (Oncovin®) (1:440, 1086)

35. Which one of the following general characteristics is *not* true for alkaloids?
   A. contain nitrogen in the molecule
   B. have good alcohol solubility
   C. have pK_as less than 7
   D. often exhibit stereoisomerisms
   E. have poor water solubility (1:430)

36. Which of the following antipsychotic drugs is available in three different salt forms for intramuscular injection?
   A. promethazine (Phenergan®)
   B. chlorpromazine (Thorazine®)
   C. fluphenazine (Prolixin®)
   D. haloperidol (Haldol®)
   E. trifluoperazine (Stelazine®) (1:1024)

37. A fused ring system *not* found in any other natural compound is characteristic of penicillins. This ring system is the
   A. isoxazolylidine
   B. allylmercapto
   C. B-lactam thiazolidine
   D. phthalimidomalonalide
   E. penicillinic (38:275, 290)

38. The various penicillins which are available differ chemically
   A. in the nature of the acyl side chain
   B. in substituents on the fused ring nucleus
   C. in spatial arrangements of atoms around an asymmetric carbon
   D. in the nature of the original (naturally occurring) nucleus
   E. only by being different salts (38:274–76)

39. The USP defines a unit of penicillin as
   A. the smallest amount of penicillin that will inhibit, in vitro, the growth of a strain of staphylococcus under specified conditions
   B. the antibiotic activity of 0.6 μg of USP Sodium Penicillin G Reference Standard
   C. equivalent to 1 mg of pure penicillin
   D. the amount of penicillin which will produce a clear ring of 1 cm diameter in the disk assay method under specified conditions
   E. the weight of penicillin which will prevent the development of turbidity in a specified fluid medium after the introduction of 1×10^8 organisms of a nonresistant strain of staphylococcus (38:273)

40. The potassium content of potassium penicillin G is ____ per million units.
   A. 0.1 mEq
   B. 0.6 mEq
   C. 1.7 mEq
   D. 5.0 mEq
   E. 5.7 mEq (17:468, 546)

41. Which of the following penicillins is most readily decomposed in an acid medium?
   A. sodium methicillin (Staphcillin®)
   B. sodium oxacillin (Bactocill®, Prostaphlin®)
   C. potassium penicillin V
   D. ampicillin (Omnipen®, Alpen®)
   E. amoxicillin (Amoxil®, Larotid®) (4:705; 38:281; 39:723)

42. Which of the following penicillins is useful for treating infections caused by staphylococci resistant to penicillin G?
   A. ampicillin (Penbritin®, Polycillin®)
   B. disodium carbenicillin (Geopen®)
   C. hetacillin (Versapen®)
   D. sodium oxacillin (Bactocill®, Prostaphlin®)
   E. penicillin V (V-Cillin®, Pen-Vee®) (4:706; 5:870; 38:281)

43. Which of the following is classified as a broad-spectrum antibiotic?
   A. ampicillin
   B. penicillin G
   C. sodium methicillin
   D. sodium cloxacillin
   E. potassium phenethicillin (4:700; 38:282–84)

44. Which of the following penicillins is used to provide a prolonged duration of action?
   A. phenethicillin potassium (Maxipen®, Syncillin®)
   B. penicillin V (Pen-Vee®, V-Cillin®)
   C. penicillin G benzathine (Bicillin®, Permapen®)
   D. ampicillin trihydrate (Amcill®, Polycillin®)
   E. hetacillin (Versapen®) (1:1131; 38:279)

45. Which of the following penicillin derivatives is both acid-stable and resistant to penicillinase?
   A. methicillin
   B. disodium carbenicillin
   C. ampicillin
   D. oxacillin
   E. penicillin V (39:723)

46. Which of the following is *not* true for Penicillamine USP?
   A. forms nondissociable complex with copper
   B. enzymatically hydrolyzes penicillin
   C. used to treat Wilson's disease
   D. a degradation product of penicillin
   E. effective when taken orally (1:1256; 38:241, 244)

47. Sulfonamides differ chemically in substitutions which are made on a fundamental structure common to all. That structure is:
   A.

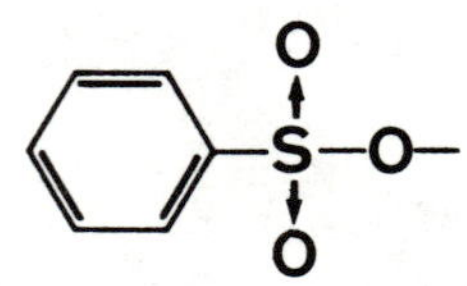

   B.

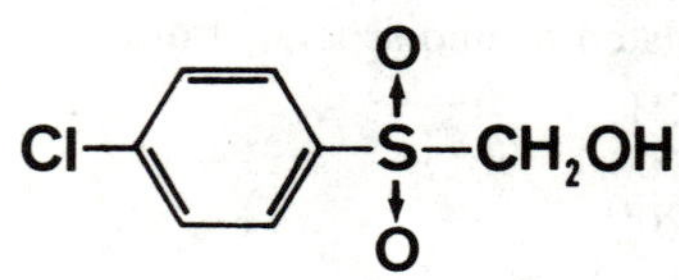

   C.

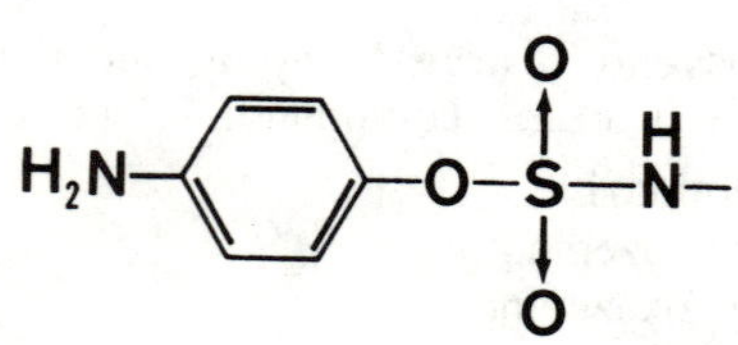

   D.

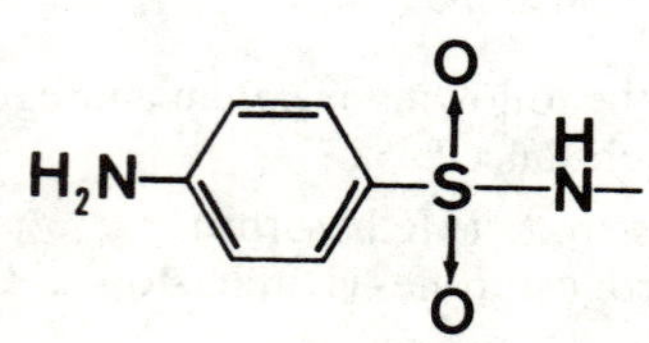

   E.

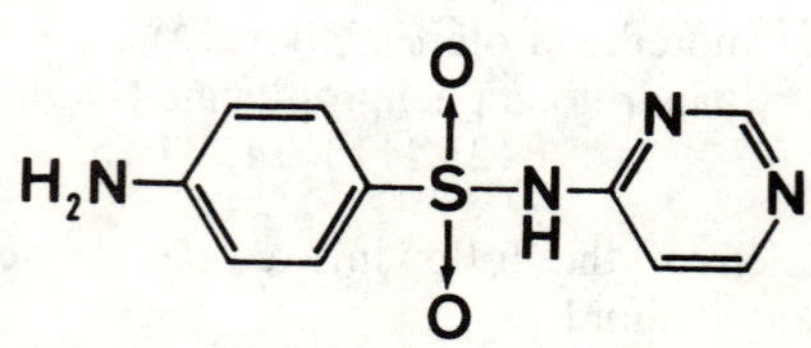

(38:204)

48. To have useful antibacterial activity, a sulfonamide molecule must possess or be capable of conversion in the body into which of the following?
   A. an alkylated aromatic amino group
   B. an alkoxy group
   C. a chloride group
   D. a nonsubstituted aromatic amino group
   E. a free sulfonic acid group (38:205)

49. An aqueous solution of the sodium salt of an antibacterial sulfonamide would be
   A. neutral
   B. strongly basic
   C. weakly acidic
   D. weakly basic
   E. strongly acidic (38:206)

50. A white precipitate will appear in an aqueous sodium sulfadiazine solution which is exposed to the atmosphere. This precipitate is
   A. sodium sulfadiazine
   B. sulfadiazine
   C. sodium oxysulfadiazine
   D. sulfanilamide
   E. acetamide (38:207)

51. Sulfonamides are metabolized by humans principally by
   A. acetylation
   B. deamination
   C. oxidation
   D. conjugation
   E. methylation (38:112–13, 206)

52. The general structure of tetracyclines is an octahydro analogue of naphthacene on which a number of substituents are possible:

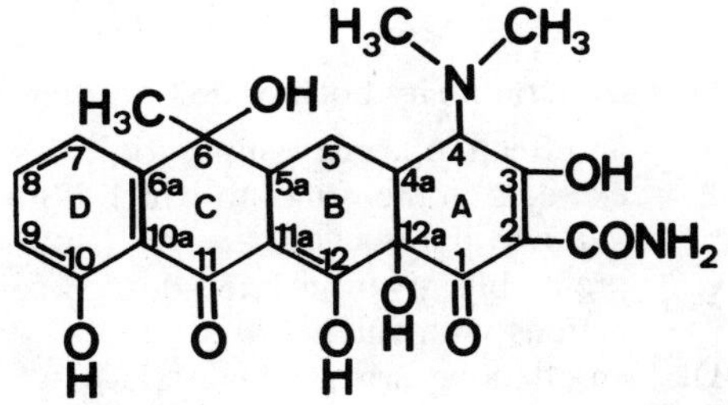

From inspection of this structure, you should expect tetracyclines to be
   A. amphoteric
   B. basic
   C. acidic
   D. neutral
   E. inert (5:1155; 38:306; 39:731)

53. Discarding outdated or improperly stored tetracyclines is especially important because they may
   A. lose all potency
   B. become more likely to cause dental pigmentation
   C. become insoluble and cannot be absorbed
   D. change into more toxic forms
   E. attain an unpleasant odor and taste (5:1175)

54. Streptomycin and other aminoglycoside antibiotics are
   A. ototoxic
   B. carcinogenic
   C. hyperglycemic
   D. hepatotoxic
   E. goiterogenic (5:653; 38:295)

55. Which of the following is *not* closely related in structure to streptomycin?
   A. kanamycin (Kantrex®)
   B. neomycin (Mycifradin®, Neobiotic®)
   C. viomycin (Vinactine®, Viocin®)
   D. gentamicin (Garamycin®)
   E. paromomycin (Humatin®) (4:813; 38:332; 39:706)

56. Linseed oil has good "drying properties" because it
   A. is not easily hydrolyzed
   B. is a monoglyceride
   C. has no double bonds in its molecular structure
   D. is resistant to development of rancidity
   E. has a high degree of unsaturation (1:423)

57. Chemically, fats are
   A. esters of glycerin and fatty acids
   B. polypeptides
   C. compounds of glycerol, fatty acids, phosphoric acid, and choline
   D. steroids with one or more hydroxyl groups
   E. esters of fatty acids with high-molecular-weight alcohols (1:422–24; 38:323)

58. Rancidity of fats may be due to
   A. reduction to alcohols
   B. impurities
   C. oxidation at double bonds
   D. saponification
   E. hydrogenation at double bonds (20b:441)

59. Surfactants are characterized by the presence of
    - A. water-solubilizing groups
    - B. negative charges
    - C. positive charges
    - D. fat-solubilizing groups
    - E. water-solubilizing and fat-solubilizing groups in the same molecule (38:222)

60. Acetone has some limited use in the pharmaceutical industry. Its disadvantages as a solvent include all of the following *except*
    - A. flammability
    - B. poor water miscibility
    - C. high toxicity
    - D. unpleasant odor
    - E. high volatility (38:963–64)

61. A polysaccharide which has been found to be of use as a plasma expander is
    - A. starch
    - B. dextrose
    - C. mannitol
    - D. sorbitol
    - E. dextran (6:767)

62. Lactulose (Cephulac®, Duphalac®) is a
    - A. synthetic disaccharide
    - B. refined lactose
    - C. milk sugar
    - D. polysaccharide
    - E. cellulose derivative (25:1668–69; 27:1338)

63. Which of the following is *not* true of aspirin?
    - A. it has antipyretic activity
    - B. it is very soluble in water
    - C. in the presence of moisture, it hydrolyzes to form salicylic acid and acetic acid
    - D. it has anti-inflammatory activity
    - E. aqueous solutions of aspirin are most stable at pH 2.5 (38:714–16)

64. The anti-inflammatory agent, sulindac (Clinoril®) has the closest structural similarity to
    - A. indomethacin (Indocin®)
    - B. aspirin
    - C. cortisone
    - D. phenylbutazone (Butazolidin®)
    - E. ibuprofen (Motrin®) (10; 25:1140A; 48:35–37)

65. Which one of the following drugs would *not* be converted in the body to the salicylate form?
    - A. aspirin
    - B. salsalate (salicylsalicylic acid, Disalcid®)
    - C. salicylamide
    - D. calcium carbaspirin (Calurin®)
    - E. salol (phenyl salicylate) (2a:126; 3:700; 25:1390; 38:714, 716)

66. Which of the following is a phenothiazine derivative?
    - A. chlorprothixene (Taractan®)
    - B. haloperidol (Haldol®)
    - C. hydroxyzine (Atarax®, Vistaril®)
    - D. thioridazine (Mellaril®)
    - E. chlorcyclizine (Perazil®) (38:388, 398, 400, 662)

67. A phenothiazine derivative that has prominent antihistaminic activity and is also commonly used as a sedative or as an adjunct to anesthetics or narcotics is
    - A. ethopropazine (Parsidol®)
    - B. promethazine (Phenergan®)
    - C. trimeprazine (Temaril®)
    - D. methdilazine (Tacaryl®)
    - E. prochlorperazine (Compazine®) (4:1110–05)

68. A thiazide diuretic can
    - A. enhance action of amphetamines
    - B. antagonize action of guanethidine
    - C. antagonize action of digitalis drugs
    - D. enhance action of oral hypoglycemics
    - E. antagonize action of tricyclic antidepressants (39:432)

69. All of the following are antineoplastic agents. Which one is *not* an alkylating agent?
    - A. chlorambucil (Leukeran®)
    - B. cyclophosphamide (Cytoxan®)
    - C. mechlorethamine hydrochloride (Mustargen®)
    - D. thiotepa
    - E. cytarabine (Cytosar®) (4:1107, 1118; 39:666)

70. Phenazopyridine hydrochloride (Pyridium®) is
    - A. an effective urinary antiseptic
    - B. excreted in the urine, to which it gives a yellow fluorescence
    - C. preferably given in fixed-dosage combinations with sulfas
    - D. an effective urinary analgesic
    - E. curative for cystitis, prostatitis, and urethritis (4:355; 38:160)

71. Piperazine citrate (Antepar®), gentian violet, pyrvinium pamoate (Povan®), and thiabendazole (Mintezol®) are all
    - A. anthelmintics
    - B. dyes

C. antiseptics
D. scabicides
E. anticholinergics (38:145–55)

72. Phenobarbital is a weak acid. To treat acute overdosage you should recommend increasing urinary excretion with
A. IV mannitol injection
B. oral doses of ascorbic acid
C. IV sodium bicarbonate injection
D. IV ammonium chloride injection
E. both A and C procedures (6:121; 39:39)

73. Which of the following is *not* soluble in or miscible with Alcohol USP?
A. ether
B. acacia
C. methanol
D. phenobarbital
E. water (38:121)

74. Which is true for alcohols?
A. water solubility increases as the molecular weight of the alcohol increases
B. water solubility increases with an increase in the number of hydroxyl groups
C. water solubility decreases with branching of the carbon chain of the alcohol
D. for a given carbon chain, boiling point is decreased as the number of hydroxyls is increased
E. polarity decreases with increase in number of hydroxyl groups (12:292)

75. Which of the following is likely to have the greatest water solubility?
A. butane
B. tertiary butanol
C. tertiary pentanol
D. n-butanol
E. n-pentanol (15:350, 351)

76. Benzaldehyde NF must be stored in well-filled, tight, light-resistant containers because it
A. is inflammable
B. reacts with carbon dioxide, adding a carboxy group
C. loses CO_2 to the air, becoming benzene
D. is hygroscopic
E. is auto-oxidized to benzoic acid by O_2 of the air (38:964)

77. Chlorobutanol (Chloretone®) is widely used as a bacteriostatic agent in pharmaceuticals intended for ophthalmic or nasal administration. Which of the following is *not* true of chlorobutanol?
A. it takes some time to make an aqueous solution because chlorobutanol dissolves slowly
B. hydrolyzes in boiling water
C. volatile at room temperature
D. available as hydrate and also in anhydrous form
E. chemically classified as a ketone (38:141)

78. White wax is primarily
A. cetyl palmitate
B. composed of high-molecular-weight hydrocarbons
C. a stearin
D. a mixture of esters of high-molecular-weight alcohols and acids
E. carnauba wax (38:962)

79. Chemically, glycerin is classified as a/an
A. fat
B. acid
C. ester
D. alcohol
E. aldehyde (38:963)

80. Simethicone is a component of several antacid formulations (Di-Gel®, Mylanta®, Silain-Gel®). Chemically, simethicone is classified as a/an
A. wax
B. surfactant
C. alcohol
D. ketone
E. silicone (1:714, 736)

81. Sodium nitrite has been used in pharmacy as a/an
A. anticorrosive agent
B. antimicrobial agent
C. chelating agent
D. cleansing agent
E. disinfectant (26:257)

82. The solubility of a chemical in a given solvent is influenced by many factors. All of the following physicochemical constants may be useful in predicting the solubility of a chemical *except*
A. dielectric constants
B. pH of solution
C. pK_a of the chemical
D. solubility parameters
E. valence of the chemical (8:40–43; 12:290–314)

83. Levarterenol (Levophed®) is

A. L-epinephrine
B. L-norepinephrine
C. isoproterenol
D. L-dopa
E. L-ephedrine (38:443)

84. Which of the following is a chemical property of acetaldehyde?

A. reduces to acetic acid
B. oxidizes to ethyl alcohol
C. polymerizes to paraldehyde
D. condenses with primary amines to form aldols
E. forms sodium salt (20b:437–38; 39:170)

85. Dimercaprol (BAL) has the formula:

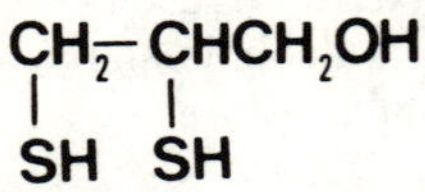

It is an effective antidote for poisoning with arsenic, gold, antimony, and mercury. Which compound would you expect this agent to form with mercury?

A.

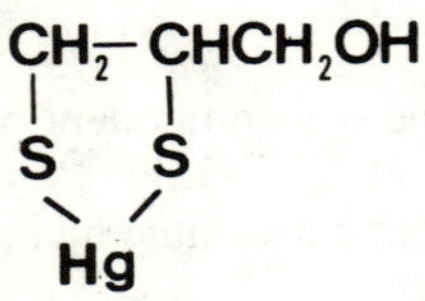

B.

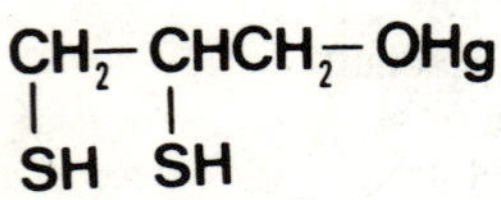

C.

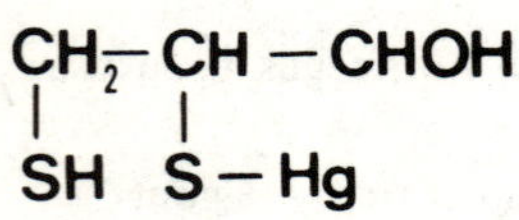

D.

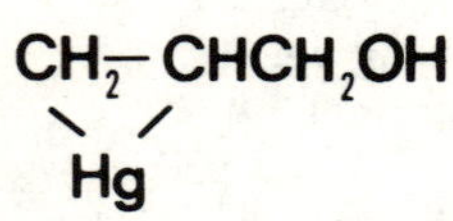

E.

HgS

(38:165; 39:418)

86. Freshly prepared aqueous solutions of the drug represented by the structural formula

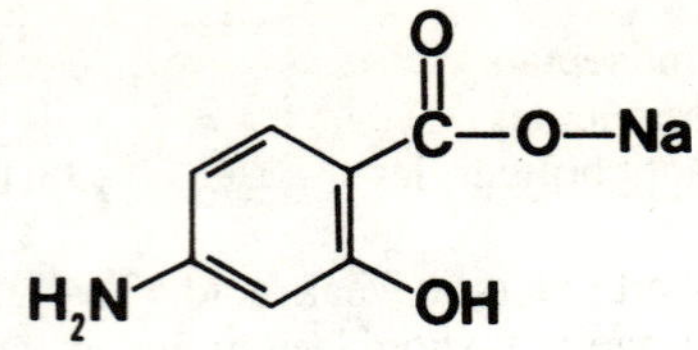

are nearly colorless, but on standing they develop an amber and eventually a dark brown to black color. Addition of 0.1% of sodium sulfite will prevent the discoloration but will not prevent another important decomposition (chemical) change from taking place. The other reaction is

A. oxidation
B. methylation
C. decarboxylation
D. deamination
E. reduction (38:145)

87. Which of the listed substances has the structure portrayed below?

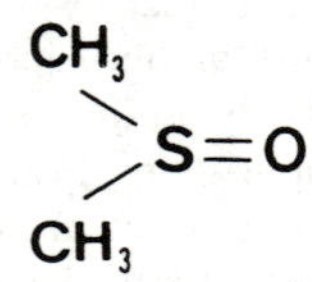

A. dimethyl sulfone
B. dimethyl sulfide
C. dimethyl sulfate
D. dimethyl sulfite
E. dimethyl sulfoxide (3:1270–71; 27:1461–63; 33b:697; 46:63)

88. Which is *not* true for camphor?

A. forms eutectic mixture with phenol
B. can be powdered by rubbing with a small amount of alcohol or ether
C. is a ketone
D. dissolves readily in water
E. has a therapeutically useful topical antipruritic action (1:720; 5:220)

89. In one test for impurities in Ether USP, potassium iodide test solution is added to ether. The formation of free iodine (colored) shows the impurity is present. The impurity is

A. ether peroxide
B. ethyl alcohol
C. acetone
D. acetaldehyde
E. acetic acid (38:351)

90. Which of the following does *not* have at least one phenolic hydroxyl group?
    A. tannic acid
    B. resorcinol
    C. hexachlorophene
    D. salicylic acid
    E. phenylpropanolamine (Propadrine®) (38:452)

91. Which of the following is *not* true of Formaldehyde Solution USP?
    A. contains methanol to prevent internal use
    B. miscible with water or alcohol
    C. has pungent characteristic odor
    D. may become cloudy on long standing, especially in the cold
    E. contains not less than 37% of formaldehyde gas (1:1090; 38:124)

92. Another acceptable chemical name for isopropyl alcohol is
    A. methanol
    B. ethanediol-1,2
    C. 2-propanol
    D. n-propanol
    E. propylcarbinol (38:123)

93. Which of the following acids is the strongest?
    A. acetic
    B. propionic
    C. 2-hydroxy propionic
    D. trichloroacetic
    E. stearic (38:969)

94. Which is *not* true for phenols? Phenols
    A. have an aromatic nucleus in which one or more hydrogen atoms has been replaced by a hydroxyl group (OH)
    B. are tertiary alcohols
    C. are acidic
    D. are particularly resistant to oxidation
    E. generally give characteristic colors with aqueous or alcoholic ferric chloride solutions (38:181–84)

95. A soap may be formed by a reaction between
    A. an alcohol and an organic (fatty) acid
    B. a phenol and an inorganic acid (such as sulfuric)
    C. an inorganic base and an inorganic acid
    D. an inorganic base and an organic acid
    E. an organic base and an inorganic acid (20b:439–40)

96. Which one of the following is *not* a soap?
    A. ethyl acetate
    B. sodium stearate
    C. potassium oleate
    D. zinc stearate
    E. triethanolamine oleate (38:238, 965, 970)

97. Which one of the following is an ester?
    A. glyceryl trinitrate
    B. sodium salicylate
    C. methyldopa hydrochloride
    D. polyethylene glycol 400
    E. methyl chloride (20b:440)

98. Which of the following is *not* a solvent for polyethylene glycols?
    A. mineral oil
    B. water
    C. ethyl alcohol
    D. glycerin
    E. chloroform (14:146; 38:236)

99. A number of drugs which have the following basic structure but differ in the nature of the R and R′ groups are marketed.

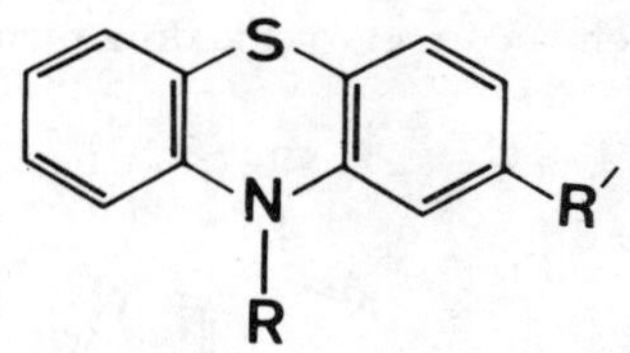

All of these drugs would be expected to have certain pharmacological properties in common. Which is *not* a typical action for this group of drugs?
    A. antiemetic
    B. anticholinergic
    C. antipsychotic
    D. antihistaminic
    E. antimalarial (38:383, 386; 39:208)

100. Which is *not* true for the substance with the following chemical structure?

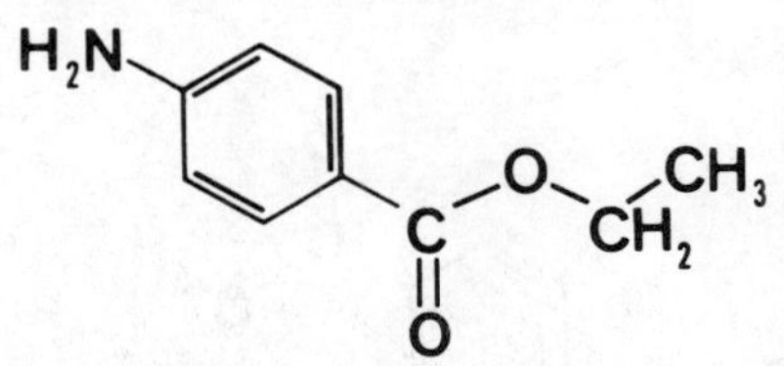

    A. insoluble in water
    B. used as a topical, local anesthetic
    C. a benzoic acid derivative
    D. readily hydrolyzed in boiling water
    E. insoluble in mineral acids (1:987; 38:630–32)

101. Chemically, methyldopa is (−)-3-(3,4-dihydroxyphenl-2-methylalanine. Dopa

stands for dihydroxyphenylalanine. What is the water-soluble form used for the commercially available aqueous injection?

A. methyldopa
B. methyldopa hydrochloride
C. sodium methyldopa
D. the ethyl ester hydrochloride of methyldopa
E. methyldopazwitterion (1:837; 39:387)

102. Polyethylene glycols are polymers represented by the formula

A. $CH_2OHCHOHCH_2OH$
B. CH_2OCH_2
C. $HOCH_2(CH_2OCH_2)_8\ CH_2O\text{-}\overset{O}{\overset{\|}{C}}\text{-}C_{17}H_{35}$
D. $C_{12}H_{25}OCH_2CH_2O\ (CH_2CH_2O)_x\ CH_2CH_2OH$
E. $H(OCH_2CH_2)_nOH$
(38:123, 231, 232, 236–37, 963)

103. Which is correct for the drug pictured below?

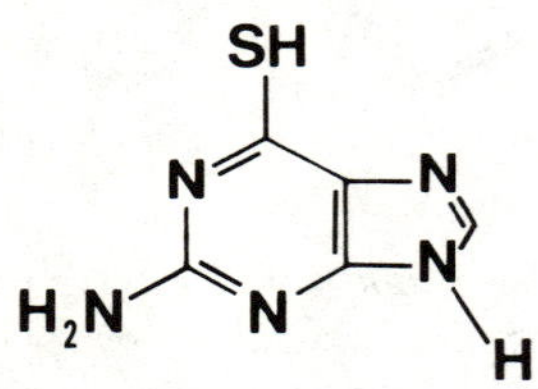

A. an antineoplastic
B. immunosuppressive
C. cytotoxic
D. an antimetabolite
E. all of the above (38:174; 39:457–58)

104. The drug with the following chemical structure has which of the given actions?

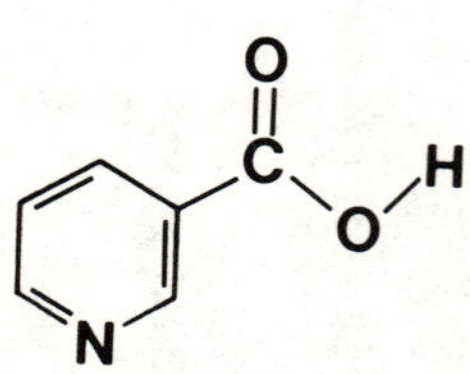

A. antiepileptic
B. anticoagulant
C. antivitamin
D. antilipemic
E. antihistaminic (39:474, 477)

105. The structure pictured below is a/an

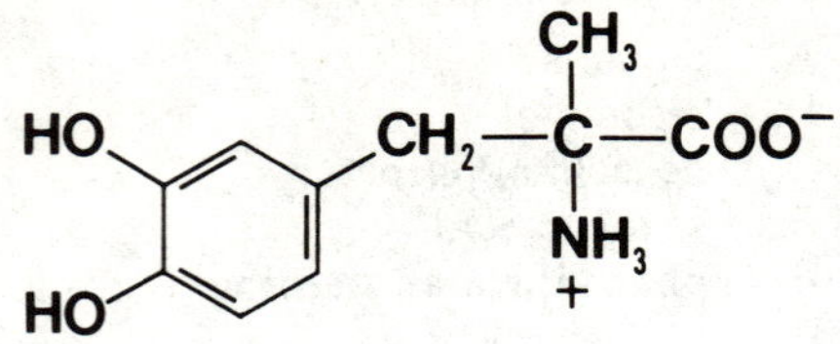

A. internal chelate
B. resonant form
C. impossibility
D. zwitterion
E. ion pair (14:298; 38:45, 602)

106. In the following general formula, X represents nitrogen, oxygen, or carbon connecting the side chain R to the nucleus.

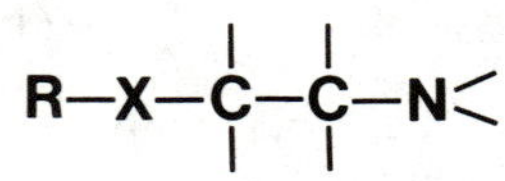

The formula represents

A. antihistamines
B. analgesics
C. synthetic penicillins
D. sympathomimetic amines
E. antipyretics (38:650, 653, 656, 658)

107. The basic structure pictured below has given rise to a number of widely used derivatives. These are called

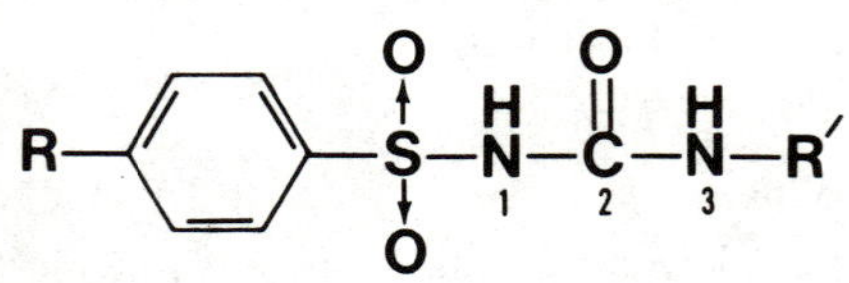

A. thiazides
B. sulfonamides
C. sulfones
D. phenylmalonylureas
E. sulfonylureas (38:615)

108. The compound pictured is 1-phenylbiguanide monohydrochloride. Which of the following is its therapeutic or pharmacological action?

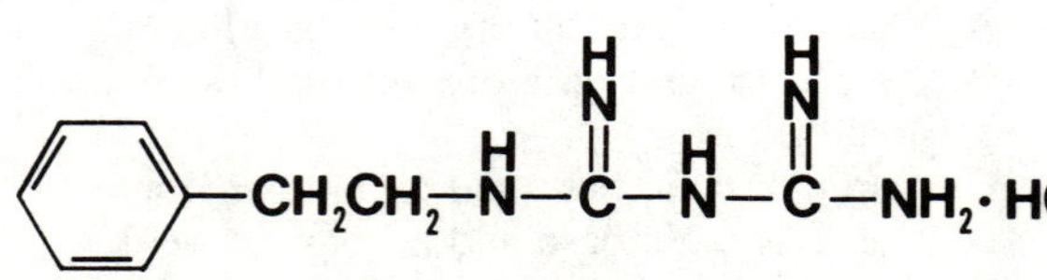

A. antitubercular
B. antidepressive
C. antidiabetic
D. antifertility
E. antipyretic (38:617)

109. Select the appropriate designation for the following compound pictured.

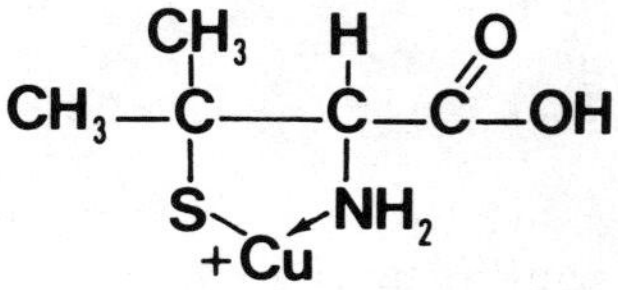

A. heterocycle
B. thiazide
C. cupramino
D. chelate
E. alkaloid (38:51)

110. Which of the following is a common therapeutic use for the compound pictured?

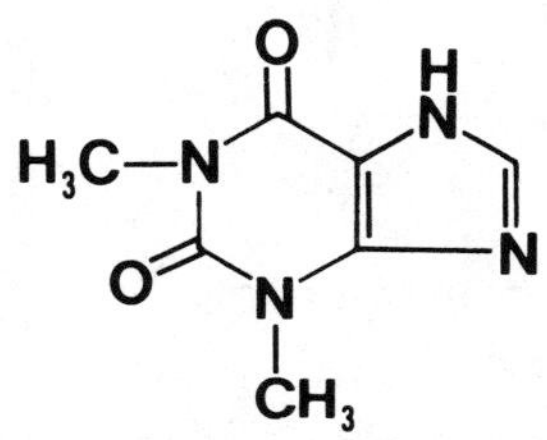

A. CNS sedative
B. antiasthmatic
C. hypoglycemic agent
D. anticoagulant
E. anthelmintic (6:375; 38:578)

111. The compound with the following structure is (–) –3– (3,4–dihydroxyphenyl)– L –alanine. Select the statement which is most appropriate.

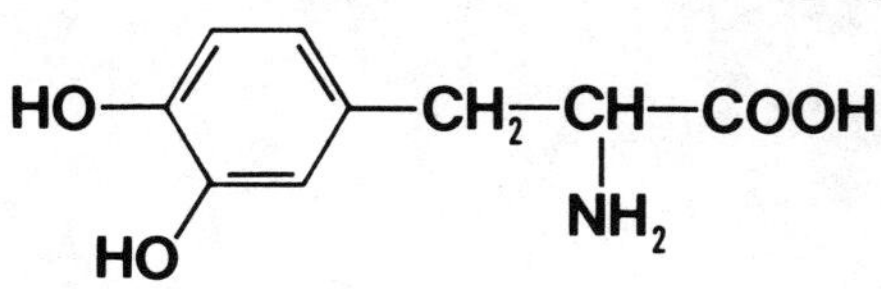

A. this is epinephrine
B. a dextrorotatory compound
C. a precursor of dopamine
D. used to treat hypertension
E. an essential amino acid (6:229; 38:847)

112. The structure pictured below is the basic one for

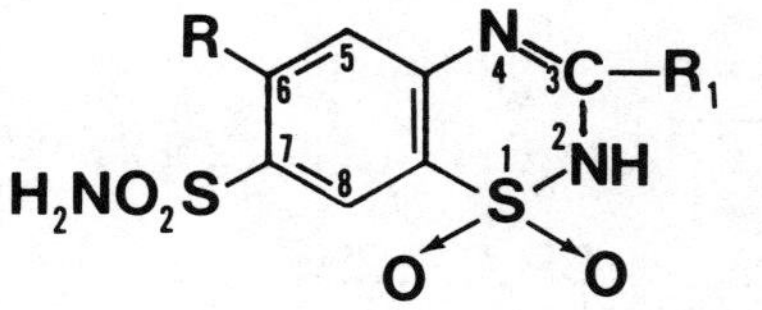

A. thiazide diuretics
B. sulfones
C. thiobarbiturate sedatives
D. antineoplastic thioguanines
E. coumadin anticoagulants (38:583)

113. The H_2 antagonist whose structure is shown below is an analogue of ____ with a modified side chain.

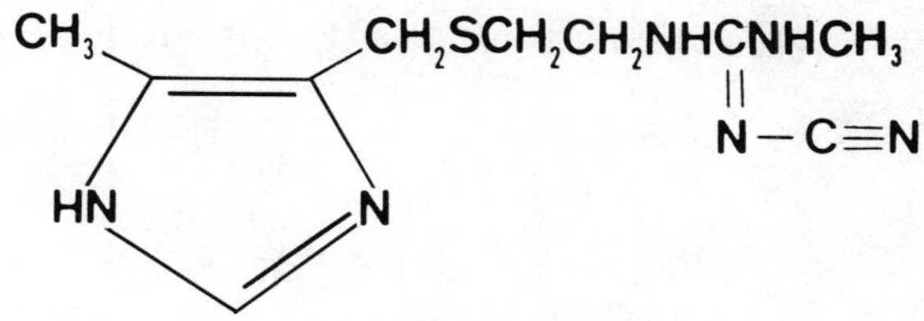

A. urea
B. histamine
C. homatropine
D. hydrocortisone
E. hydralazine (17:193; 38:648)

114. Sodium aminosalicylate (various brands) has the formula:

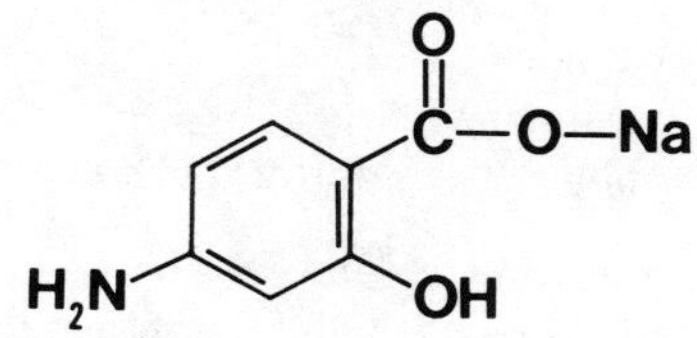

The drug

A. is more effective than isoniazid (Nydrazid®), streptomycin, or ethambutol (Myambutol®) in the treatment of tuberculosis
B. yields an acetylated metabolite that tends to precipitate in alkaline urine
C. activity against *M. tuberculosis* cannot be reversed by administration of p-aminobenzoic acid
D. is effective only against growing bacilli
E. speeds up development of resistance to streptomycin and isoniazid if used with them (1:1150; 38:144–45; 39:710)

115. The sympathomimetic amine structure in the following picture can be modified by substituting at the alpha and beta carbons. Which of the following effects will result if the R group on the alpha carbon is methyl rather than hydrogen?

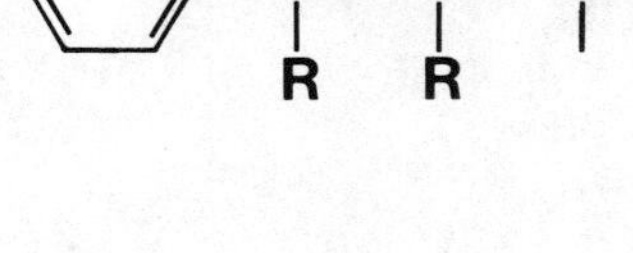

A. activity following oral ingestion
B. increased pressor activity
C. less toxicity
D. less CNS stimulation
E. activity after parenteral injection only (38:441)

116. The following structure is the active ingredient in

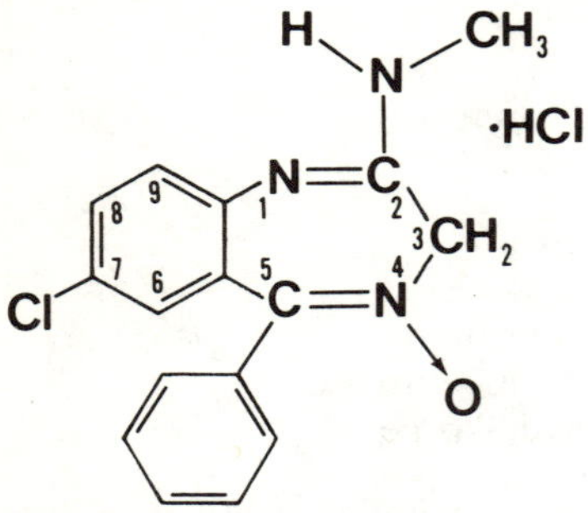

A. Valium®
B. Librium®
C. Serax®
D. Dalmane®
E. none of the above (18:80; 38:374–77)

117. The following structure is a hormone. By which of the following is this hormone elaborated?

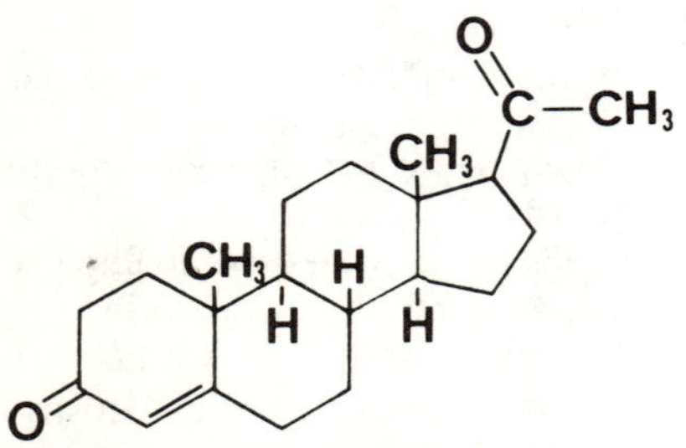

A. corpus luteum
B. testis
C. posterior pituitary
D. anterior pituitary
E. pancreas (38:740, 743–44, 755–57)

118. The phenylpropionic acid derivative in the following picture is now available in this country. It will have to prove to be better than ____ for its therapeutic indication.

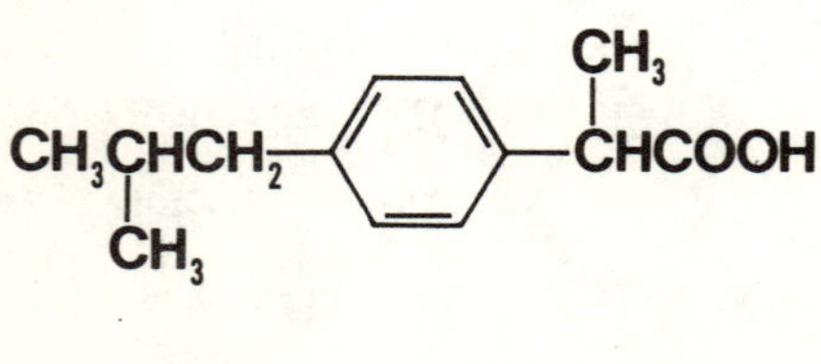

A. morphine
B. phenobarbital
C. atropine
D. epinephrine
E. aspirin (6:343; 25:1765; 39:550)

119. A large number of derivatives have been prepared with the general structure in the following picture. If the R_1 is hydrogen and the R_5 groups are ethyl and phenyl, the compound is

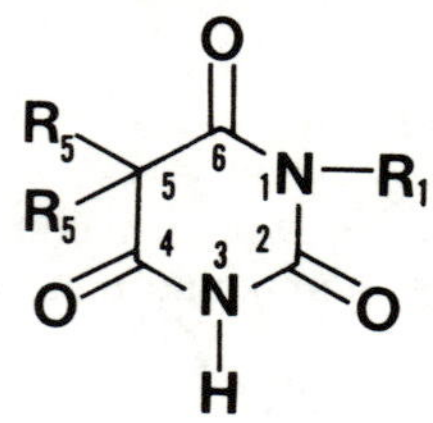

A. phenytoin
B. phenobarbital
C. phenurone
D. phenylmalonylurea
E. phenmetrazine (38:356–59)

120. A part of the drug structure portrayed below is shaded. This structural feature is believed to contribute significantly to the therapeutic activity of the drug.

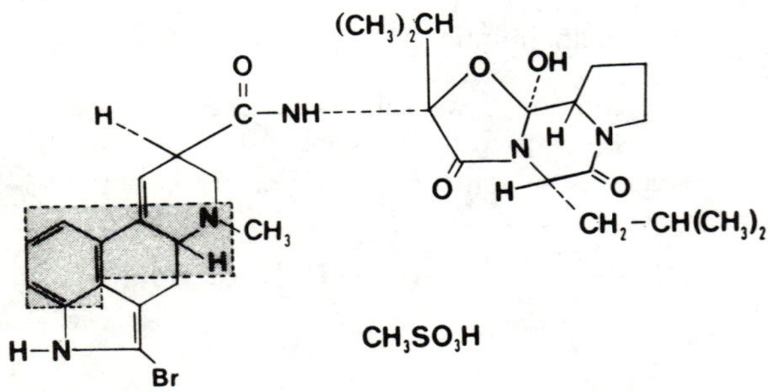

Which of the following substances has this structure?

A. merbromin (Mercurochrome®)
B. bromocriptine mesylate (Parlodel®)
C. bromopheniramine maleate (Dimetane®)
D. bromelains (Ananase®)
E. bromisovalum (Bromural®)
25:1402, 1481-82; 27:1729-31; 38:365 46.53-54)

121. The structure portrayed below is

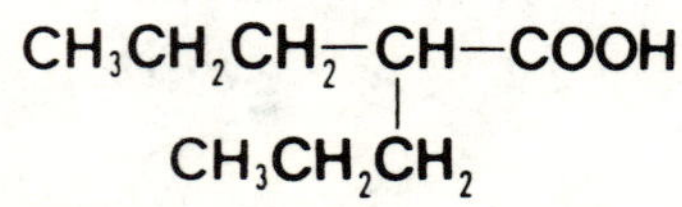

A. valeric acid
B. Valium®
C. Visine®

D. valproic acid
E. Veronal® (3:928–29; 46:51)

Directions: Each set of the following questions consists of several numbered items followed by a list of five lettered words or phrases. MATCH the lettered words or phrases most closely associated with the numbered item. Use each letter once only unless otherwise indicated.

Questions 122 to 126
MATCH the lettered common or brand name with the related numbered chemical name.

122. hydromorphone
123. methylmorphine
124. diacetylmorphine
125. ethylmorphine
126. oxymorphone

A. heroin
B. codeine
C. Numorphan®
D. Dilaudid®
E. Dionin® (38:673, 692–94)

Questions 127 to 131
Each group of numbered chemical structures is followed by a list of lettered names. MATCH the lettered name most closely associated with the structure.

127.

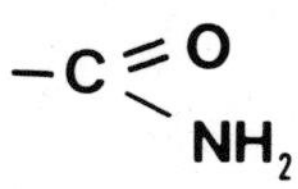

128.

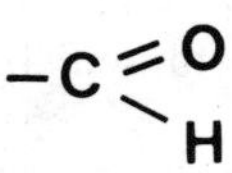

129.

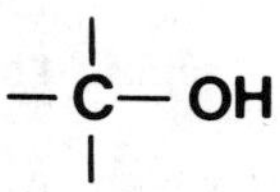

130.

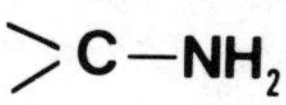

131.

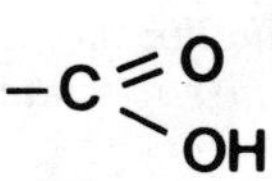

A. aldehyde
B. amide
C. alcohol
D. amine
E. carboxyl (1:399, 405)

(Questions 132 to 136)

132. —OH
133. —CH_3
134. $C_6H_5CH_2$—
135. CH_3—CO—
136. CH_3CH_2—

A. methyl
B. acetyl
C. ethyl
D. benzyl
E. hydroxyl (1:405–06)

(Questions 137 to 141)

137.

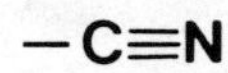

138.

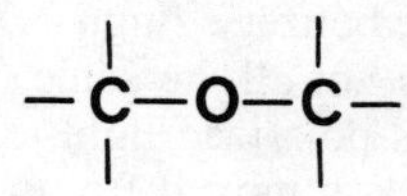

139.

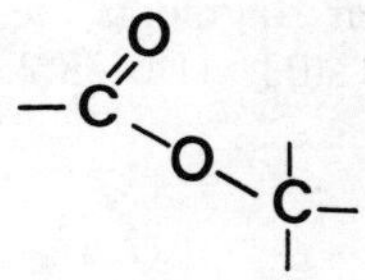

140.

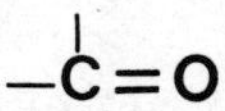

141.

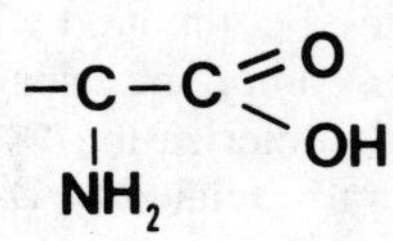

A. ester
B. ketone
C. ether
D. nitrile
E. amino acid (1:399, 400)

Questions 142 to 145
Each of the numbered organic nitrogenous compounds in the following series of questions may be considered to have been derived from ammonia by substitution of hydrogen with one of the lettered functional groups given below. MATCH the lettered functional group with the associated numbered type of compound.

142. quaternary amine
143. amide
144. imide

145. carbamate

A. —OH
B. —COOH
C. HCO—
D. $(CH_3—)_4$
E. $(HCO—)_2$ (1:405, 455)

Questions 146 to 155
Each group of numbered prefixes used in chemistry is followed by a list of lettered phrases which define or identify the prefixes. MATCH the lettered phrase most closely associated with the numbered prefix.

146. levo-
147. ortho-
148. poly-
149. hetero-
150. anhydro-

A. signifies the neighboring or 1,2 positions on the benzene ring
B. means not all the same
C. rotates polarized light to the left
D. water is removed from a compound
E. indicates several identical molecules or molecular fragments are joined together (1:403, 412; 38:236–37, 308–09)

151. sub-
152. desoxy-
153. nor-
154. meta-
155. D-

A. denotes removal of oxygen from a molecule
B. indicates a compound which is related to another compound, generally by alkylation or isomerization
C. structurally related to D-glyceraldehyde
D. a basic salt
E. the 1,3 positions on the benzene ring (1:403, 404; 22:54; 38:93, 418; 39:76)

Questions 156 to 159
The group of numbered names of acids given below is followed by a list of lettered chemical formulas. MATCH the lettered formula with the corresponding numbered name.

156. acetic acid
157. stearic acid
158. oleic acid
159. formic acid

A. $CH_3(CH_2)_7CH{=}CH(CH_2)_7COOH$
B. $HCOOH$
C. $CH_3(CH_2)_5CH(OH)CH_2CH{=}CH(CH_2)_7COOH$
D. $CH_3(CH_2)_{16}COOH$
E. CH_3COOH (1:1247; 38:82, 953, 966, 969)

Questions 160 to 163
The group of numbered names of oils which is given below is followed by a lettered list of synonyms for oils. MATCH the lettered synonym with the corresponding numbered oil.

160. theobroma oil
161. castor oil
162. olive oil
163. peanut oil

A. oleum ricini
B. cocoa butter
C. teel oil
D. arachis oil
E. sweet oil (1:741, 1241, 1247, 1268; 38:953)

Questions 164 to 167
The group of numbered types of chemical reactions given below is followed by a list of lettered definitions of chemical reactions. MATCH each lettered definition with the corresponding numbered type of reaction.

164. saponification
165. hydrolysis
166. esterification
167. neutralization

A. reaction of a fat or oil with alkali to form soaps and glycerol
B. reaction of acids with bases to form salt(s) and water
C. reaction of salts or esters with water to form acids and bases or alcohols
D. reaction in which the hydroxyl of an organic acid is replaced by an alkoxy group (RO)
E. reaction in which hydrogen atoms are added across a double bond (1:281, 399, 423, 537)

Questions 168 to 175
Each group of generic or chemical names given below is followed by a list of lettered chemical structures for the side chains of penicillin molecules. MATCH the lettered chemical structure with the appropriate numbered name.

168. benzyl penicillin (penicillin G)
169. methicillin
170. ampicillin

171. cloxacillin

A.

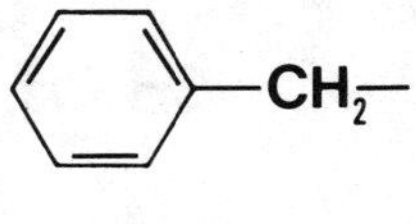

B.

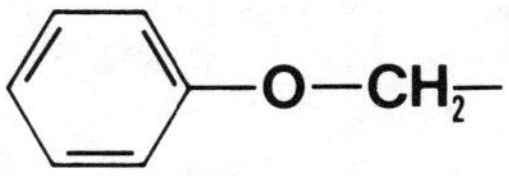

C.

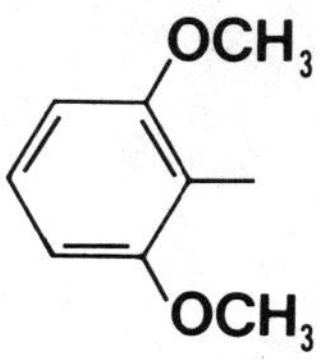

D.

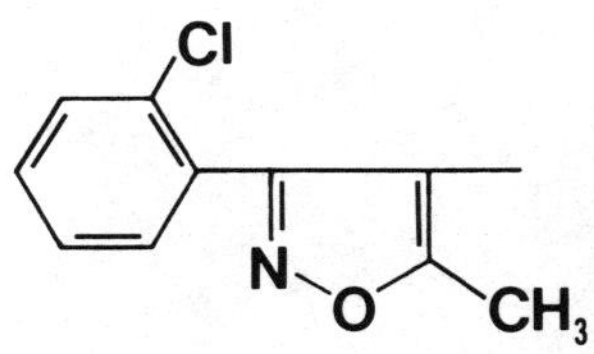

E.

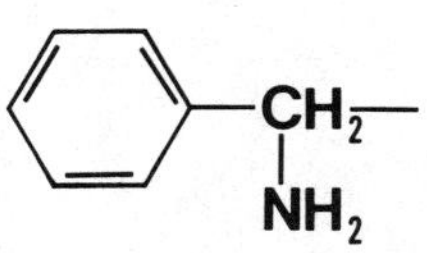

(38:274–75, 278–83)

172. nafcillin
173. oxacillin
174. phenethicillin penicillin
175. amoxicillin

A.

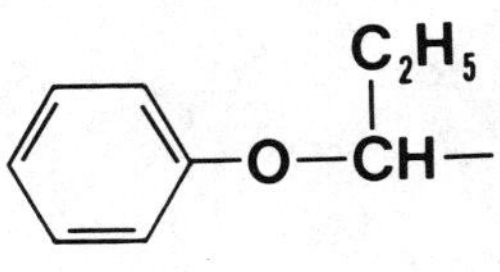

B.

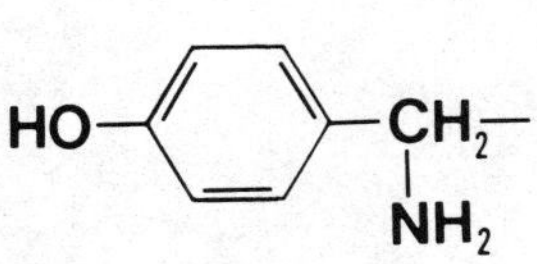

C.

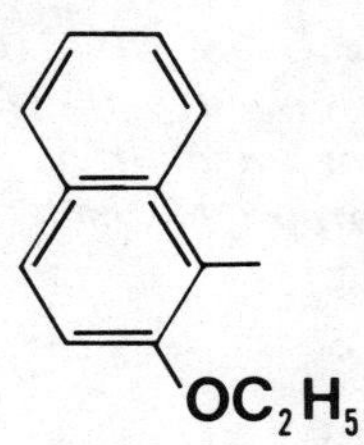

D.

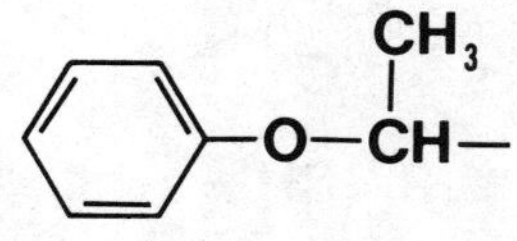

E.

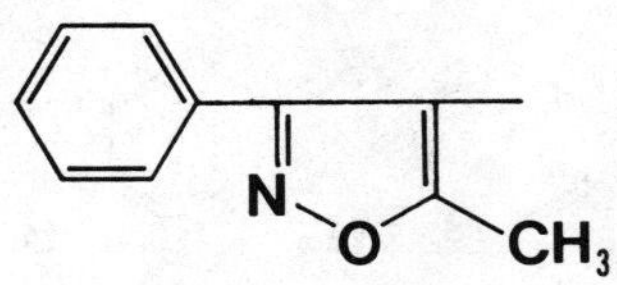

(38:280–84)

Questions 176 to 179
MATCH the lettered category of surfactant with the associated numbered chemical structure.

176. $CH_3\ (CH_2)_{10}CH_2OSO_3Na$

177.

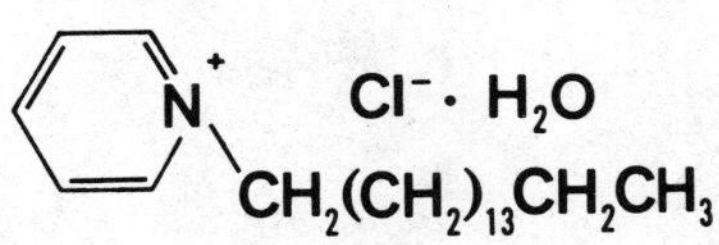

178.

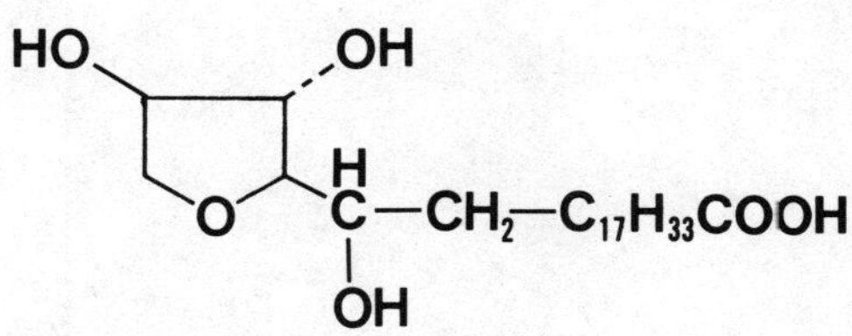

179.

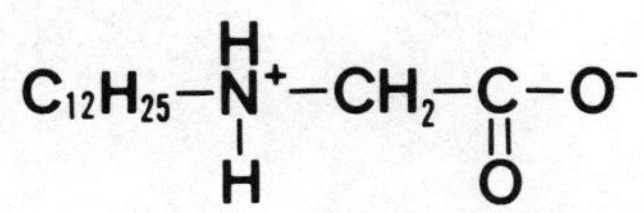

A. cationic
B. ampholytic
C. nonionic
D. lympholytic
E. anionic

(38:225, 229, 232, 235)

Questions 180 to 182
Each numbered structure is the basic structure for several derivatives which have in common the therapeutic use as a major tranquilizer. MATCH the lettered name with the appropriate numbered chemical structure.

180.

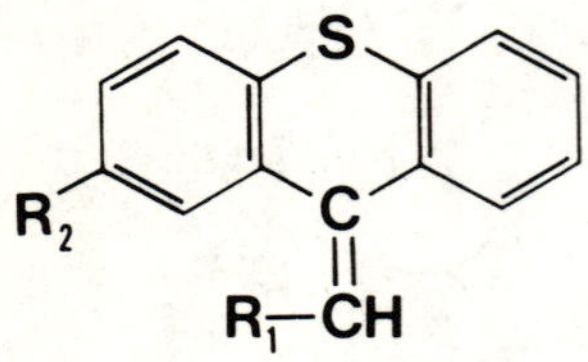

181.

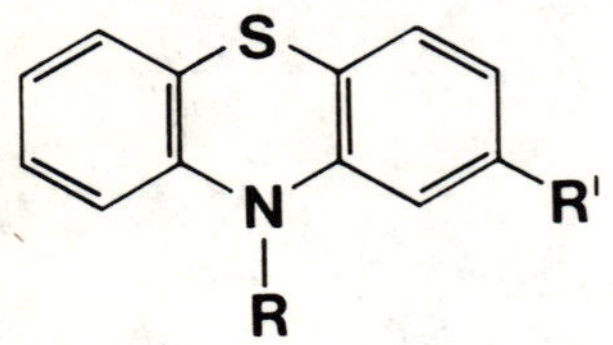

182.

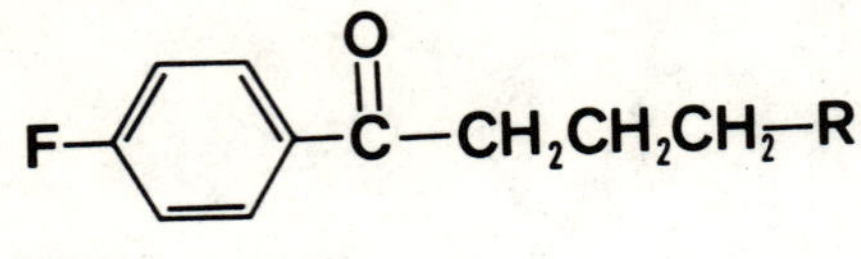

A. phenothiazine
B. thioxanthene
C. thiuram
D. flurandelide
E. flurobutyrophenone (38:383, 398, 400)

Answers and Commentary

1. **D.** Diazoxide is a nondiuretic thiazide derivative useful in the treatment of hypertensive crisis. It can be used effectively only by rapid intravenous injection and generally produces a fall in blood pressure within five minutes. (1:783; 33b:198)

2. **E.** DBI® (Meltrol®, phenformin) is a biguanide. In 1977 its use was discontinued in the United States because of its reported association with lactic acidosis. However, it is still being used in other countries. (37:764–65)

3. **D.** Benzalkonium chloride is a cationic surface active agent. In the presence of anionic agents such as soaps, benzalkonium chloride and similar cationic agents are inactivated because of the combination of large cations with large anions of soaps to form an inactive product. (6:1001–02)

4. **B.** Diphenoxylate is similar in structure to meperidine (Demerol®) and exhibits some of the addicting properties of this compound. (38:681, 698)

5. **A.** Cyclopropane is a gaseous anesthetic. (38:349–52)

6. **A.** Aminophylline consists of theophylline which has been reacted with ethylenediamine to improve its water solubility. Upon exposure to air, carbon dioxide is absorbed and free theophylline will form. Addition of small amounts of ethylenediamine will redissolve these crystals. A note in the monograph for Aminophylline Injection USP states, "Do not use the Injection if crystals have separated." (1:1067–68; 18:25–26)

7. **A.** All these drugs are antimalarials, each having its own particular advantages and disadvantages. Chloroquin, a 4-aminoquinoline, is an effective erythrocytic schizontocide and is also useful in the treatment of extraintestinal amebiasis.
   B. Quinacrine, a 9-aminoacridine, is an erythrocytic schizontocide and gametocide but is now primarily used as an anthelmintic against intestinal tapeworms.
   C. Proguanil, a biguanide, is schizontocidal and also effective against the exoerythrocytic stage of *P. falciparum;* rapid development of resistant organisms has limited its use.
   D. Quinine, which has a quinoline nucleus, acts only as an erythrocytic schizontocide.
   E. Pyrimethamine, a pyrimidine derivative, has both schizontocidal and sporontocidal activity. (38:255–58)

8. **A.** Quinine bisulfate is soluble in 10 parts of water, while the sulfate requires 810. However, because of the bitter taste of quinine salts, solutions are not the usual oral dosage forms. Capsules, tablets, or suspensions are used.
   B. Quinine is one of the most intensely bitter-tasting substances known.
   C. The heptahydrate salt effloresces (loses water of crystallization) readily at room temperature, so the dihydrate, which is stable under normal conditions of storage, has been the official form for some time.
   E. When exposed to light, quinine sulfate acquires a brown tint. (1:1158; 38:255)

9. **B.** Quinine is an alkaloid (nitrogenous base) extracted from cinchona bark. The quinidine molecule differs from quinine only in spatial configuration of groups at one asymmetric carbon and is therefore an optical isomer. The isomers are equivalently effective as antimalarials, but quinidine has its major therapeutic use in the management of certain irregularities of the heartbeat. (38:252, 254)

10. **E.** Paraldehyde is a cyclic ether formed by the polymerization of acetaldehyde. The reaction is slowly reversible (catalyzed by exposure to light). Acetic acid is produced when the liberated acetaldehyde is oxidized by atmospheric oxygen. USP packaging and storage requirements call for well-filled, tight, light-resistant containers holding not more than 30 ml, at a temperature not exceeding 25°C. The USP also requires that the label of all containers of paraldehyde, including those dispensed by the pharmacist, must include a statement directing the user to discard the unused contents of any container that has been open for more than 24 hours. (18:358; 38:370)

11. **B.** Petrolatum is a colloidal dispersion of aliphatic liquid hydrocarbons (C_{18} to C_{24}) in solid hydrocarbons (C_{25} to C_{30}). It is therefore a nonpolar substance and will dissolve in or mix with other nonpolar substances. The hydroxyl group in ethyl alcohol makes the molecule too polar to permit solvation of petrolatum. (38:961)

12. **A.** Phosgene, CCl_2O, is a highly reactive gas which hydrolyzes in the lung tissues to hydrogen chloride, producing pulmonary edema. Since ethyl alcohol reacts with phosgene to form nontoxic diethylcarbonate, 0.5 to 1% alcohol is added to chloroform to prevent phosgene formation. (38:962)

13. **C.** The glucose oxidase test is quite specific for glucose, in contrast to the Benedict's test, which relies on the reduction of cupric ions in alkaline solution to reddish-orange insoluble cuprous oxide. The latter reaction can be elicited by reducing substances such as ascorbic acid and by a number of drugs which may occur in the urine from time to time. (1:588, 601; 8:450–52)

14. **D.** Tes-Tape® contains glucose oxidase and therefore is specific for glucose. Clinistix® and Diastix® also use the glucose oxidase method. Ascorbic acid, levodopa, salicylates, and phenazopyridine (Pyridium®) may produce false-negative results with these agents. (3:1671; 44:283)
A. C. Benedict's qualitative test and Clinitest® tablets are based on the copper reduction method. (44:283–84)
B. Acetest® tablets and Ketostix® are used to detect the presence of ketones in the urine. Levodopa and phenazopyridine may interfere. (3:1670; 8:462)

15. **B.** Acetazolamide (Diamox®) is a potent inhibitor of the enzyme, carbonic anhydrase. The normal function of this enzyme in kidney tubule cells is to facilitate the formation of HCO_3^- and H_3O^+ by the reaction:

$$H_2O + CO_2 \underset{\text{anhydrase}}{\overset{\text{carbonic}}{\rightleftharpoons}} H_2CO_3$$

$$H_2CO_3 \rightleftharpoons HCO_3^- + H_3O^+$$

When this reaction is inhibited, there is a deficiency of H_3O^+ to exchange for the Na^+ in the urine. Na^+ and HCO_3^+ are excreted along with the necessary additional water, thereby producing diuresis. A systemic acidosis is produced, and the urine may reach a pH of 8.2. Other disadvantages of the carbonic anhydrase inhibitors as diuretics are the need for intermittent administration, because patients become refractory to them, and the increased excretion of K^+. The major therapeutic use for acetazolamide is to reduce intraocular pressure in glaucoma. (39:423, 425)

16. **C.** Lactic acid is added to infant formulas as a digestive aid. It is used as a spermatocidal agent in contraceptives. (38:967, 972)
Choice A is oxalic acid. (38:83)
Choice B is tartaric acid. (38:967)
Choise D is acetic acid. (38:966)
Choice E is maleic acid. (1:1223; 38:972)

17. **D.** Mineral oil, being nonpolar, is miscible with most fixed oils but is immiscible with water, alcohol, or castor oil, all of which exhibit a higher degree of polarity due to the hydroxyl radicals in their structures. (1:744)
A. Up to 10 ppm of dl-alpha-tocopherol may be used as an antioxidant to prevent conversion of unsaturated aliphatic contaminants to peroxides, which impart an undesirable odor and taste. (38:952)

18. **A.** A chelate is a complex formed between a multivalent metal and a compound containing two or more potential ligands. A ligand is either a specific atom or a molecule that contains an atom which can attach itself to a metal. The formation of chelates is a common way of treating poisonings involving heavy metals such as lead or mercury. (38:50, 239)

19. **C.** The most common and most stable chelate rings are those made up of five or six atoms. (38:50)
A. Three-membered rings apparently do not occur.
B. Four-membered rings are known, and those containing sulfur may be quite stable.
D., E. Chelate rings containing eight or 10 atoms have not been identified.

20. **A.** The magnitude of the magnetic moment of a proton (hydrogen atom) is dependent on its magnetic environment (i.e., on the atoms surrounding it in the molecule). An NMR spectrum is a display of energy absorption peaks versus magnetic field strength for various protons in different magnetic environments. Interpretation of a plot of resonant frequencies versus an arbitrary intensity scale yields information about the spatial arrangement of the hydrogen atoms and the carbons to which they are bonded. (1:647–49; 39:87–88)

21. **D.** Free rotation about single bonds in acyclic (open chain) compounds does not exist because energy barriers to rotation arise from interactions of nonbonded atoms. The atoms tend to position themselves in space with no two atoms directly facing (i.e., eclipsed). The favored conformation is usually the one in which the larger groups are separated from one another by as great a distance as possible (i.e., staggered). The accompanying diagrams illustrate these conformations for ethane (CH_3—CH_3). (38:26; 39:77, 82–84)

Conformations of Ethane

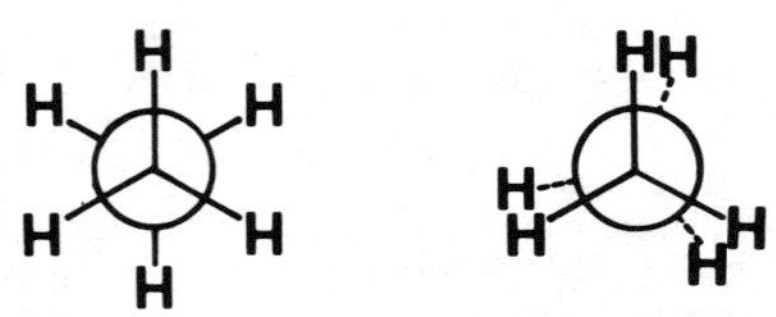

Staggered **Eclipsed**

C. A compound which is optically inactive due to this type of internal compensation is a meso-compound; i.e., mesotartaric acid. (39:77)

22. **D.** (38:26; 39:85)
A. The other six hydrogens are parallel with the axis of the ring, three being above the plane of the molecule and three below. The accompanying diagrams illustrate these conformations. (39:85)

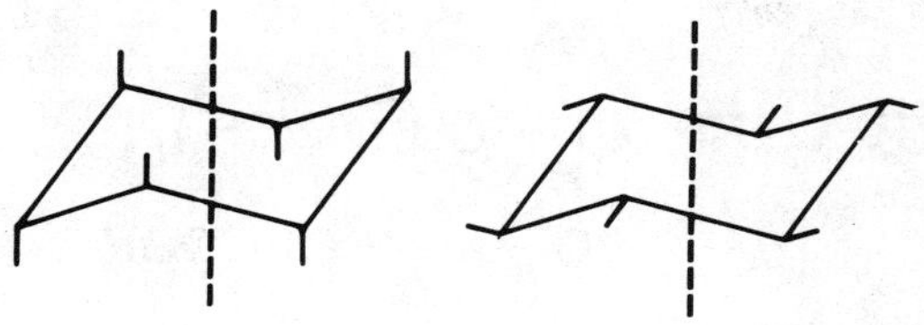

Axial bonds **Equatorial bonds**

23. **B.** Oleic acid is

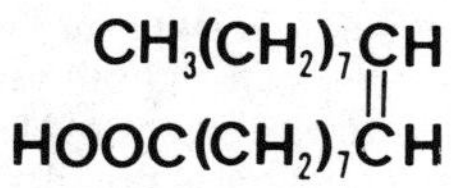

Elaidic acid is the transisomer and has the following formula:

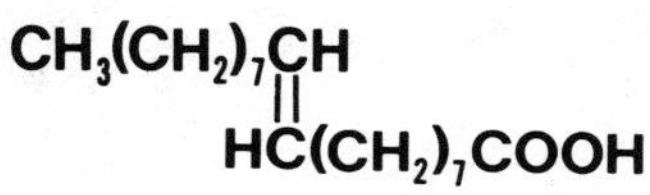

Other geometric isomers of this type are maleic (cis) and fumaric (trans) acids. (38:27)

24. **C.** Molecules whose mirror images are not superimposable are called optical enantiomorphs, enantiomers, or optical antipodes.The structure shown are for (+)–epinephrine and (–)–epinephrine. These are mirror images, differing in the spatial arrangement of the hydroxyl group at the alpha carbon of the side chain. Optical enantiomorphs usually have identical chemical and physical properties except for their ability to rotate the plane of polarized light. However, they often show differences in biological activity. For example, (–)–epinephrine is 12 to 15 times more active as a vasoconstrictor than is (+)–epinephrine. (38:31–33)
B. Stereoisomers which are not mirror images of each other are called diastereoisomers. (1:179)

25. **D.** The prostaglandins (PGs) are a group of 20-carbon, unsaturated, lipid-soluble carboxylic acids with a cyclopentane ring. At least 14 have been identified. The six main classes, A, B, C, D, E, and F, are distinguished by the substituents on the cyclopentane ring of the molecule. A further subdivision according to the number of double bonds in the side chains is indicated by subscript 1, 2, or 3. Isomers in the F class are identified by subscript α or β. The E and F series are the most abundant (especially E_2 and F_2) and are sometimes considered the "primary prostaglandins." (6:641; 33b:667–70; 39:30)

26. **A.** All these drugs lower levels of lipids in the blood. For most of them, the mechanism of action is not definitively known. (3:502–13; 6:746–51)

27. **E.** Dissociation constants are always less than one and are expressed as exponential notations. To provide whole numbers for ease of comparison and calculation, the reciprocal log of the dissociation constant $\left(\frac{1}{\log K_a}\right)$ or ($-\log K_a$) is used to express acid strength. For example, the K_a of acetic acid is $1.75 \times 10_5$. The pK_a of acetic acid may be calculated as:

$$
\begin{aligned}
pK_a &= -\log K_a \\
&= -(\log 1.75 \times 10^{-5}) \\
&= -(\log 1.75 + \log 1 \times 10^{-5}) \\
&= -(0.24 - 5) \\
&= -(-4.76) \\
&= 4.76
\end{aligned}
$$

(12:192)

28. **C.** Hydrochloric acid is classified as a strong acid. Strong acids ionize almost completely into hydronium ions and the corresponding anions. Other strong acids are sulfuric and nitric. These acids do not have pK_a values listed since the values would be close to 0. The fact that all of the other acids listed in the question have pK_as indicates that they are weaker acids (less ionization) than hydrochloric acid. (12:208)

29. **C.** Stronger acids have larger ionization constants than weaker acids. The pK_a is the reciprocal of the ionization constant, so stronger acids have lower pK_as than weaker acids. Of the acids listed, boric acid has the highest pK_a and is the weakest of these acids. Salicylic acid, which has the lowest pK_a on the list, is the strongest. (12:208)

30. **D.** A buffer system consists of a weak acid or base and its corresponding strong salt. In preparing a buffer system, one should choose an acid or base with a pK_a value close to the desired pH. For example, lactic acid and sodium lactate can be combined to obtain a pH of exactly 4.0. The molar concentration of each needed may be calculated by using the Henderson-Hasselbalch equation. (12:249)

31. **B.** For a weak acid and its salt, the Henderson-Hasselbalch equation can be stated as

$$pH = pK_a + \log \frac{[\text{dissociated}]}{[\text{undissociated}]}$$

If the values for pH and pK_a which are supplied are used in this equation, it can be seen that the ratio of the dissociated form of the drug to the undissociated form will be the antilog of 2, which is equal to 100. (1:269)

32. **C.** Loxapine succinate (Loxitane®) is a tricyclic dibenzoxazepine compound which is indicated in schizophrenia. Although side effects and adverse effects are qualitatively similar to those produced by the phenothiazines, loxapine succinate may be of value in

those patients who do not respond to other antipsychotic drugs. (38:400)

33. **B.** Dydrogesterone (Duphaston®, Gynorest®) is a synthetic steroid structurally related to progesterone. It is used to treat primary and secondary amenorrhea. When taken orally from day 15 to day 25 of the menstrual cycle it will produce progestational secretory changes in the estrogen-primed endometrium. It is also indicated for treatment of abnormal uterine bleeding caused by hormonal imbalance. It is a pure progestogen, i.e., without estrogenic, androgenic, or anabolic activity. Progestational agents should not be taken during the first four months of pregnancy (to prevent abortion) because of the risk of harming the fetus. (23:1113–14; 37:756)

34. **E.** Vincristine (Oncovin®) is an alkaloid derivative of Vinca rosea. It appears to exert its cytotoxic effect by arresting progression of the mitotic cycle. It has been used with considerable success in combination with prednisone for induction of remission of acute leukemia in children. (1:440, 1086)

35. **C.** Most alkaloids have pK_as as above 7; therefore, they are weak bases that form salts with acids (eg., pilocarpine hydrochloride, morphine sulfate). (1:430) D. Stereoisomerism is common in alkaloidal structures and large differences in therapeutic activity can be expected among isomers. (1:430)

36. **C.** While all of the drugs mentioned are available for intramuscular injection, only fluphenazine is available as the hydrochloride, eninthate, and decanoate salts. The latter two salts are relatively insoluble and are very slowly absorbed after injection. Intramuscular injection need only be given at two-week intervals if the enanthate salt is used, and perhaps at even longer intervals if the decanoate salt is used. (1:1024)

37. **C.** The thiazolidine ring appears in other natural compounds, but the four-membered-lactam ring is unique to penicillins and cephalosporins. Cephalosporins contain a six-membered dihydrothiazine ring rather than the five-membered thiazolidine.

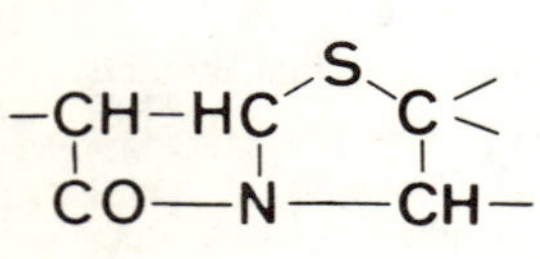

β-lactam thiazolidine

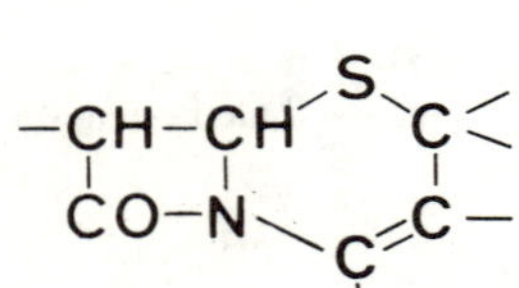

β-lactam dihydrothiazine

(38:275, 290)

38. **A.** Penicillins differ in the nature of the acyl side chains; i.e., the R group varies in the structural formula that follows:

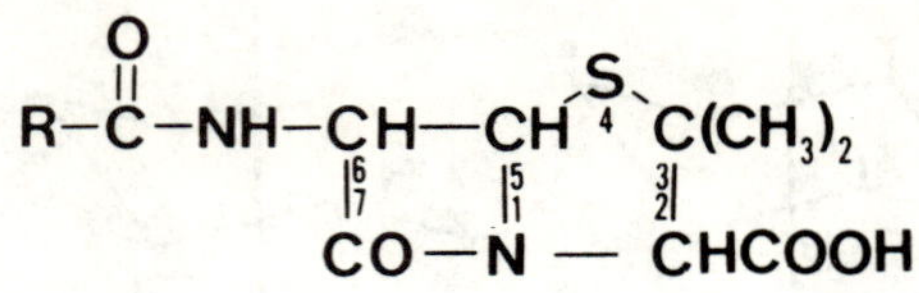

They may also differ in salt or ester formation. (38:274–76)

39. **B.** The availability of pure crystalline penicillin makes it possible to determine antibiotic activity by comparison of the sample with the reference standard. The weight-unit relationship will vary with the nature of the penicillin side chain and salt as shown in the table below. A. defines the Oxford Unit, which was used with the impure extracts originally available.

Penicillin	Units/mg
Sod. Pen. G	1667
Pot. Pen. G	1595
Procaine Pen. G	1009
Pot. Pen. V	1530

(38:273)

40. **C.** Most penicillins are dispensed as the sodium or potassium salt of the free acid. Although the potassium content of potassium penicillin G is not ordinarily a factor in its use, the use of large doses of this preparation will provide quantities of potassium that may be of therapeutic significance. Severely elevated potassium levels interfere with neuromuscular function to produce weakness and paralysis. Abdominal distention and diarrhea may also occur. As potassium levels rise, the ECG (electrocardiogram) reflects impaired conduction, which may progress to ventricular fibrillation and cardiac arrest. (17:468, 546)

41. **A.** Sodium methicillin is stable in the dry form, but like most penicillins, it is very sensitive to moisture and pH. Penicillins generally are most stable at pHs between 6.0 and 6.8 and are therefore susceptible to acid hydrolysis in the stomach. Oral forms of penicillin G are buffered in order to raise the gastric pH to levels at which the drug is more stable. Methicillin is so unstable at acid pH (i.e., it is acid-labile) that it cannot be taken orally and must be given only by injection. All of the other penicillins in this listing are classified as acid-resistant, which means that the rate of hydrolysis at gastric pHs is sufficiently low that an acceptable amount of drug escapes inactivation in the stomach. See Table I for other acid-resistant penicillins. Some authorities consider acid-resistant penicillins to have no therapeutic advantage for control of organisms equally susceptible to large doses of the less expensive oral forms of buffered penicillin G. (4:705; 38:281; 39:723)

Table I

Penicillin	Acid-Stable	Penicillinase-Resistant
Penicillin G & salts	0	0
Penicillin V & salts	X	0
Phenethicillin & salts	X	0
Sodium Methicillin	0	X
*Sodium Oxacillin	X	X
*Sodium Cloxacillin	X	X
*Sodium Dicloxacillin	X	X
*Sodium Nafcillin	X	X
Ampicillin	X	0
Hetacillin	X	0
Disodium Carbenicillin	0	0
Carbenicillin Indanyl Sodium	X	0
Amoxicillin	X	0

X = yes, 0 = no

*Acid-resistance greater than that of penicillin G and less than of penicillin V or phenethicillin (38:280–89; 39:723)

42. **D.** Resistance to penicillin G is denoted by the requirement for therapeutically unrealistic high concentrations of the drug to control infections caused by certain strains of *Staphylococcus*. Recent reports indicate up to 20% of *S. aureus* organisms isolated from outpatients are fully resistant to penicillin G and alpha-phenoxyalkyl derivatives (e.g., penicillin V), and that 90 to 95% of nosocomial strains are totally resistant. Resistant organisms elaborate betalactamase enzymes (penicillinase) capable of opening the beta-lactam ring through hydrolysis to form therapeutically inactive penicilloic acids. Semisynthetic penicillins (oxacillin and others—see Table I) which are penicillinase-resistant have an amide side chain consisting of an aromatic ring structure substituted at one or both ortho positions with groups that sterically block the attack on the ring. (4:706; 5:870; 38:281)

43. **A.** Because it is more active than other penicillins against some gram-negative bacteria and enterococcal infections, and also retains activity against gram-positive organisms (though less effective than penicillin G), ampicillin has been called a broad-spectrum antibiotic. Perhaps the alpha-amino group in the side chain confers an ability to cross cell wall barriers that are impenetrable to other penicillins. Amoxicillin, which is p-hydroxy-ampicillin, also has a broad (extended) spectrum. Carbenicillin, which has a side chain alpha-carboxyl group, has the widest range of antimicrobial activity of any currently available penicillin. Appropriate side-chain modification has achieved the long sought goal of extending the range of penicillin effectiveness. (4:700; 38:282–84)

44. **C.** Penicillin G benzathine (Bicillin®, Permapen®) is a salt with a large cation (N,N′—dibenzylethylenediamine). It therefore is quite insoluble (1 g in about 5000 ml of water). Insolubility gives it great stability, and prolonged duration of effect. It can be administered orally without buffers. Upon intramuscular injection, penicillin is released slowly. Sustained but low blood levels can be demonstrated for as long as four weeks. Prolonged duration is also obtained from procaine penicillin G (soluble 1 g in 250 ml of water). An oil suspension gelled with 2% aluminum monostearate is used to further prolong the duration of action of procaine penicillin G injections. Repository penicillin dosage forms reduce cost, local trauma, and the need for repeated injections. (1:1131; 38:279)

45. **D.** (See Table I)
A., B., C., E. Ampicillin and penicillin V are acid-stable but are not resistant to penicillinase. Methicillin and carbenicillin are resistant to penicillinase but are not acid-stable. The indanyl sodium salt of carbenicillin (Geocillin®) is acid-stable. (39:723)

46. **B.** (1:1256; 38:241, 244)
A., C. Penicillamine is a chelating agent capable of forming nondissociable complexes (chelates) with metals such as lead, gold, mercury, and copper. Tying up the metal prevents its toxic reaction and urinary excretion of the complex reduces the metal level in the body. Wilson's disease is characterized by high tissue and serum copper levels. Other chelating agents used as antidotes for heavy metal poisonings are Calcium Sodium Edetate USP, Dimercaprol USP, and Disodium Edetate USP.
D. Penicillamine is prepared by acid hydrolysis of penicillin. (1:1256; 38:244)

47. **D.** The fundamental radical is designated as a sulfanilamido group. (38:204)

48. **D.** The bacteriostatic activity of the sulfonamide type is shown only by molecules which have a free amino group on an aromatic ring in the position para to the sulfonamido group. Some groups (acylamido, nitro, azo) can be converted to a free amino group in the body. Sulfonamides with such groups will be active in vivo, but not in vitro. (38:205)

49. **B.** Sulfonamides are weak acids (pK_as vary from 4.77 to 10.43; most are between 6 and 8). Salts made with sodium hydroxide, a strong base, would be expected to hydrolyze in water to produce strongly alkaline solutions. The high pH of sodium sulfonamide solutions makes them damaging to tissues and limits their usefulness. (38:206)

50. **B.** The alkaline aqueous solution (pH 9 to 10) will absorb carbon dioxide from the air. As acidity increases, sufficient sulfadiazine will form to exceed its limited solubility in water. (38:207)

51. **A.** Sulfonamides are metabolized to N^4 – acetyl compounds and in general are excreted as such. The extent of the acetylation varies markedly with the sulfonamide used. Also, there appear to be geneti-

cally determined "rapid acetylators" and "slow acetylators." Most, but not all, of the acetylated derivatives are less soluble than the unacetylated compounds and crystalluria (precipitation of crystals in the urine in the renal tubules) may occur. To decrease the possibility of crystalluria, patients should be advised to drink large quantities of water. Sodium bicarbonate was taken concurrently with earlier sulfonamides (sulfathiazole) to alkalinize the urine, thus increasing the solubility of the weakly acidic metabolites. (38:112–13, 206)

52. **A.** Tetracyclines are amphoteric compounds capable of forming salts with either acids or bases. Acid salts, such as the commonly available hydrochlorides, are formed through protonation of the dimethylamino group on carbon number 4. These salts are soluble in water and form acid solutions that are fairly stable. In parenteral products, generally an acid (such as ascorbic acid) is incorporated to minimize precipitation of free tetracyclines, which normally occurs above pH 4.0. (5:1155; 38:306; 39:731)

53. **D.** Upon aging, especially under unfavorable storage conditions (high humidity, elevated temperature), tetracyclines degrade to an amber-to-brown semisolid which contains two toxic substances, epianhydrotetracycline and anhydrotetracycline. These cause nausea, vomiting, and renal damage with symptoms of reduced kidney function, acidosis, proteinuria, glycosuria, and aminoaciduria. This "Fanconi syndrome" is reversible. Citric acid, once regarded as an adjuvant to absorption, was found to contribute to the degradation process. (5:1175)

54. **A.** Damage to the cochlear and vestibular portions of the eighth cranial nerve is a serious adverse reaction to the aminoglycosides. Tinnitus, dizziness, vertigo, and auditory loss are symptoms which may occur following parenteral administration or even after oral use of these drugs. Concomitant use with other ototoxic drugs should be avoided. Because these drugs are excreted through the kidney, the danger of ototoxicity is greatly enhanced when there is severe or even moderate renal impairment. In this connection, it is worth noting that aminoglycosides may themselves cause serious kidney damage. (5:653; 38:295)

55. **C.** Viomycin has a polypeptide structure, while streptomycin and the other antibiotics listed are aminoglycosides. Viomycin, although structurally different, does share some properties with streptomycin. For example, both have antituberculosis activity, with usefulness limited by rapid development of resistant strains. All the aminoglycosides (and also vancomycin) are poorly or not at all absorbed when given orally. The major adverse reactions are damage to the cochlear and vestibular portions of the auditory nerve, and renal damage. (4:813; 38:332; 39:706)

56. **E.** A drying oil forms a hard film when spread and exposed to air. These oils (linseed, hempseed, tung, walnut, poppyseed, sunflower seed) are high in their content of linoleic (two double bonds) and linolenic (three double bonds) acids. Cottonseed, corn, soybean, and sesame oils are "semidrying"; they contain oleic (one double bond) and linoleic acid moieties. Nondrying oils contain large quantities of oleic bonds, e.g., olive, palm, peanut, and coconut oils. Drying oils are used in paints. (1:423)

57. **A.** These esters are known as glycerides. (1:422–24; 38:323)
B. Polypeptides are chains of amino acids joined in amide linkages. (38:323)
C. Compounds listed in choice C are phospholipids, or, more specifically, lecithins. (1:422)
D. Steroids described in choice D (and lacking carbonyl or carboxyl groups) are sterols. Cholesterol is an example. (1:424)
E. This is a definition of waxes. (1:422)

58. **C.** Rancidity of fats may be due to either oxidative or, less commonly, hydrolytic processes. Oxidative processes consist of addition of atmospheric oxygen across double bonds and/or oxidation of methylene groups to peroxides. Short-chain acids, aldehydes, and ketones with unpleasant tastes and odors are produced. Light, heat, moisture, presence of metals, and exposure to air influence the rate and degree of rancidity production. Antioxidants such as propyl gallate or tocopherols may be added to prevent or delay rancidity. (20b:441)

59. **E.** A surfactant has both hydrophilic (water-solubilizing) and lipophilic (fat-solubilizing) properties in a proper balance; i.e., not completely in either direction. The HLB (hydrophile-lipophile balance) system is a semiquantitative classification of surfactants. (38:222)

60. **B.** Acetone is miscible with both water and alcohol as well as with many organic solvents. It is used as a solvent for fats and resins. (38:963–64)

61. **E.** Dextran is a branched polysaccharide containing about 200,000 glucose units with a molecular weight of about 40 million. By partially hydrolyzing this huge molecule, polysaccharides having a wide range of molecular weights can be produced. Dextrans having an average molecular weight of 40,000 and

75,000 have been used effectively to expand blood volume temporarily in patients who have experienced a loss of blood and plasma. (6:767)

62. **A.** Lactulose is a synthetic disaccharide (galactopyranosyl-D-fructofuranose). When taken orally it is not affected by disaccharidase in the small intestine and is not absorbed systemically. Saccharolytic bacteria in the colon break it down into acetic and lactic acids, which stimulate bowel movements and exert a local osmotic effect in the colon. It can be used to treat chronic constipation. A more important use is for reduction of blood ammonia concentration in the treatment of portal-systemic encephalopathy. The fatty acids trap NH_3 in the colon in the form of nonabsorbable NH_4^+ and create a concentration gradient favoring diffusion of NH_3 from the blood into the colon. The laxative action helps to remove the NH_4^+. (25:1668–69; 27:1338)

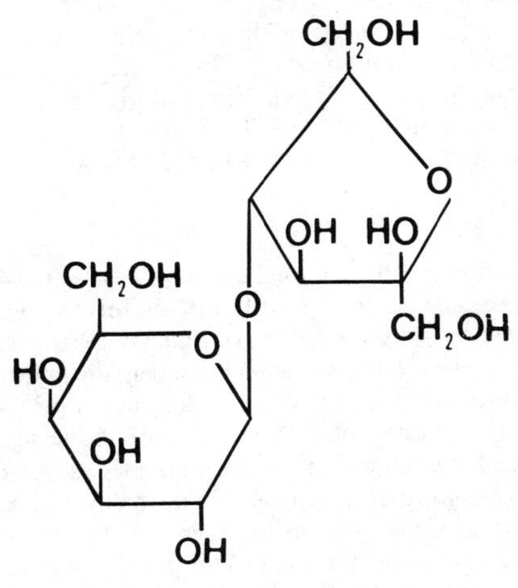

Lactulose

63. **B.** Aspirin is only slightly soluble in water (1 g in 300 ml at 25°C), but is quite soluble in alcohol (1 g in 5 ml at 25°C). (38:71–16)

64. **A.** Comparison of their structures (see next column) shows the alterations made in the indomethacin molecule to produce sulindac. Replacing the N-acylindole moiety (circled) with benzylidene indene (circled) was expected to reduced the CNS effects that occur with indomethacin. The methoxy group was replaced by fluoride to enhance potency. Water solubility was increased by replacing chlorine with a methylsulfinyl group. The sulindac structure turned out to be inactive as such. It is a "prodrug," requiring metabolic conversion to an active form, the sulfide. The inactivity of the sulindac structure per se is assumed to account for its causing less gastrointestinal irritation than does indomethacin. (10; 25:1140A; 47:35–37)

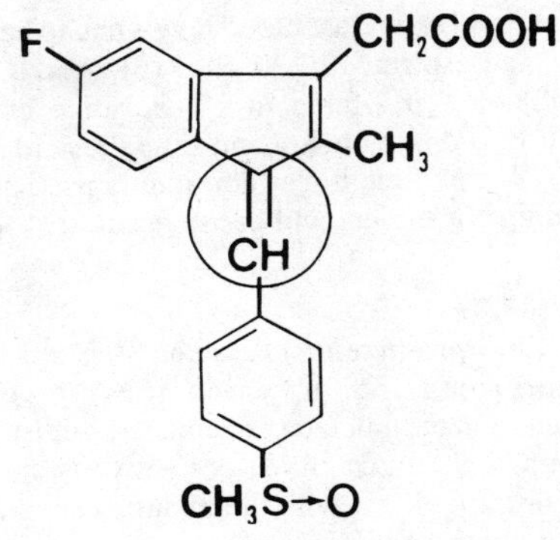

Sulindac

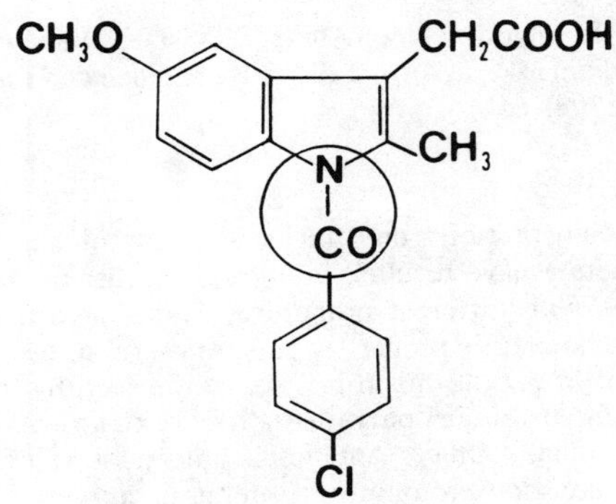

Indomethacin

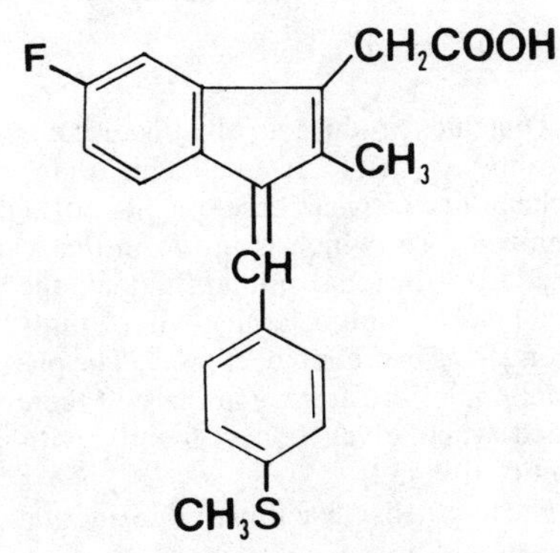

Sulindac Sulfide Metabolite

65. **C.** Salicylamide is chemically similar to the other salicylates but is not converted to a salicylate in the body. Instead, its analgesic activity is believed due to the salicylamide molecule. (2a:126)
B. Salsalate does not dissolve in gastric acid. Upon absorption in the small intestine, each ester molecule of salsalate is hydrolyzed into two salicylate moieties. (25:1390)
D. This is a complex of calcium aspirin and urea which is more soluble than aspirin and is said to give

more rapid salicylate blood levels and to be less irritating than aspirin. (3:700; 38:716)
E. Salol is insoluble in gastric juice but is slowly hydrolyzed into phenol and salicylic acid in the intestine. At one time it was commonly used as an enteric coating for tablets and capsules. (38:714)

66. **D.** (38:388)
A. Chlorprothixene (Taractan®) is an isostere of chlorpromazine in which the nitrogen of the phenothiazine nucleus is replaced with a methylene group. This thiozanthine derivative is classified as a major tranquilizer with therapeutic uses similar to the phenothiazines. (38:398)
B. Haloperidol (Haldol®) is a fluorobutyrophenone. (38:400)
C., E. Hydroxyzine (Atarax®, Vistaril®) and chlorcyclizine (Perazil®) are diphenylmethane derivatives. (38:398, 662)

67. **B.** Substitutions on the basic phenothiazine ring structure have resulted in a great number of derivatives with different properties. Some have marked anticholinergic properties and are useful in the treatment of parkinsonism in spite of the fact that many PTZs produce parkinson-like extrapyramidal symptoms. Others antagonize the actions of histamine and serotonin and are used as antipruritic agents (e.g., trimeprazine and methdilazine). Still others (e.g., prochlorperazine) are most useful in the treatment of nausea and vomiting. (4:1100–05)

68. **A.** Thiazides produce an alkaline urine (shift urinary pH from 6.0 → 7.4). In an alkaline urine, more of the amphetamine (a weak base, $pK_a \cong 10$) will be in the unionized form which is the form that can be reabsorbed from the renal tubular fluid into the blood. The blood levels of amphetamine will be higher and more prolonged as excretion decreases. The pharmacological actions of the amphetamine will therefore be enhanced when given concomitantly with a thiazide diuretic. (39:432)
B. The hypotensive action of thiazides enhances that of guanethidine.
C. Thiazides cause hypokalemia which enhances both toxicity and action of digitalis drugs.
D. The hyperglycemic effect of thiazides is antagonistic to oral hypoglycemic agents.
E. Like amphetamines, the tricyclic antidepressants are weak bases and their action will be *enhanced* by thiazide diuretics by the same mechanism. (39:432)

69. **E.** Cytarabine, a synthetic nucleoside, acts by inhibiting DNA polymerase. In combination with thioguanine, it is the treatment of choice for acute myeloblastic leukemia. Alkylating agents have high reactivity with and affinity for DNA, probably causing cross-linking, depurination, and scission of these macromolecules which are essential for cell division. A basic structure for the alkylating agents is

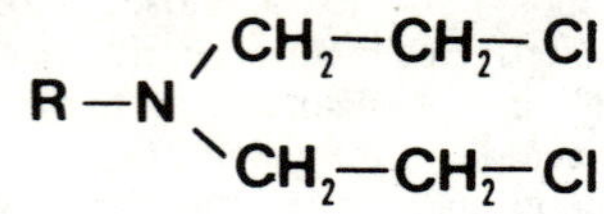

They are used primarily to treat chronic leukemias, lymphomas, and myelomas. (4:1107, 1118; 39:666)

70. **D.** Phenazopyridine hydrochloride is rapidly excreted in urine and has topical anesthetic activity capable of relieving pain in cystitis, prostatitis, and urethritis. However, it has no antibacterial action and is not curative. It is an azo dye (as is amaranth) and colors urine red to orange. Patients should be warned to expect this. Phenazopyridine is available in fixed dosage combinations with urinary antiseptics (Azo Gantrisin®, Suladyne®). However, medical authorities suggest that it is better to give it separately and to eliminate it from the regimen as soon as the symptoms are controlled. (4:355; 38:160)

71. **A.** Although all are anthelmintics, they show varying degrees of activity against different worms. Piperazine salts are effective against pinworms and roundworms. Gentian violet is used against pinworms and threadworms. Pyrvinium pamoate is principally useful for pinworms. Thiabendazole is the agent of choice for threadworms and for cutaneous larva migrans (creeping eruption) and is probably the best all around agent of this group. Gentian violet and pyrvinium pamoate are dyes. The purple stains of the former and the red of the latter are difficult to remove. During treatment with pyrvinium pamoate, the feces will be stained bright red to reddish-brown. The pharmacist should warn the patient of this as well as telling him or her not to chew the tablets. (38:145–55)

72. **E.** IV sodium bicarbonate will alkalinize the urine to a pH of 7.8 to 8.0. Phenobarbital is a weak acid ($pK_a = 7.4$). The percentage of drug existing in the ionized lipid-insoluble form will be increased in alkaline fluid as shown in Table II. The ions cannot pass through the kidney tubule cell membranes back into the blood. The normal reabsorption of the barbiturate from urine is decreased; excretion of the drug is increased. Mannitol injection acts as an osmotic diuretic. The combination of diuresis and alkalinization has been shown to reduce the period of barbiturate coma compared with untreated patients. (6:121)

Table II

Calculated Percent Unionized Phenobarbital at Various pH Values (39:39)

pH	% Unionized
4.0	99.96
6.0	96.17
7.0	71.53
8.0	20.07
10.0	0.25

73. **B.** Gums are not soluble in alcohol. Neither are most inorganic and organic salts or proteins. (38:121)

74. **B.** The hydroxyl group of the alcohols permits hydrogen bonding with water molecules. Water solubility increases therefore, as the number of hydroxyl groups is increased and the carbon content is held constant. On the other hand, as the carbon content increases, the molecule becomes more nonpolar and loses water solubility. (12:292)

75. **B.** Water solubility decreases with increases in the number of carbons in an alkane chain. Therefore, the butanols will be more soluble than the pentanols. Since side chains tend to improve water solubility, tertiary butanol would be more soluble than n-butanol. (15:351)
A. The absence of hydroxyl groups in butane would indicate poor water solubility. (15:350)

76. **E.** Auto-oxidation is oxidation by atmospheric oxygen. Benzaldehyde absorbs O_2 from air rather rapidly to form a peroxide which decomposes to form benzoic acid. Crystals of benzoic acid are seen at the neck of bottles of benzaldehyde that are not full or not tightly stoppered. (38:964)

77. **E.** Chlorobutanol is tertiary trichlorobutyl alcohol. In addition to its antibacterial properties, it is effective as a hypnotic and sedative and also has some local anesthetic action. (38:141)

78. **D.** White wax is yellow wax (beeswax) from which the color has been bleached. By definition, waxes are esters of high-molecular-weight alcohols and acids. In beeswax, the alcohols and acids contain 24 to 34 carbon atoms.
A. Cetyl palmitate is the primary constituent of spermaceti, the waxy substance obtained from the head of the sperm whale.
E. Carnauba wax has higher molecular weight esters than beeswax. These confer characteristics of hardness and high gloss, which make it pharmaceutically useful in polishing mixtures for coated tablets. (38:962)

79. **D.** Glycerin (trihydroxypropane) is a triol since each molecule has three alcoholic hydroxyl groups. Glycols are representative of pharmaceutically useful alcohols which are classified as diols. (38:963)

80. **E.** Silicones are polymers consisting of chains of alternating oxygen and silicone atoms with substituent organic groups (generally methyl or phenyl) attached to the silicone atoms. Chain length, substituents, and degree of cross-linking between chains can be varied to yield a wide range of properties. Because simethicone is an excellent surfactant, it is able to disrupt the liquid films of gas bubbles in the froth which may develop in the stomach. It is often incorporated with antacids in formulations intended to relieve gaseous discomfort as well as hyperacidity. (1:714, 736)

81. **A.** Sodium nitrite is present in Antirust® tablets. The tablet also contains sodium carbonate. Four tablets are dissolved in 1 quart of zephiran chloride solution 1:750. This disinfectant solution is used to store metal instruments. (26:257)

82. **E.** Valences of atoms do not reflect the solubility characteristics of a chemical. (8:40–43)
A., D. Both dielectric constants and solubility parameters of solutes and solvents reflect relative polarities. The closer the solute and solvent values, the greater the potential solubility. (12:298; 302)
B., C. The pK_a of a weak acid or base and the pH of the final solution will determine the species of chemical that will be present and the corresponding degree or extent of solubility. (8:42–43; 12:309–14)

83. **B.** (38:443)

84. **C.** Acetaldehyde in the presence of a small amount of concentrated sulfuric acid will polymerize to the liquid trimer, paraldehyde $(CH_3\text{—}CHO)_3$. (39:170)
A. The conversion of acetaldehyde to acetic acid is an oxidation reaction. (20b:437; 39:170)
B. The conversion of acetaldehyde to ethyl alcohol is a reduction reaction. (20b:438)
D. Aldols are formed by condensation with other aldehydes. (20b:438)

85. **A.** Mercury (Hg) and other heavy metals poison by tying up—SH groups in tissues, thus interfering with enzyme groups which depend on free—SH groups for their activity. Synthetic dithiol compounds remove

the metal by forming a ring compound that is relatively nontoxic and rapidly excreted. (38:165; 39:418)

86. **C.** Decarboxylation of sodium para-amino-salicylate to m-aminophenol will take place. The sodium sulfite prevents the typical oxidation of phenols to colored quinone structures. The amber color is not necessarily a sign of extensive decomposition, but the USP monograph does have a caution to prepare solutions within 24 hours of administration and that under no circumstances should a solution be used if its color is darker than that of a freshly prepared solution. (38:145)

87. **E.** Dimethyl sulfoxide (DMSO) is a colorless hydroscopic viscous liquid that is miscible with water and alcohol and most organic solvents but not with mineral oil. It is a highly polar substance and is widely used as an industrial solvent. In the early 1960s DMSO received great publicity in the lay press when it was found to penetrate intact human skin rapidly, producing a number of pharmacological actions including reduction of inflammation, local analgesia, and dissolution of collagen. It was used experimentally for the treatment of arthritis and also as a carrier of other substances through the skin. Generally, aqueous solutions or gels containing 60 to 90% DMSO were applied. In 1965 the drug was withdrawn even from investigational use when large doses given orally to dogs and monkeys caused lens opacities. In 1978 DMSO was approved for use in the United States in the form of a 50% aqueous solution for direct instillation into the bladder. It affords smptomatic relief of intersitial cystitis by producing analgesia and reducing urinary frequency. Rimso-50® is marketed in 50-ml containers since that is the usual volume put into the bladder each time. (3:1270–71; 27:1461–63; 33b:697; 46:63)
A., B. Dimethylsulfoxide is partially excreted unchanged in the urine and some is oxidized to dimethylsulfone, which is much more slowly excreted in the urine. About 3% is converted to dimethyl sulfide and excreted in the lungs. Because of the latter metabolite, patients may note a garlic-like taste within a few minutes after instillation. Also a garlic odor may persist on the breath and skin for as long as 72 hours. (27:1462)

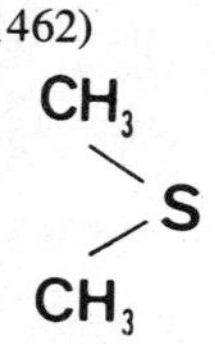

Dimethyl Sulfide

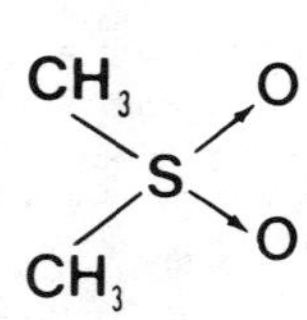

Dimethyl Sulfone

88. **D.** Camphor is soluble in alcohol or organic solvents but is only slightly soluble (1 g in 800 ml) in water. (1:720; 5:220)

89. **A.** The formation of iodine from iodide requires an oxidizing agent. The only effective oxidizing agent in the list given is ether peroxide. Nonvolatile peroxides may form in ether upon long standing in contact with air in partially filled containers. They will remain as a residue when ether is evaporated and will explode with terrific force when heated. (38:351)

90. **E.** All the chemicals except phenylpropanolamine are phenolic in nature and show the general phenol characteristics in varying degrees. For example, all have some antiseptic activity. All except hexachlorophene are quite easily oxidized. (38:452)

91. **A.** Formaldehyde solution does contain methanol, which is added to prevent polymerization to paraformaldehyde. Because cold increases formation of insoluble polymers, the solution should be stored at temperatures above 15°C. A common name for the official 37% solution is formalin. The solution is used full-strength or diluted for disinfection of inanimate objects. (1:1090; 38:124)

92. **C.** The 2- in the name identifies the hydroxyl group as being attached to the second carbon of the three-carbon (propyl) radical.
D. In n-propanol, the hydroxyl is in the "normal" position of being attached to a terminal carbon of the propyl radical. (38:123)

93. **D.** Introduction of halogen atoms into an acid increases the acidic properties. Acetic acid, like most carboxylic acids, is a weak acid. Trichloroacetic acid (TCA) is as strong as hydrochloric acid. Because of its corrosive action on the skin, TCA is used in aqueous solutions to remove warts and moles. (38:969)

94. **D.** Phenols are susceptible to oxidation by atmospheric oxygen and by other oxidizing agents, often producing colored end products. The presence of alkalinity accelerates the oxidation. Polyphenols such as epinephrine are so readily oxidized that special storage conditions and stabilizers (bisulfites, hydrosulfites) are needed. Although the hydroxyl group(s) attached to the aromatic nucleus give(s) the molecules the general nature of tertiary alcohols and the capability of undergoing many chemical reactions characteristic of alcohols, phenols are actually acidic and able to form salts with bases. Phenol (monohydroxybenzene) is weakly acidic (pK_a = 10). Introduction of electron-attracting groups on the nucleus will increase the acidity. Trinitrophenol (picric acid), for example, is about as strong as the mineral acids. (38:181–84)

95. **D.** The usual soaps are ammonium, potassium, or sodium salts of fatty acids containing eight or more carbon atoms. Potassium oleate and sodium stearate are examples. Also other metal salts (e.g., zinc and lead) and amine salts (e.g., triethanolamine) are classified as soaps. Aqueous soap solutions are generally quite alkaline and are decomposed by acids which liberate the free fatty acids. (20b:439–40)

96. **A.** Ethyl acetate is an ester formed by reaction between an alcohol and an organic acid. A soap is a salt

of an organic (fat) acid. Inorganic acids also form esters with alcohols. Salts of monovalent metals generally have detergent properties, may be mildly antiseptic, and are alkaline in aqueous solution. (38:965)
D. Zinc stearate is a water-repellent powder used as a tablet lubricant. Its use in dusting powders was discontinued when it was found to cause pulmonary inflammation on inhalation. (38:970)
E. Triethanolamine oleate, an amine salt, is the emulsifying agent in Benzyl Benzoate Lotion NF. (38:238)

97. **A.** An ester is a salt of an alcohol and either an organic or inorganic acid. In the presence of moisture most esters are gradually hydrolyzed to the corresponding acids and alcohols. (20b:440)

98. **A.** The polyethylene glycol molecule contains a high proportion of oxygen atoms and thus, in spite of their high molecular weights, polyethylene glycols are soluble in polar solvents but not in the nonpolar aliphatic hydrocarbons found in mineral oil. (38:236)
E. Chloroform is classified as a nonpolar solvent but sometimes may be considered semipolar because of the inductive effect. The highly charged chlorine atoms attract electron pairs away from the hydrogen atom. In effect, the entire molecule becomes polarized—weakly so, but enough to allow polyethylene glycols to mix with it. (14:146; 38:236)

99. **E.** The basic structure is the phenothiazine nucleus. The nature and the position of the substituents strongly influence activity. In a given derivative, one or more of the possible actions may predominate and overshadow others. In addition to the typical actions listed in the question, individual phenothiazines also may have effects that are antiadrenergic, antiserotonin, cardiovascular, respiratory, and muscle relaxant. Phenothiazines lower body temperature in humans and animals. The ability of phenothiazines to enhance or to antagonize effects of other drugs is well documented. (38:383, 386; 39:208)

100. **E.** The compound ethyl aminobenzoate (benzocaine) is one of the several benzoic acid esters that exhibit local anesthetic activity. All are insoluble in water, but will react with mineral acids such as hydrochloric acid to form soluble salts. However, aqueous solutions of these salts are too irritating to use because of the acidity caused by extensive hydrolysis. (38:632)
A. Benzocaine is insoluble in water and soluble in alcohol, vegetable oils, and several organic solvents. (38:631)
B. Many products marketed for use to relieve surface pain or itching contain benzocaine in concentrations of 1 to 20%. (38:632)
D. Hydrolysis yields alcohol and p-aminobenzoic acid. (1:987)

101. **D.** Methyldopa (Aldomet®) is only sparingly soluble in water, so the water-soluble hydrochloride of the ester salt (methyldopate hydrochloride, Aldomet Ester Hydrochloride®) is used for the injection. It is sufficiently stable to be marketed as an aqueous solution (50 mg/ml) but is rapidly hydrolyzed in vivo to methyldopa. (1:837; 39:387)

102. **E.** Polyethylene glycols are available in a range of molecular weights. Polyethylene Glycol 400 USP is a viscous colorless liquid, has an average molecular weight of 400, and n in the given formula varies from 8.2 to 9.1. Polyethylene Glycol 4000 USP is a waxy solid with an average molecular weight of 4000, and n varies from 68 to 84. Polyethylene Glycol Ointment USP is a 60:40 mixture of the 400 and 4000. (38:236–37)
Choice A is glycerin. (38:963)

Choice B is ethylene oxide, 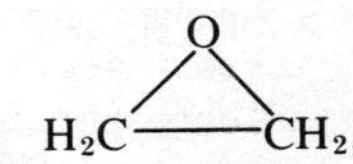, which can be polymerized to prepare polyethylene glycols. (38:123, 236)
Choice C is polyethylene glycol monostearate, a stearic acid ester of polyethylene glycol, which is a nonionic surfactant. (38:231)
Choice D is a polyoxyalkylene fatty ether of the Brij® series, commercially used as a surfactant in preparing lotions and creams. (38:232)

103. **E.** Mercaptopurine (Purinethol®) is the 6-thio analogue of adenine, a constituent of one of the nucleotides forming the deoxyribonucleic acid (DNA) chains necessary for protein synthesis and cellular reproduction. It is believed to act as an antimetabolite, replacing adenine in pathways leading to nucleic acid formation. The drug is therefore cytotoxic and useful against leukemia. Because it blocks the biosynthesis of antibodies by cells of the reticuloendothelial system in response to foreign cells (the immune response), mercaptopurine is used to prevent rejection of renal and other transplants. Thioguanine, a close relative of mercaptopurine, has similar uses. (38:174; 39:457–58)

104. **D.** The drug is nicotinic acid (niacin). In large doses (3.0 to 6.0 g daily) the antilipemic effect is observed in terms of lowered serum levels of cholesterol, phospholipid, free fatty acid, and triglyceride. Side effects include flushing, gastric irritation, and pruritis. (39:474, 477)

105. **D.** The compound is methyldopa (Aldomet®). Depending on pH it will exist as an anion or cation or as a zwitterion with no net charge. The pH at which the zwitterion exists is the isoelectric point for the molecule. At a pH below the isoelectric point the cation is formed and at the higher pH, the negative form, the anion, predominates. (14:298; 38:45, 602)

106. **A.** Molecules with this general structure combine with tissue receptor sites to block attachment of histamine to the sites and thus diminish or prevent the pharmacological actions of histamine. Diphenhydramine hydrochloride (Benadryl®) has the oxygen

connector, tripelennamine citrate (Pyribenzamine®), the nitrogen, and chlorpheniramine maleate (Chlor-Trimeton®), the carbon connector. (38:650, 653, 656, 658)

107. **E.** The sulfonylurea oral hypoglycemics are urea derivatives with an arylsulfonyl group in the 1-position and an aliphatic group at the 3-position. Maximum activity occurs when the R′ group contains three to six carbons; apparently this carbon chain length confers appropriate liposolubility. (38:615)

108. **C.** Phenformin hydrochloride (DBI®) is an oral hypoglycemic agent of the biguanide group. (38:617)

109. **D.** The structure pictured is the 1:1 copper chelate of penicillamine. It is probably the 2:1 chelate, which possesses two ionizable and water-solubilizing carboxyl groups, that acts as the sequestering agent in the removal of copper from the body in the treatment of Wilson's disease. (38:51)

110. **B.** The compound pictured, theophylline, is classified as a xanthine along with caffeine and theobromine. Of these compounds, theophylline is the most used for its action as a bronchodilator in the treatment of asthma. (6:375; 38:578)

111. **C.** The compound pictured is levodopa (Dopar®, Larodopa®, Levopa®). Levodopa can cross the blood-brain barrier and, presumably, is converted to dopamine in the basal ganglia. It is used in the treatment of parkinsonism. (38:847)
D. Although therapeutic doses of levodopa cause significant orthostatic hypotension, it is usually asymptomatic, and tolerance develops within a few months. The drug is not useful as an antihypertensive. (6:229)

112. **A.** A large number of thiazide diuretics are marketed; they differ chemically in the nature of the R and R_1 groups at the carbons numbered 3 and 6. Chlorothiazide is an example. In hydrochlorothiazide, the C_3 double bond is removed by hydrogenation. (38:583)

113. **B.** Cimetidine (Tagamet®) has the structure shown. Its evident relationship to histamine (see below) is believed to account for its ability to attach to H_2 receptors, thus blocking histamine stimulation of parietal cell secretion of gastric acid. (17:193; 38:468)

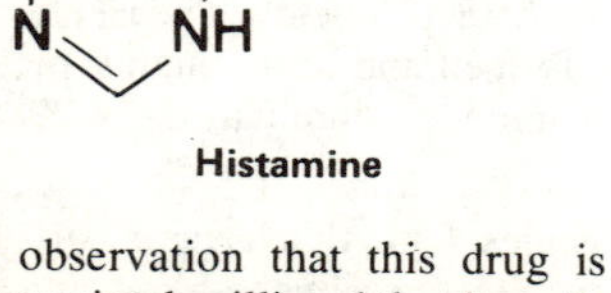

Histamine

114. **D.** The observation that this drug is active only against growing bacilli and that its action *is* reversed by p-aminobenzoic acid indicates a sulfonamide-like mechanism of action. Sodium aminosalicylate is much less effective than isoniazid or streptomycin but is used in combination with them because it delays the development of strains resistant to the more potent drugs. The free acid has been used, but it produces an acid urine from which its major metabolite, the acetylated form, may crystallize out of solution. The sodium salt produces a neutral or slightly alkaline urine in which the metabolite is sufficiently soluble. (1:1150; 38:144–55; 39:710)

115. **A.** The phenylethylamine derivatives such as epinephrine are inactive on oral administration, whereas the phenylpropylamine derivatives such as amphetamine and ephedrine are orally active drugs. (38:441)
B., C., D. Generally, the methyl substitution on the alpha carbon will decrease pressor activity, increase toxicity, and increase the CNS stimulating action in comparison with the parent compound. (38:441)

116. **B.** All of the drugs listed are benzodiazepine derivatives. The structure shown is for chlordiazepoxide hydrochloride (Librium®, 7-chloro -2- (methylamino -5- phenyl -3H-1,4- benzodiazepine -4- oxide hydrochloride). The USP categorizes this drug as a sedative. (18:80; 38:374–77)

117. **A.** Progesterone is produced by the corpus luteum and also by the adrenal glands and the placenta. It has multiple biological functions in the body. Synthetic derivatives (progestins) are components of oral contraceptives. (38:740, 743–44, 755–57)

118. **E.** Ibuprofen (Motrin®, (±)-2-(p-isobutyl-phenyl) propionic acid) is a nonsteroidal anti-inflammatory agent with analgesic and antipyretic activities. It is indicated in the chronic symptomatic treatment of rheumatoid arthritis and osteoarthritis and consequently must be compared with aspirin, which has been the standard drug for these conditions for many years. (6:343; 25:1765; 39:550)

119. **B.** The barbiturates are widely used sedative-hypnotic drugs. All are colorless crystalline solids which are not very soluble in water. They are weak acids. The sodium salts are water soluble but undergo extensive hydrolysis to yield strongly alkaline solutions from which the insoluble molecular form may precipitate. (38:356–59)

120. **B.** Bromocriptine mesylate (Parlodel®) is said to act as a direct dopamine receptor agonist. The structural feature that is shaded is phenethylamine; dopamine is *d*ihydr*o*xy*p*henethyl*a*mine. This fixed dopamine-like conformation presumably enables bromocriptine to fit and to act upon the dopamine receptor. The bromine atom at the 2-position significantly reduces the vasoconstrictive and oxytocic activity shown by the parent compound, the ergot alkaloid, alpha-ergocryptine. Stimulation of dopamine receptors causes inhibition of the release of prolactin by the pituitary. Bromocriptine is used to treat the galactorrhea-amenorrhea syndrome associated with hyperprolactinemia. (27:1729–31; 46:53–54)

C. Bromopheniramine maleate (Dimetane®) is an antihistamine used to alleviate allergic conditions. (25:1402)
D. Bromelains (Ananase®) is a concentrate of proteolytic enzymes derived from the pineapple plant. It is marketed as enteric tablets with claims for anti-inflammatory activity. (25:1481–82)
E. Bromural® is 2-bromoisovalerylurea, a sedative-hypnotic now of historical interest only. (38:365)

121. **D.** Valproic acid is alpha propyl valeric acid. It is chemically unlike other anticonvulsants in that it lacks nitrogen and aromaticity. (3:928–29; 46:51)
A. Valeric acid (pentoic acid, propylacetic acid) is an oily liquid with an unpleasant odor. The disputed sedative properties of the now medicinally obsolete valerian root were attributed to its valeric acid constituent. According to the 23rd edition of the *U.S. Dispensatory* (1944), p. 1214, the juice of the fresh root was once claimed to be an anticonvulsant useful in epilepsy.

122. **D.** (38:673, 693)

123. **B.** (38:673, 692)

124. **A.** (38:673, 693)

125. **E.** (38:673, 693)

126. **C.** (38:673, 694)

127. **B.** (1:405)

128. **A.** (1:399)

129. **C.** (1:399)

130. **D.** (1:399)

131. **E.** (1:405)

132. **E.** (1:405)

133. **A.** (1:406)

134. **D.** (1:405)

135. **B.** (1:405)

136. **C.** (1:405)

137. **D.** (1:400)

138. **C.** (1:399)

139. **A.** (1:399)

140. **B.** (1:400)

141. **E.** (1:399)

142. **D.** (1:455)

143. **C.** (1:455)

144. **E.** (1:405)

145. **B.** (1:405)

146. **C.** l-ephedrine is an example. d-glucose rotates polarized light to the right. (1:403)

147. **A.** Ortho-hydroxybenzoic acid, for example. (1:403)

148. **E.** Polyethylene glycols are polymers of ethylene oxide and water represented by the formula $H(OCH_2CH_2)_nOH$. (38:23–37)

149. **B.** In a heterocyclic organic compound, one or more of the atoms in the ring is not carbon; the five-membered heterocyclic isoxazole ring has three carbons, one oxygen, and one nitrogen. (1:412)

150. **D.** Strong acids dehydrate tetracycline to the inactive anhydrotetracycline. (38:308–09)

151. **D.** A *sub* salt is a basic salt such as aluminum subacetate, $Al(OH)(C_2H_3O_2)_2$. It may be thought of as an incompletely neutralized base, $Al(OH)_3$ in the example cited. (1:404; 22:54)

152. **A.** Desoxyephedrine (methamphetamine) is ephedrine less an oxygen atom. (1:403; 38:418)

153. **B.** Epinephrine has an N-methyl group which norepinephrine lacks. (1:403; 38:93)

154. **E.** Meta-dihydroxybenzene is an example. (1:403)

155. **C.** The terms D- and L- refer to the absolute configuration of an asymmetric center; optical rotation, left or right, is denoted by l- or d- or by (−) or (+). It is possible to have a D(−) or an L(+) isomer. (39:76)

156. **E.** (38:966)

157. **D.** (38:969)

158. **A.** (1:1247)

159. **B.** (38:82)
Choice C is ricinoleic acid. Ricinolein, the triglyceride of this acid, is the major component of castor oil. The hydroxyl group and the double bond confer some polarity upon the castor oil molecule. Consequently, castor oil, unlike most vegetable oils, is miscible with alcohol and immiscible with hydrocarbon solvents such as mineral oil. (38:953)

160. **B.** (1:1268)

161. **A.** (1:741; 38:953)

162. **E.** (1:1247)

163. **D.** (1:1241)
C. Teel oil is a synonym for sesame oil. (1:1241)

164. **A.** (1:423)

165. **C.** (1:281)

166. **D.** (1:399)

167. **B.** (1:537)
Choice E is hydrogenation, a process which is used to convert liquid oils to solid fats. (1:423)

168. **A.** Benzylpenicillin is a natural penicillin; the others are semisynthetics. (38:274, 278)

169. **C.** This side chain confers resistance to hydrolysis by penicillinase. (38:274, 281)

170. **E.** This side chain confers activity against some gram-negative organisms, so this penicillin has an extended spectrum of antimicrobial activity. It is readily hydrolyzed by penicillinase. (38:275, 282)

171. **D.** This bulky side chain also confers resistance to hydrolysis by penicillinase. (38:275, 282)
B. Phenoxymethyl penicillin is Penicillin V. It is resistant to hydrolysis by acid but is not resistant to penicillinase. (38:274, 280)

172. **C.** This side chain confers resistance to hydrolysis by either acid or penicillinase. (38:282)

173. **E.** This penicillin also is acid- and penicillinase-resistant. (38:281)

174. **D.** Phenethicillin is acid-resistant but not penicillinase-resistant. (38:280)

175. **B.** This new penicillin is acid-resistant and has an extended spectrum of antibiotic activity. It is not penicillinase-resistant. (38:283–84)

176. **E.** Sodium lauryl sulfate (Duponol®) is a mixture of sodium alkyl sulfates, mostly the one illustrated. The *anion* which has the surfactant qualities has the lipophilic (nonpolar) 12-carbon chain and the highly hydrophilic (polar) sulfate group. (38:225)

177. **A.** The quarternary nitrogen of the hetrocyclic ring structure is the hydrophilic part of the *cation* and the long aliphatic carbon chain is lipophilic. The compound, cetylpyridinium chloride (Ceepryn®), is used as a local anti-infective. (38:229)

178. **C.** Sorbitan monooleate (Span® 80) is a *non-ionic* oleic acid ester of sorbitan, an inner ether of sorbitol. The oleic acid portion of the molecule is lipophilic; the hydroxyl groups provide the hydrophilic character. This is useful for making w/o emulsions, especially in combination with Tweens®. (38:232)

179. **B.** Dodecyl glycine, representing the ampholytes, has the $C_{12}H_{25}$ nonpolar carbon chain and both a cationic and an anionic hydrophilic group. At a low pH, the positive group will predominate and confer cationic activity. At a higher pH, the anionic activity will predominate, and, at some intermediate point, the surfactant will act as though it were nonionic. The high cost has limited the use of these versatile agents. (38:235)

180. **B.** An example is chlorprothixene (Taractan®) in which R_1 is a dimethylaminoethyl group and R_2 is chlorine. (38:398)

181. **A.** One of the many available phenothiazine derivatives is chlorpromazine (Thorazine®), in which R is a dimethylaminoethyl group and R′ is chlorine. (38:383)

182. **E.** Haloperidol (Haldol®), in which R is the 4-(p-chlorophenyl) 4-hydroxypiperidino radical, as an example of a fluorobutyrophenone. (38:400)

CHAPTER 3

Pharmacology

From its inception in 1940, reference 6 in this book has been known to successive classes of pharmacy students simply as "Goodman and Gilman." In this new edition, on page 1, there is this statement: "In its entirety, *pharmacology* embraces the knowledge of the history, source, physical and chemical properties, compounding, biochemical and physiological effects, mechanisms of action, absorption, distribution, biotransformation and excretion, and therapeutic and other uses of drugs. Since a *drug* is broadly defined as any chemical agent that affects living processes, the subject of pharmacology is obviously quite extensive."

The test items in this chapter deal with some of these areas of pharmacology. Others are in the chapters on pharmaceutical chemistry, biopharmaceutics and pharmacokinetics, and clinical pharmacy.

Directions: Each of the questions or incomplete statements below is followed by five suggested answers or completions. Select the BEST answer in each case.

1. Xanthines such as caffeine and theophylline exert all of the following pharmacological effects *except*

   A. cardiac stimulation
   B. diuresis
   C. relaxation of smooth muscle
   D. peripheral vasoconstriction
   E. central nervous system stimulation (6:368–69)

2. Which of the following is *not* true of epinephrine?

   A. therapeutically effective after oral or parenteral administration
   B. will tend to elevate arterial blood pressure
   C. is a bronchodilator
   D. may be administered by inhalation
   E. will cause vasoconstriction in mucous membranes (6:483–90)

3. Heparin does *not*

   A. inhibit blood clotting
   B. inhibit formation of fibrin clots
   C. inhibit activation of the fibrin-stabilizing factor
   D. lyse existing clots
   E. prolong clotting time (1:583, 766)

4. Papaverine is used primarily for its ability to produce

   A. cough suppression
   B. analgesia
   C. skeletal muscle relaxation
   D. vasodilation
   E. emesis (6:735)

5. Which of the following is a vasodilating drug with marked platelet-suppressing activity?

   A. nitroglycerin
   B. nylidrin (Arlidin®)
   C. pentaerythritol tetranitrate (Peritrate®)
   D. dipyridamole (Persantine®)
   E. hydralazine (Apresoline®) (6:1365–66)

6. Urokinase (Abbokinase®) is a drug indicated for the treatment of

   A. hyperuricemia
   B. peptic ulcer disease
   C. carcinoma of the bladder
   D. dermal ulcers
   E. pulmonary emboli (25:502, 503, 917)

7. The ergot alkaloids have been found to be useful in the treatment of migraine headaches and are also used extensively as

   A. nasal decongestants
   B. oxytocics
   C. skeletal muscle relaxants
   D. local anesthetics
   E. antineoplastic agents (6:874, 879)

8. Which of the following metals has been found useful in the treatment of rheumatoid arthritis?

   A. platinum
   B. gold
   C. copper
   D. silver
   E. mercury (6:931–34)

9. As an antiarrhythmic drug, procainamide is most similar in action to which of the following agents?

   A. lidocaine
   B. phenytoin
   C. propranolol
   D. quinidine
   E. benzocaine (6:694)

10. Acetylcysteine is an agent used clinically as a

   A. laxative
   B. cough suppressant
   C. hemostatic
   D. mucolytic
   E. diagnostic agent (6:955)

11. Oxtriphylline (Choledyl®) can best be classified pharmacologically as a/an

   A. digestive enzyme
   B. skeletal muscle relaxant
   C. CNS depressant
   D. bronchodilator
   E. antipsychotic (6:374)

12. Which of the following agents may be added to local injections of lidocaine HCl in order to prolong its effect?

   A. epinephrine
   B. sodium carboxymethylcellulose
   C. atropine sulfate
   D. norepinephrine
   E. succinylcholine chloride (6:389)

13. Cholestyramine resin is most commonly used to treat

   A. hyperkalemia
   B. hyperglycemia
   C. hypernatremia
   D. hyperlipidemia
   E. hyperchlorhydria (6:748–49)

14. Which of the following drugs does *not* lower plasma lipoprotein concentrations?

   A. nicotinamide
   B. clofibrate
   C. ethinyl estradiol
   D. heparin
   E. dextrothyroxine (6:749, 1353)

15. Which of the following has *not* been used extensively for the treatment of parkinsonism?

   A. Thorazine®
   B. Cogentin®
   C. Artane®
   D. Kemadrin®
   E. Akineton® (6:169)

16. A drug that has been shown to have a high level of antagonism for both histamine and 5-hydroxytryptamine (5-HT) is

   A. chlorpheniramine (Chlor-Trimeton®)
   B. tripelennamine (Pyribenzamine®)
   C. promethazine (Phenergan®)
   D. pyrilamine
   E. cyproheptadine (Periactin®) (6:623)

17. Idoxuridine (Stoxil®, Herplex®, Dendrid®) is an effective treatment for dendritic keratitis, which is caused by

   A. *E. coli*
   B. herpes simplex
   C. *Staphylococcus aureus*
   D. helminthosporium siccans
   E. *Pseudomonas aeruginosa* (6:1242)

18. Retinoic acid is used therapeutically

   A. as a urinary acidifier
   B. as an antifungal agent
   C. in the topical treatment of acne
   D. in the treatment of tuberculosis
   E. as an ophthalmic irrigant (6:1577)

19. An agent that would be most likely to cause drug-induced bronchospasm is

   A. propranolol
   B. hydrochlorothiazide
   C. isoproterenol
   D. reserpine
   E. aminophylline (6:550)

20. Dopamine (Intropin®) is

   A. an alpha and beta agonist
   B. primarily a beta agonist
   C. primarily an alpha agonist
   D. a beta-blocking drug
   E. an alpha-blocking drug (10)

21. Terbutaline sulfate (Brethine®) is a/an

   A. beta-receptor agonist
   B. alpha-receptor agonist
   C. beta-receptor antagonist
   D. alpha-receptor antagonist
   E. alpha- and beta-receptor agonist (10)

22. Which of the following is a pharmacological action of histamine?

    A. capillary constriction
    B. stimulation of gastric secretion
    C. elevation of blood pressure
    D. skeletal muscle paralysis
    E. none of the above (6:591–94)

23. Which of the following would *not* be an expected effect of inhaling the smoke of cannabis (marihuana)?

    A. anorexia
    B. increase in pulse rate
    C. perceptual changes
    D. vascular congestion of the eyes
    E. all of the above are expected effects (6:307)

24. Of the following glucocorticoids, which one has the greatest anti-inflammatory potency?

    A. cortisol (Cortef®)
    B. prednisone (Meticorten®)
    C. triamcinolone (Aristocort®)
    D. dexamethasone (Decadron®)
    E. methylprednisolone (Medrol®) (6:1491)

25. Which of the following hormones is released from the posterior pituitary gland?

    A. adrenocorticotropic hormone (ACTH)
    B. oxytocin
    C. thyroid-stimulating hormone (TSH)
    D. follicle-stimulating hormone
    E. growth hormone (6:868)

26. At ovulation there will be the highest hormonal levels of

    A. follicle-stimulating hormone (FSH)
    B. luteinizing hormone (LH)
    C. both FSH and LH
    D. progesterone
    E. both progesterone and LH (2a:195)

27. A phenothiazine derivative commonly used for its antihistaminic effect is

    A. chlorpromazine
    B. promazine
    C. promethazine
    D. prochlorperazine
    E. thioridazine (6:610)

28. An active metabolite of the anticonvulsant drug primidone (Mysoline®) is

    A. phenobarbital
    B. dopamine
    C. phenytoin
    D. methsuximide
    E. trimethadione (6:210–11)

29. Carbamazepine (Tegretol®) is indicated for the treatment of

    A. enuresis
    B. trigeminal neuralgia
    C. endometriosis
    D. psoriasis
    E. minimal brain dysfunction (10; 17:311–12)

30. Of the following antianxiety agents, the one which possesses the greatest degree of antihistaminic action is

    A. diazepam (Valium®)
    B. hydroxyzine HCl (Atarax®)
    C. meprobamate (Miltown®, Equanil®)
    D. chlordiazepoxide (Librium®)
    E. oxazepam (Serax®) (10; 6:192)

31. Which of the following is *not* true of aminophylline?

    A. relaxes the smooth muscle of the respiratory tract
    B. an ethylenediamine complex of theophylline
    C. increases the contractile force of the heart
    D. causes central nervous system depression
    E. stimulates the production of gastric secretions (6:368, 374)

32. Penicillins are believed to exert their antibacterial effect by which of the following mechanisms?

    A. detergent effect on the bacterial cell membrane
    B. inhibition of bacterial cell wall synthesis
    C. destruction of the bacterial cell nucleus
    D. inhibition of protein synthesis
    E. none of the above mechanisms (6:1134)

33. The antibacterial mechanism of the penicillins is most similar to that of

    A. lincomycin (Lincocin®)
    B. tetracycline HCl (Achromycin®)
    C. neomycin (Mycifradin®)
    D. cephalexin (Keflex®)
    E. gentamicin (Garamycin®) (6:1134)

34. Which of the following agents may be administered with ampicillin and other penicillins to achieve higher blood levels of the penicillin?

    A. aspirin
    B. streptomycin
    C. probenecid (Benemid®)

D. nitrofurantoin (Furadantin®)
E. epinephrine (6:863)

35. One milligram of pure potassium penicillin G is equivalent to approximately ____ Penicillin Units of activity.

A. 37
B. 600
C. 1600
D. 250,000
E. 600,000 (6:1133)

36. Which of the following agents is most similar in action to ampicillin?

A. amoxicillin (Amoxil®)
B. nafcillin (Unipen®)
C. penicillin V (Pen Vee®)
D. dicloxacillin (Pathocil®)
E. benzyl penicillin (6:1145)

37. Penicillamine is a drug used therapeutically

A. in the treatment of gram-positive infections
B. as a diagnostic agent for penicillin allergy
C. as a chelator of various metals
D. in the treatment of gram-negative infections
E. as an antifungal agent (6:919–20)

38. Polymyxin B is pharmacologically and microbiologically similar to

A. ampicillin
B. colistin (Coly-Mycin S®)
C. kanamycin (Kantrex®)
D. penicillin G
E. tetracycline (Achromycin®) (6:1232)

39. A potentially fatal aplastic anemia is a toxicity associated with

A. demeclocycline (Declomycin®)
B. chloramphenicol (Chloromycetin®)
C. nitrofurantoin (Furadantin®)
D. clindamycin (Cleocin®)
E. cephalothin (Keflin®) (6:1196)

40. Which of the following agents is effective against penicillinase-producing staphylococci?

A. sodium methicillin
B. penicillin
C. phenethicillin
D. potassium hetacillin
E. amoxicillin (6:1143, 1153)

41. Which of the following antagonizes the action of sulfonamides?

A. streptomycin
B. penicillin G
C. morphine
D. p-aminobenzoic acid
E. all of the above (8:166)

42. Which of these tetracyclines has the longest duration of action?

A. tetracycline (Achromycin®, many others)
B. doxycycline (Vibramycin®)
C. demeclocycline (Declomycin®)
D. methacycline (Rondomycin®)
E. minocycline (Minocin®) (4:741–42)

43. Which of the following types of adverse drug reactions are *not* believed to be dose-related phenomena?

A. side effects and toxic reactions
B. toxic reactions and hypersensitivity
C. side effects and hypersensitivity
D. hypersensitivity and idiosyncracy
E. side effects and idiosyncracy (30:203)

44. The parietal cells of the stomach secrete

A. hydrochloric acid
B. pepsin
C. both hydrochloric acid and pepsin
D. intrinsic factor
E. both hydrochloric acid and intrinsic factor (2a:3)

45. The most prevalent side effect of the chronic use of aluminum hydroxide gel is

A. nausea and vomiting
B. constipation
C. flatulence
D. diarrhea
E. gastrointestinal bleeding (2a:7)

46. The anatomical center for hunger control (the appetite center) is believed to be located in the

A. adrenal medulla
B. hypothalamus
C. pancreas
D. pituitary
E. thyroid (2a:178)

47. Which of the following anorectic drugs is more likely to cause CNS depression than stimulation?

A. diethylpropion HCl (Tenuate®)
B. fenfluramine HCl (Pondimin®)
C. phentermine HCl (Ionamin®)
D. phendimetrazine tartrate (Plegine®)
E. phenmetrazine HCl (Preludin®) (25:1414–15)

48. An acne type of rash would most likely be associated with a chronic overdose of
    A. aspirin
    B. phenacetin
    C. tripelennamine
    D. sodium bromide
    E. aminophylline (6:126)

49. Which of the following is most likely to cause tinnitus in high doses?
    A. ibuprofen (Motrin®)
    B. aspirin
    C. indomethacin (Indocin®)
    D. mefenamic acid (Ponstel®)
    E. phenylbutazone (Butazolidin®) (6:327)

50. Which one of the following statements concerning salicylamide is *not* true?
    A. analgesic activity in humans is less than that of acetaminophen
    B. antipyretic activity in humans is less than that of aspirin
    C. most aspirin-sensitive patients can tolerate salicylamide
    D. salicylamide will increase prothrombin time
    E. salicylamide is present in some over-the-counter sleep aids (2a:126)

51. A uricosuric drug is one that
    A. decreases flow of urine
    B. increases flow of urine
    C. blocks excretion of uric acid in the urine
    D. promotes excretion of uric acid in the urine
    E. aids in the reabsorption of uric acid (6:862)

52. Which of the following can exert a uricosuric effect?
    A. colchicine
    B. aspirin
    C. hydrochlorothiazide
    D. allopurinol
    E. acetaminophen (6:331)

53. Which of the following diuretics has uricosuric activity?
    A. spironolactone
    B. furosemide
    C. chlorothiazide
    D. chlorthalidone
    E. ticrynafen (10)

54. Gluconeogenesis occurs primarily in the
    A. adrenal cortex
    B. liver
    C. kidney
    D. skeletal muscle
    E. thyroid (16:404)

55. A drug found to be useful in reducing elevated serum cholesterol in primary hypercholesterolemia is
    A. streptokinase (Streptase®)
    B. hytakerol
    C. mazindol (Sanorex®)
    D. probucol (Lorelco®)
    E. sodium polystyrene sulfonate (Kayexalate®) (25:843–44)

56. Nerves in the human body that transmit their impulses by releasing acetylcholine are known as ____ nerves.
    A. adrenergic
    B. choleretic
    C. axillary
    D. cholinergic
    E. neurogenic (6:419)

57. Which of the following is *not* true of methadone?
    A. available commercially under the name Dolophine®
    B. can be given orally or parenterally
    C. a narcotic antagonist
    D. an addicting drug
    E. has significant analgesic activity (6:268–69)

58. Naloxone and nalorphine are similar in that they both fall into the therapeutic category known as
    A. non-narcotic analgesic
    B. narcotic analgesic
    C. cough suppressant
    D. narcotic antagonist
    E. hallucinogen (6:273)

59. Which of the following is *not* a pharmacological effect of morphine?
    A. smooth muscle stimulation
    B. cough suppression
    C. diarrhea
    D. respiratory depression
    E. nausea and vomiting (6:253)

60. Etidronate disodium (Didronel®) is an agent primarily indicated for the treatment of
    A. Paget's disease
    B. Meniere's syndrome
    C. Crohn's disease
    D. Hansen's disease
    E. Parkinson's disease (46:63–64)

61. An agent used for the same indication as etidronate disodium (Didronel®) is
   A. methocarbamol (Robaxin®)
   B. salmon calcitonin (Calcimar®)
   C. carmustine (BiCNU®)
   D. sodium nitroprusside (Nipride®)
   E. bretylium tosylate (Bretylol®) (46:63–64)

62. Which of the following is *not* an action of digitalis on the myocardium?
   A. increased force of contraction
   B. slowed AV conduction
   C. prolonged refractory period of the AV node
   D. decreased rate of the SA node
   E. increased oxygen consumption of the heart (6:655–65)

63. The antiarrhythmic action of disopyramide (Norpace®) most closely resembles that of
   A. lidocaine
   B. phenytoin
   C. quinidine
   D. propranolol
   E. bretylium (10; 25:A49, 1580–82)

64. Which of the following cardiac glycosides is most completely absorbed after oral administration?
   A. digoxin (Lanoxin®)
   B. lanatoside (Cedilanid®)
   C. digitoxin (Crystodigin®, Purodigin®)
   D. ouabain
   E. gitalin (Gitaligin®) (6:673)

65. Lactulose (Cephulac®, Duphalac®) acts by
   A. inhibiting diarrhea
   B. inhibition of ammonia absorption from the GI tract
   C. destroying colonic bacteria responsible for the production of ammonia
   D. causing systemic acidosis
   E. binding with ammonia in the GI tract (10; (10; 25:1197–98; 27:1338)

66. The active laxative principle formed by hydrolysis of castor oil in the GI tract is
   A. pyruvic acid
   B. mandelonitrile
   C. ricinoleic acid
   D. benzaldehyde
   E. carvone (6:982)

67. Which of the following is classified as a systemic antacid?
   A. sodium bicarbonate
   B. aluminum hydroxide
   C. magnesium trisilicate
   D. calcium carbonate
   E. magnesium hydroxide (6:960–61)

68. The early diuretic effect of alcoholic beverages is due to
   A. the increased fluid load that must be handled by the kidneys
   B. suppression of ADH release from the posterior pituitary gland
   C. both A and B
   D. competitive inhibition of ADH at renal receptor sites
   E. inhibition of sodium reabsorption in the proximal tubule (6:141)

69. The primary site of action of triamterene (Dyrenium®) and spironolactone (Aldactone®) is the
   A. proximal tubule
   B. descending loop of Henle
   C. ascending loop of Henle
   D. distal tubule
   E. glomerulus (6:837–38)

70. Which of the following drugs is most useful in the relief of acute attacks of gout?
   A. probenecid
   B. aspirin
   C. meperidine (Demerol®)
   D. colchicine
   E. allopurinol (Zyloprim®) (6:352)

71. Prolonged use of phenylbutazone (Butazolidin®, Azolid®) is usually contraindicated because of its potential for producing
   A. damage to the auditory nerve
   B. blood dyscrasias
   C. damage to the optic nerve
   D. precipitation of an acute attack of gout
   E. electrolyte depletion (6:340)

72. After oral administration, the greatest amount of iron absorption occurs in the
   A. duodenum
   B. stomach
   C. sigmoid portion of the large intestine
   D. transverse portion of the large intestine
   E. ascending portion of the large intestine (6:1310)

73. Following oral administration of usual doses, iron is primarily absorbed
   A. in the ferric state
   B. by an active transport process
   C. by passive diffusion

D. as ferritin
E. in the ferric state by active transport, then in the ferrous state by passive diffusion (6:1310)

74. Which of the following insects neither bites nor stings humans?
A. bedbugs
B. fleas
C. lice
D. mites
E. ticks (2a:265)

75. Which of the following drugs is/are excreted primarily by renal tubular secretion?
A. gentamicin (Garamycin®)
B. kanamycin (Kantrex®)
C. tetracycline (Achromycin®)
D. carbenicillin (Geopen®, Pyopen®)
E. A and B (6:1146, 1171–79)

76. Which of the following is the usual route of administration of amyl nitrite?
A. intramuscular
B. inhalation
C. sublingual
D. intravenous
E. oral (6:729)

77. Stage IV of general anesthesia is generally referred to as the stage of
A. respiratory paralysis
B. delirium
C. stimulation
D. surgical anesthesia
E. analgesia (6:60–61)

78. Which is characteristic of prostaglandins?
A. stored in many tissues
B. primarily found in semen
C. a limited range of functions in the body
D. all have qualitatively the same pharmacological actions, differing only in degree
E. rapidly synthesized in the body (6:641, 644)

79. Timolol maleate is a drug used in the treatment of glaucoma. Which of the following best describes the action it exerts on the eye?
A. miotic
B. increases the outflow of aqueous humor
C. interferes with the enzyme carbonic anhydrase
D. acts as an osmotic diuretic
E. none of the above (47:39, 40)

80. Demecarium bromide, echothiophate iodide, and isoflurophate are all classified as long-acting anticholinesterase agents for glaucoma. Maximum activity for these drug solutions occurs in approximately how many hours after instillation into the eye?
A. four
B. eight
C. 12
D. 24
E. 48 (4:928)

81. Which of the following is *not* an effect of atropine on the human body?
A. cardiac stimulation
B. diminished sweating
C. stimulation of gastric secretion
D. reduction of gastrointestinal tone
E. mydriasis (6:518–21)

82. Which of the following statements best describes the mechanism of action of antihistaminic drugs?
A. they interfere with the synthesis of histamine in the body
B. they form inactive complexes with histamine
C. they block the receptor sites on which histamine acts
D. they stimulate the metabolism of endogenous histamine
E. none of the above (6:595)

83. The pain associated with angina pectoris is caused by
A. spasm of the aorta
B. electrolyte imbalance on the myocardial surface
C. ventricular tachycardia
D. aortic stenosis
E. ischemia of some area of the myocardium (6:737)

84. Agents useful in the treatment of bronchial asthma usually
A. block both alpha- and beta-adrenergic receptors
B. stimulate alpha receptors but block beta receptors
C. stimulate beta receptors but block alpha receptors
D. stimulate alpha and/or beta receptors
E. none of the above (4:627–28)

85. Intravenous administration of furosemide (Lasix®) usually results in diuresis in
   A. less than 30 minutes
   B. one hour
   C. two to four hours
   D. eight hours
   E. 12 to 24 hours (6:833)

86. Advantages of acetaminophen over aspirin include all of the following *except*
   A. no alteration of bleeding time
   B. greater anti-inflammatory action
   C. no occult blood loss
   D. no appreciable uricosuric antagonism
   E. less gastric irritation (1:1048)

87. Which of the following is true of propoxyphene HCl (Darvon®)?
   A. it has about the same analgesic activity as an equivalent dose of codeine
   B. it has significant analgesic and antipyretic properties
   C. it has analgesic and anti-inflammatory properties but has no antipyretic properties
   D. the analgesic property of this drug resides only in the levorotatory isomer (1-propoxyphene)
   E. none of the above (6:270)

88. Although classified as antibiotics, dactinomycin (Cosmegen®) and mithramycin (Mithracin®) are used in cancer chemotherapy because they have a/an
   A. immunosuppressant effect
   B. antiviral effect
   C. cytotoxic effect
   D. anabolic effect
   E. ability to "sterilize" the blood (6:1288, 1292)

89. Which of the following cancer chemotherapeutic agents is/are classified as (an) antimetabolite(s)?
   A. nitrogen mustard (Mustargen®)
   B. cyclophosphamide (Cytoxan®)
   C. fluorouracil
   D. chlorambucil (Leukeran®)
   E. all of the above (6:1250–51)

90. Although it has not been proved, it has been recently suggested that the anti-inflammatory effect of aspirin may be due to
   A. an anticoagulant effect
   B. an antigen-antibody reaction
   C. inhibition of the synthesis of prostaglandins
   D. increased membrane permeability of inflamed tissue
   E. stimulation of endogenous hydrocortisone (6:332, 647)

91. Carbon monoxide exerts its toxic effects primarily by
   A. reacting with body enzymes to produce acidic substances
   B. paralyzing the muscles of the diaphragm
   C. reacting with amino acids in the body to form ammonia
   D. inhibiting the gag reflex
   E. decreasing the oxygen-carrying capacity of the blood (6:900)

92. The most serious potential consequence of ingestion of a liquid hydrocarbon such as kerosine or gasoline is
   A. dissolution of the mucoid coat of the esophagus
   B. the corrosive action of the poison on the stomach lining
   C. the paralysis of peristaltic motion of the GI tract
   D. the aspiration of the poison into the respiratory tract
   E. the destruction of body enzymes by the poison (6:907–08)

93. A specific antidote for the treatment of poisoning due to the oral ingestion of silver nitrate would be the oral administration of
   A. potassium permanganate solution
   B. vegetable oil
   C. acetic acid solution
   D. normal saline
   E. sodium bicarbonate (6:930)

94. Antihistaminic drugs such as diphenhydramine and its congeners show other important pharmacological effects as well. Which of the following is *not* one of these effects?
   A. CNS depression
   B. local anesthetic activity
   C. anti-inflammatory activity
   D. anticholinergic activity
   E. CNS stimulation (6:603–11)

95. Which of the following agents is classified pharmacologically as a carbonic anhydrase inhibitor?
   A. furosemide (Lasix®)
   B. spironolactone (Aldactone®)
   C. chlorothiazide (Diuril®)
   D. acetazolamide (Diamox®)
   E. triamterene (Dyrenium®) (6:826)

96. The thiazide diuretics may reduce the excretion of
    A. sodium
    B. urea
    C. uric acid
    D. bicarbonate
    E. creatinine (6:830–31)

97. The renal excretion of amphetamines can be diminished by alkalinization of the urine. Which of the following would tend to diminish the excretion rate of amphetamine sulfate?
    A. methenamine mandelate
    B. acetazolamide
    C. tetracycline HCl
    D. ammonium chloride
    E. niacin (6:499, 828)

98. Which of the following drugs inhibits the metabolism of ethanol?
    A. phenylbutazone
    B. disulfiram
    C. chlorpheniramine
    D. metronidazole
    E. B and D (8:97, 151, 216)

99. Which of the following is *not* an enzyme inhibitor?
    A. pargyline
    B. glutethimide
    C. isocarboxazid
    D. tranylcypromine
    E. phenelzine (6:180–84)

100. Which of the following is a microsomal enzyme inducer?
    A. indomethacin
    B. clofibrate
    C. tolbutamide
    D. glutethimide
    E. ibuprofen (8:47)

101. The thiazide derivative, diazoxide (Hyperstat®)
    A. is a stronger diuretic than hydrochlorothiazide
    B. is a weaker diuretic than hydrochlorothiazide
    C. produces about the same diuretic response as an equal dose of hydrochlorothiazide
    D. is not a diuretic
    E. produces diuresis in normotensive subjects only (6:714)

102. Which of the following is an ultrashort-acting barbiturate?
    A. phenobarbital
    B. amobarbital
    C. thiopental sodium
    D. pentobarbital sodium
    E. metharbital (6:117–18)

103. Aminocaproic acid (Amicar®) is a synthetic compound that is an effective
    A. antineoplastic agent
    B. anticoagulant
    C. inhibitor of fibrinolysis
    D. antifungal agent
    E. anthelmintic (10; 6:1365)

104. Phenylbutazone (Butazolidin®) is
    A. an active metabolite of oxyphenbutazone (Tandearil®)
    B. an inactive metabolite of oxyphenbutazone
    C. hydroxylated to oxyphenbutazone which is an active metabolite
    D. excreted unchanged in the urine
    E. metabolized to an anti-inflammatory steroid (6:340)

105. A pharmacist receives a prescription order for phenylbutazone (Butazolidin®). He should consult with the physician if the medication record indicates that the patient
    A. has gout
    B. has arthritis
    C. is hypertensive
    D. has insomnia
    E. has a peptic ulcer (4:369)

106. The sulfonylureas (i.e., Orinase®, Diabinese®) are believed to exert their hypoglycemic effect by
    A. stimulating the release of insulin from the pancreas
    B. inhibiting the breakdown of endogenous insulin
    C. enhancing the effectiveness of small amounts of insulin that the diabetic can produce
    D. increasing the peripheral utilization of glucose
    E. all of the above mechanisms (37:743)

107. Which of the following oral hypoglycemic drugs has the longest serum half-life?
    A. acetohexamide (Dymelor®)
    B. chlorpropamide (Diabinese®)
    C. tolazamide (Tolinase®)
    D. tolbutamide (Orinase®)
    E. all of the above have about the same serum half-life (6:1521)

108. Vidarabine (Vira-A®) is an antiviral agent indicated for the treatment of

   A. rubella
   B. herpes simplex encephalitis
   C. influenza
   D. rubeola
   E. smallpox (25:1324–25)

109. Which of the following statements regarding methenamine mandelate is *not* true?

   A. after oral ingestion formaldehyde is formed in acid urine
   B. it is maximally effective at a urinary pH below 5.5
   C. it should be given with sulfonamides to enhance effectiveness of therapy
   D. it is contraindicated in renal insufficiency
   E. ammonia is produced in acid urine after its oral ingestion (6:1006–07)

110. Inactivation of the proteolytic activity of pepsin will aid in the healing of ulcers. Pepsin activity will be destroyed if the stomach pH is raised to a minimum pH of

   A. 4.0
   B. 6.0
   C. 7.0
   D. 8.0
   E. 10.0 (2a:6)

111. An agent that has been shown to have a high order of antagonism for both histamine and 5-hydroxytryptamine (5-HT) is

   A. phenylephrine HCl
   B. guaifenesin
   C. cyproheptadine
   D. tubocurarine
   E. theophylline (6:622–23)

112. Cromolyn sodium (Intal®, Aarane®) is an antiasthmatic drug that is

   A. effective in acute asthmatic attacks
   B. a synthetic corticosteroid
   C. a histamine antagonist
   D. a stabilizer of sensitized mast cells
   E. a theophylline derivative (6:602)

Directions: EACH set of the following questions consists of several numbered items followed by a list of five lettered words or phrases. MATCH the lettered words or phrases most closely associated with the numbered item. Use each letter once only unless otherwise indicated.

Questions 113 to 117
Some drugs are assayed by biological techniques, especially when more conventional chemical methods will not reflect the pharmacological action of the drug. MATCH the lettered animal with the appropriate drug for which the animal or parts of the animal is employed for assay purposes. Note: lettered answers may be used more than once.

113. cod liver oil
114. insulin injection
115. heparin injection
116. oxytocin injection
117. protamine sulfate

   A. chicken
   B. dog
   C. rabbit
   D. rat
   E. sheep (1:574–76)

Questions 118 to 122
MATCH the lettered drug with the numbered antihypertensive mechanism most closely associated with it.

118. ganglionic blocking agent
119. catecholamine depleter
120. false neurotransmitter
121. direct action on arterioles
122. direct action on central nervous system

   A. methyldopa (Aldomet®)
   B. hydralazine (Apresoline®)
   C. reserpine (Serpasil®)
   D. mecamylamine (Inversine®)
   E. veratrum alkaloids (6:557, 570–73, 707–10, 716–17)

Questions 123 to 127
The next group of numbered names of diseases is followed by a list of lettered names which are used for these same diseases. MATCH the lettered name with the corresponding numbered name.

123. Cooley's disease
124. Down's syndrome
125. Hansen's disease
126. Herpes zoster
127. St. Vitus' dance

   A. chorea
   B. familial erythroblastic anemia
   C. leprosy
   D. mongolism
   E. shingles (11:407, 457, 707, 1519, 1593)

Questions 128 to 137
MATCH the lettered adverse drug reaction most closely associated with the use of the numbered drug name.

128. Inderal®
129. Serpasil®

130. Ritalin®
131. Achromycin®
132. Loridine®

A. depression
B. nephrotoxicity
C. photosensitivity
D. bradycardia
E. nervousness (17:94, 105, 302, 552, 556)

133. Lasix®
134. Decadron®
135. Amcill®
136. Chloromycetin®
137. Aldactone®

A. fluid retention
B. aplastic anemia
C. hyperkalemia
D. hypokalemia
E. urticaria (17:357, 364, 533, 544, 716)

Questions 138 to 149
MATCH the lettered side effect, adverse effect, or hypersensitivity reaction with the associated numbered drug.

138. spironolactone (Aldactone®)
139. guanethidine (Ismelin®)
140. methyldopa (Aldomet®)
141. sulfisoxazole (Gantrisin®)

A. positive Coombs' test
B. Stevens-Johnson syndrome
C. gynecomastia
D. peripheral neuritis
E. orthostatic hypotension (17:110, 577; 6:709)

142. rifampin (Rifadin®)
143. demethylchlortetracycline (Declomycin®)
144. gentamicin (Garamycin®)
145. chlorpromazine (Thorazine®)

A. nephrotoxicity, ototoxicity
B. discoloration of urine and sweat
C. oculocutaneous pigmentation
D. gingival hyperplasia
E. photosensitization
6:163) (17:571, 558, 540; 6:163)

146. isoniazid (INH®)
147. erythromycin estolate (Ilosone®)
148. phenytoin (Dilantin®)
149. diazoxide (Hyperstat®)

A. photosensitization
B. gingival hyperplasia
C. cholestatic jaundice
D. hyperglycemia
E. peripheral neuritis (17:310, 392, 571, 581)

Questions 150 to 165
MATCH the lettered pharmacologic category with the associated numbered drug.

150. thiothixene (Navane®)
151. protriptyline (Vivactil®)
152. trimethadione (Tridione®)
153. oxazepam (Serax®)

A. anticonvulsant
B. antianxiety agent
C. antidepressant
D. antiemetic
E. antipsychotic (17:231, 259, 295, 312)

154. trimethobenzamide (Tigan®)
155. isocarboxazid (Marplan®)
156. hydrochlorothiazide (Hydrodiuril®)
157. tripelennamine (Pyribenzamine®)

A. anticholinergic
B. antiemetic
C. antihypertensive
D. antihistamine
E. monoamine oxidase inhibitor (17:160, 186, 190, 192, 304)

158. phenylbutazone (Butazolidin®)
159. benztropine (Cogentin®)
160. lidocaine (Xylocaine®)
161. procarbazine (Matulane®)

A. antiarrhythmic
B. anti-inflammatory
C. antineoplastic
D. anticholinergic
E. hypoglycemic (17:153, 291, 292, 322, 486)

162. sulfinpyrazone (Anturane®)
163. tolnaftate (Tinactin®)
164. flurazepam (Dalmane®)
165. acetohexamide (Dymelor®)

A. uricosuric
B. hypnotic
C. diuretic
D. antifungal
E. hypoglycemic (17:239, 386, 440, 587)

Questions 166 to 185
MATCH the lettered therapeutic indication most closely corresponding to the numbered brand name.

166. Tinactin®
167. Pro-Banthine®
168. Dilantin®
169. Lasix®
170. Dimetapp®

A. tinea pedis
B. grand mal

C. peptic ulcer
D. nasal congestion
E. congestive heart failure
(17:77, 192, 309, 587, 716)

171. Zyloprim®
172. Ismelin®
173. Elixophyllin®
174. Cordran®
175. Dopar®

A. bronchial asthma
B. parkinsonism
C. hypertension
D. inflammation
E. gout (17:110, 124, 318, 360, 490)

176. Macrodantin®
177. Percodan®
178. Tofranil®
179. Isordil®
180. Nilstat®

A. pain
B. urinary tract infection
C. depression
D. vulvovaginal candidiasis
E. angina pectoris
(17:121, 278, 294, 586, 588)

181. Dalmane®
182. Atarax®
183. Drixoral®
184. Cytomel®
185. Tolinase®

A. anxiety
B. diabetes mellitus
C. acute rhinitis
D. insomnia
E. hypothyroidism
(10: 17:239, 262, 346, 389)

Questions 186 to 188
Deficiencies of certain substances may result in disease. MATCH the lettered substance believed to be deficient in the body with the numbered resulting disease.

186. pellagra
187. pernicious anemia
188. scurvy

A. ascorbic acid
B. cyanocobalamin
C. niacin
D. riboflavin
E. thiamine (11:85, 1152, 1393)

Questions 189 to 193
MATCH the lettered antimicrobial agent with the numbered disease for which it would be most likely to be used.

189. gonococcus
190. leprosy
191. *Candida albicans*
192. tinea capitis
193. tuberculosis

A. nystatin
B. griseofulvin
C. streptomycin
D. penicillin G
E. dapsone (6:1097, 1101, 1103)

Questions 194 to 205
MATCH the lettered mechanism of action with the most closely associated numbered drug. A letter may be used more than once.

194. erythromycin
195. sulfisoxazole (Gantrisin®)
196. polymyxin B (Aerosporin®)
197. actinomycin (Cosmegen®)
198. ampicillin
199. cephalothin (Keflin®)
200. nystatin (Mycostatin®)
201. amphotericin B (Fungizone®)
202. rifampin (Rifadin®)
203. chloramphenicol
204. methacillin (Staphcillin®)
205. tetracycline

A. inhibition of growth by means of competitive antagonism
B. inhibition of cell wall synthesis
C. inhibition of cell membrane function
D. inhibition of protein synthesis
E. inhibition of nucleic acid synthesis
(6:1091)

Questions 206 to 211
The group of numbered laxatives below is followed by a list of lettered mechanisms by which laxatives act. MATCH the lettered mechanism with the numbered laxative. Letters may be used more than once.

206. bisacodyl
207. magnesium citrate
208. mineral oil
209. poloxamer 188
210. psyllium
211. sodium biphosphate

A. draws water into intestinal tract by osmosis
B. forms bulk by absorbing water
C. softens stools by lubrication
D. softens stools by lowering surface tension
E. stimulates intestinal wall (2a:41–44)

Questions 212 to 216
MATCH the lettered narcotic compound most closely associated with the numbered description. Letters may be used more than once or not at all.

212. has the greatest analgesic activity
213. has the weakest analgesic activity
214. used as an ophthalmic solution
215. specific antidote in the treatment of acute narcotic intoxication
216. available in a suppository dosage form

A. ethylmorphine HCl
B. hydromorphone
C. morphine
D. nalorphine HCl
E. oxymorphone HCl (1:1040–42)

Questions 217 to 221
MATCH the lettered antihypertensive agent with the numbered adverse effect with which it is most closely associated.

217. syncope after first dose
218. drug-induced SLE
219. positive Coomb's reaction
220. drug-induced inhibition of ejaculation
221. sodium retention

A. methyldopa (Aldomet®)
B. prazocin (Minipress®)
C. hydralazine (Apresoline®)
D. guanethidine (Ismelin®)
E. diazoxide (Hyperstat®)
(3:469, 473, 484; 6:556; 10)

Answers and Commentary

1. **D.** Since the xanthines are direct-acting smooth muscle relaxants, coronary, pulmonary, and general systemic blood vessels are dilated. This effect tends to decrease blood pressure but is minimized by the pressor effects of medullary and cardiac stimulation. (6:368–69)

2. **A.** Epinephrine will elicit little or no response when taken orally for a number of reasons such as inactivation by digestive secretions, local vasoconstriction which will inhibit systemic absorption, and rapid enzymatic inactivation in the systemic circulation. (6:483–90)

3. **D.** (1:583, 766)

4. **D.** Papaverine is a nonspecific, smooth muscle relaxant derived from crude opium. It is capable of relaxing the smooth muscle of blood vessels, thereby causing a moderate degree of vasodilation. (6:735)

5. **D.** Dipyridamole (Persantine®) is a coronary vasodilator that has been shown to inhibit platelet aggregation. It has been used in conjunction with oral anticoagulants and with aspirin (which also decreases platelet aggregation) for the prophylactic treatment of thromboembolic disorders. (6:1365–66)

6. **E.** Urokinase (Abbokinase®) is an enzyme indicated for the intravenous treatment of acute, massive pulmonary emboli. Unlike heparin and other anticoagulants that prevent the propagation of thrombi, urokinase promotes their dissolution. A similar action has been proposed for the enzyme streptokinase (Streptase®). Since both agents are fibrinolytic enzymes, they may cause serious bleeding and are therefore contraindicated in patients who have had surgery, a liver or kidney biopsy, or an intra-arterial diagnostic procedure within the previous 10 days. (25:502, 503, 917)

7. **B.** Oxytocic agents stimulate the motility of the uterus. Ergot alkaloids such as ergonovine (Ergotrate®) and methylerfonovine (Methergine®) are commonly used for their ability to control postpartum hemorrhage by virtue of their oxytocic activity. These agents appear to posses relatively greater oxytocic activity than do other available ergot alkaloids. (6:874, 879)

8. **B.** Gold compounds have been used for many years in the treatment of rheumatoid arthritis. Although the mechanism of action of gold in this disease is not fully elaborated, gold compounds have been shown to be capable of altering the properties of collagen and of inhibiting the formation of glucosamine-6-phosphate in connective tissue. (6:931–34)

9. **D.** Procainamide is a drug used to treat cardiac arrhythmia (disturbances of cardiac rhythm). It is quite similar in action to quinidine. Both of these drugs will affect the electrical properties of cardiac fibers, exert a local anesthetic effect, and directly depress the mechanical activity of the heart. (6:694)

10. **D.** Acetylcysteine (Mucomyst®) is an agent which liquefies mucus and DNA (the agent in pus responsible for its viscosity) but does not affect blood clots or living tissue. It exerts its mucolytic activity by opening the disulfide bonds of mucoproteins and thereby lowering their viscosity. Its activity as a mucolytic is greatest at a pH of 7 to 9 and it may be administered by inhalation or by direct application. (6:955)

11. **D.** Oxtriphylline (Choledyl®) is the choline salt of theophylline. It is more water soluble, more stable, better absorbed from the GI tract, and less irritating to the gastric mucosa than aminophylline. It is available in tablet and elixir dosage forms. (6:374)

12. **A.** Epinephrine will cause local vasoconstriction, which will delay transportation away from the injection site and thereby prolong the local action of the lidocaine. (6:389)

13. **D.** Cholestyramine resin (Cuemid®, Questran®) is an orally administered anion exchange resin that binds bile acids in the intestine and prevents their reabsorption. The reduction in bile acid concentration causes an increase in the rate of conversion of cholesterol to bile acids in the liver. The drug is quite safe, since it is not absorbed from the gastrointestinal tract. It has the disadvantage, however, of interacting with many other drugs which are adsorbed by it. (6:748–49)

14. **A.** It has been shown that nicotinic acid (niacin) but not nicotinamide will lower plasma triglyceride levels. It is believed that this effect of nicotinic acid is due to inhibition of triglyceride formation in the liver and, subsequently, diminished release of triglycerides into the plasma. (6:749)
D. Heparin has a definite lipid-clearing effect that is probably due to stimulation of the enzyme lipoprotein lipase. It is not clinically useful for this purpose because of its short duration of action and the danger of hemorrhage. (6:1353)

15. **A.** Thorazine® is a phenothiazine derivative that may cause extrapyramidal effects such as muscular trem-

ors and may thereby aggravate parkinsonism. (6:169)

16. **E.** Cyproheptadine (Periactin®) is an agent having a structure quite similar to that of some ergot alkaloids. The drug has the unique ability to antagonize strongly the action of histamine and also of 5-HT, a substance that is also capable of eliciting many of the physiological responses produced by histamine. (6:623)

17. **B.** Idoxuridine is one of the few available antiviral agents. It acts as an antimetabolite. Ophthalmic ointments and solutions are available. The solutions require refrigeration. (6:1242)

18. **C.** Retinoic acid or vitamin A acid is a component in a number of commercial preparations used in the topical treatment of acne (Retin-A®, etc.) It acts to accelerate the production of epithelial cells in the skin, thereby promoting the healing of acne lesions. (6:1577)

19. **A.** Propranolol is a beta-adrenergic blocking agent that affects many structures in the body. Since adrenergic bronchodilation is mediated by beta receptors, the administration of propranolol consistently increases airway resistance. While this has no clinical significance in most patients, propranolol may cause severe bronchospasm in asthmatic patients. (6:550)

20. **B.** Dopamine is the immediate precursor of norepinephrine. Like norepinephrine, it activates primarily beta receptors. The net result of this positive inotropic effect is an increase in cardiac output. Another important action of dopamine is its ability to dilate renal vessels and produce sodium diuresis. (10)

21. **A.** Terbutaline is a beta-receptor agonist that is claimed to exert a preferential effect on $beta_2$ adrenergic receptors such as those located in bronchial smooth muscle. Clinical studies on this oral bronchodilator indicate proportionally greater changes in pulmonary function parameters than in heart rate or blood pressure. While this suggests some preference for $beta_2$ receptors in humans, it should be emphasized that the usual cardiovascular effects associated with sympathomimetic agents were also observed with terbutaline. (10)

22. **B.** Histamine stimulates the glands of the gastrointestinal tract (gastric, salivary, pancreatic). It has been suggested that the rate of gastric secretion is directly proportional to the rate of blood flow to the secretory area. Since histamine tends to increase such blood flow by dilation of local blood vessels, such stimulation of gastric secretion is logical. (6:591–94)

23. **A.** After oral ingestion or inhalation, cannabis often causes a marked increase in appetite, especially for sweets. (6:307)

24. **D.** The anti-inflammatory potency of the synthetic glucocorticoids is usually compared with the naturally occurring steroid cortisol. Using this basis of comparison the following relative potencies have been established: cortisol 1, prednisone 4, methylprednisolone 5, triamcinolone 5, dexamethasone 25. (6:1491)

25. **B.** The others are secreted from the anterior pituitary gland. (6:868)

26. **C.** The levels of follicle-stimulating hormone (FSH) and luteinizing hormone (LH) are at their maxima just before ovulation. The FSH has stimulated follicular growth, but eventually the matured follicle secretes estrogen, which inhibits further production of FSH. The LH stimulates the ruptured follicle into forming the corpus luteum, which then secretes progesterone, which in turn decreases further production of LH. Thus, after ovulation there is a steady decline in levels of FSH and LH. The matured corpus luteum continues the secretion of estrogens and progesterone to maintain the endometrium. If conception does not occur within 12 days after ovulation, sloughing of the endometrium occurs and menstruation starts. (2a:195)

27. **C.** Promethazine (Phenergan®) is the prototype phenothiazine for the management of allergic conditions. Its prominent sedative effects and its value in treating motion sickness have also been recognized. (6:610)

28. **A.** Primidone is very similar in chemical structure to phenobarbital. Primidone is converted in the body to two metabolites, phenobarbital and phenylethylmalonamide (PEMA). Both of these metabolites accumulate in the plasma within several days of the initiation of primidone therapy. It is believed that the anticonvulsant effects produced by this drug can be attributed both to the parent drug and to its metabolites. (6:210, 211)

29. **B.** Carbamezepine (Tegretol®) is considered to be generally equivalent to phenytoin in its pharmacological effects and has been approved for use as an anticonvulsant in some epileptic disorders in which the patient has not responded to safer drugs such as phenobarbital or phenytoin. It has been shown to be superior to phenytoin in preventing the paroxysms of terrible pain in trigeminal neuralgia. (10; 17:311–12)

30. **B.** Hydroxyzine HCl is an antianxiety drug which also possesses antiemetic and antihistaminic effects. It is, therefore, quite useful in treating allergic dermatoses, postoperative nausea and vomiting, and motion sickness. (10; 6:192)

31. **D.** Aminophylline, as is the case with other xanthine derivatives (i.e., caffeine, theophylline), acts to stimulate the central nervous system, thereby possibly producing restlessness, irritability, and insomnia. (6:368, 374)

32. **B.** Penicillins act by inhibiting cell wall synthesis. Since human cells do not have cell walls, penicillins exert very little toxicity to human cells. (6:1134)

33. **D.** Both the penicillins and cephalosporins such as cephalexin act by inhibiting cell wall synthesis of the bacterial cell. The other agents exert other actions on bacterial cells (inhibition of protein synthesis, etc.). (6:1134)

34. **C.** Probenecid interferes with the renal tubular secretion of penicillins, thereby causing higher blood levels to be reached. This is the rationale for formulations such as Polycillin-PRB® in which ampicillin is combined with probenecid intentionally to prolong high ampicillin blood levels. (6:863)

35. **C.** Each mg of potassium penicillin G exerts about 1600 units of penicillin activity. This equivalent is more commonly expressed as 250 mg = 400,000 U and represents a method of assuring a consistent standard of biological activity for penicillin preparations manufactured throughout the world. (6:1133)

36. **A.** Amoxicillin is a chemical analogue of ampicillin, having a similar spectrum of antimicrobial activity. (6:1145)

37. **C.** Penicillamine is a degradation product of penicillin hydrolysis. It has been found to be an effective chelator of copper, mercury, zinc, and lead and promotes the excretion of these metals in the urine. It is most commonly used in the treatment of Wilson's disease, which is characterized by the deposition of toxic amounts of copper in various tissues. It is available under the brand name Cuprimine® (6:919–20)

38. **B.** Polymyxin B and colistin are the least toxic and most widely used polypeptide antibiotics in this country. They act by disrupting the cytoplasmic membrane of the organism, thereby causing immediate cell death. They are effective against many gram-negative organisms. They are both potentially nephrotoxic. (6:1232)

39. **B.** Chloramphenicol is the drug most often implicated as causing aplastic anemia. Fatal cases involving this reaction do not appear to be dose-related and occur once in every 50,000 to 100,000 cases treated. This infrequent but important reaction dictates that this agent be used only for serious infections and when it offers distinct advantages over other drugs which could be given. (6:1196)

40. **A.** Methicillin was the first penicillin introduced that had antistaphylococcal activity against those strains which produced penicillinase. It is unstable in acid solutions and cannot, therefore, be given orally. Since it is less active than penicillin G in treating nonpenicillinase-producing staph infections, it should be used only in infections caused by penicillinase-producing staph. (6:1143, 1153)

41. **D.** Sulfonamides produce bacteriostasis by a competitive replacement of PABA in an enzyme system essential to the growth of the susceptible organism. They interfere with the synthesis of folic acid coenzymes by occupying receptor sites normally occupied by PABA. (8:166)

42. **B.** The major determinant of duration of action for these drugs is their rate of excretion, and this is reflected in their half-life in serum. Approximate serum half-lives are given as: chlortetracycline, 5.5 hours; tetracycline, 8.5 hours; oxytetracycline, 9.5 hours; methacycline, 15 hours; demeclocycline, 12 hours; minocycline, 17 to 19 hours; doxycycline, 15 to 17 hours. Long-acting agents can be given in lower doses and less frequently. For example, the adult oral dose of tetracycline is 1 to 2 g daily, administered in four equally divided doses, while for doxycycline it is 200 mg initially, with a maintenance dose of 100 mg daily, which may be given as a single dose or as 50 mg every 12 hours. (4:741–42)

43. **D.** Side effects and toxic reactions to drugs are both related to the amount of drug administered. As the dose is increased, we can predict that characteristic side effects and/or toxicity will develop at some dosage level. Hypersensitivity reactions are believed to be brought about as a result of the development of antibodies in an individual against a particular drug. Idiosyncratic reactions are usually severe, unpredictable, and difficult to diagnose. They often mimic pathological states that are usually caused by factors unrelated to drugs. It does not appear, however, that either hypersensitivity or idiosyncracy are related to dosage. (30:203)

44. **E.** The gastric mucosa that lines the fundus and body of the stomach contains several types of cells, including surface mucous and parietal cells. The mucous cells secrete the mucous liquid that protects and lubricates the stomach lining. The parietal cells secrete both hydrochloric acid and intrinsic factor. Intrinsic factor is essential for the absorption of extrinsic cyanocobalamin (vitamin B_{12}). The hydrochloric acid reacts with pepsinogen to form the proteolytic enzyme pepsin. (2a:3)

45. **B.** Aluminum ion exerts an astringent effect on mucous membranes. In the GI tract, this astringency tends to have a constipating effect. Magnesium ion tends to exert a mild laxative effect and is, therefore, often combined with aluminum in antacid formulations to provide a balanced null effect on the GI tract. (2a:7)

46. **B.** Animal studies have indicated that centers in the hypothalamus influence appetite. A "satiety center" discourages overeating, while the "appetite center" assures a desire for food. There may be a feedback inhibition of the appetite center by impulses from the satiety center after food ingestion. It has been postulated that amphetamines affect the satiety center, decreasing the desire for food. (2a:178)

47. **B.** Fenfluramine HCl (Pondimin®) is a sympathomimetic amine which differs from other amphetamine-like drugs used to treat obesity in that it appears to produce more CNS depression than stimu-

lation. As with other anorectic drugs, fenfluramine is to be used for only a few weeks as an adjunct to a regimen of weight reduction based on caloric restriction. (25:1414–15)

48. **D.** Chronic overdose of bromides may often precipitate a series of toxic reactions known collectively as bromism. An acne type of rash is one of the symptoms so exhibited. (6:126)

49. **B.** Tinnitus, or ringing of the ears, is a symptom of salicylate toxicity and is presumably due to damage to the auditory nerve by the elevated salicylate levels in the serum. (6:327)

50. **D.** Unlike aspirin, salicylamide does not appear to have any effect upon prothrombin times. (2a:126)

51. **D.** Uricosuric agents increase the renal excretion of uric acid by decreasing its tubular reabsorption. Examples are probenecid and sulfinpyrazone. (6:862)

52. **B.** Salicylates are capable of increasing the excretion of urates, but the effect is markedly dose-dependent. Low doses (1 to 2 g/day) may actually decrease urate excretion, while large doses (over 5 g/day) induce uricosuria. Because such high doses of salicylate are poorly tolerated, it is not routinely used as a uricosuric agent. (6:331)

53. **E.** Ticrynafen (Selacryn®) is an agent that has diuretic, antihypertensive, and uricosuric properties. Its uricosuric activity makes it unique, since other diuretic agents currently available tend to increase serum uric acid levels. The drug, which was first marketed in May 1979, was recalled in January 1980 because of strong evidence that it can cause severe hepatic injury. (10)

54. **B.** The liver is a unique organ in that it is capable of synthesizing new glucose (gluconeogenesis) from glycogenic amino acids released into the circulation from muscle. When extrinsic sources of glucose enter the body via the diet, the liver may manufacture and store glycogen for future demands upon the body's glucose reserves. (16:404)

55. **D.** Probucol (Lorelco®) is one of several drugs indicated for use as adjunctive therapy in addition to diet and other measures in the treatment of hypercholesterolemia. While its exact mechanism of action is not known, it has been shown that probucol does not affect the later stages of cholesterol synthesis in the body. Reduction of serum cholesterol with drug therapy has not been shown to have a beneficial or detrimental effect on the morbidity or mortality due to atherosclerosis or coronary artery disease. The use of such agents is based, therefore, on the presumption that they may be useful. (25:843–44)

56. **D.** Cholinergic nerves release acetylcholine at nerve endings to transmit their impulses. Adrenergic nerves transmit their impulses by releasing norepinephrine at nerve endings. (6:419)

57. **C.** Methadone is a narcotic that has addicting properties. The advantage of using methadone in controlled withdrawal is that withdrawal symptoms are significantly milder with methadone than with other commonly abused narcotic agents. (6:268–69)

58. **D.** Both naloxone and nalorphine antagonize the action of many narcotic agents. (6:273)

59. **C.** Morphine administration increases the nonpropulsive rhythmic contractions of the small and large intestines but also decreases the propulsive contractions, thereby prolonging the residence time of intestinal contents and producing constipation. (6:253)

60. **A.** Etidronate disodium (Didronel®) is an agent that is administered orally and can modify the crystal growth of calcium hydroxyapatite by chemisorption onto developing apatite crystals during bone formation. Depending on its serum concentration, etidronate disodium may either inhibit crystal reabsorption or crystal growth.

Paget's disease, which is characterized by a localized increase in bone resorption followed by an abnormal pattern of bone formation, results in a greater tendency for bone deformation and fracture. Didronel®, while effective in many patients with Paget's disease, can cause pain and fractures when administered in high doses. (46:63–64)

61. **B.** Calcitonin is a polypeptide hormone secreted by the parafollicular cells of the thyroid gland in mammals and by the ultimobranchial gland of birds and fish. It opposes the action of parathyroid hormone and thereby reduces serum calcium levels by inhibiting both bone resorption and renal tubular reabsorption of calcium and phosphorus. Salmon calcitonin has actions which are identical to mammalian calcitonin but potency per mg is greater and it has a longer duration of action. While mechanistically and structurally calcitonin differs from etidronate disodium, both are indicated for the treatment of Paget's disease of the bone. (46:63–64)

62. **E.** Digitalis enables the failing heart to contract more forcefully and more efficiently. The heart can do more work without increased consumption of oxygen. The increased force of contraction is due to a direct action on ventricular muscle and is demonstrable on normal as well as failing hearts.

B. Digitalis slows conduction through the specialized tissue connecting the atria and the interventricular septum (i.e. the AV node and the bundle of His).

C. The refractory period of the AV node is usually not clinically apparent unless there is a rapid atrial rate. In this situation, a prolonged refractory period will reduce the number of impulses activating the AV node.

D. The rate of the normal pacemaker is depressed by the cardiac glycosides. With small doses, this effect is due primarily to vagal stimulation. Larger doses of digitalis directly depress the activity of the SA node. (6:655–65)

63. **C.** Disopyramide (Norpace®) is a relatively new anti-arrhythmic agent similar in action to procainamide and quinidine. At therapeutic doses this drug shortens the sinus node recovery time, lengthens the effective refractory period of the atrium, and has a minimal effect on the AV nodal conduction time. Disopyramide also possesses anticholinergic properties which may result in adverse effects on the gastrointestinal or urogenital systems or both. (10; 25:A49, 1580–82)

64. **C.** Digitoxin is very lipid soluble and is rapidly and essentially completely absorbed after oral administration. The other commonly used glycosides are absorbed to varying degrees, but the fraction is constant for a given preparation. The highly water-soluble strophanthins such as ouabain are poorly and irregularly absorbed and cannot be used orally. (6:673)

65. **B.** Lactulose is indicated for the treatment of portal-systemic encephalopathy, a condition characterized by an increase in blood ammonia levels. The drug is administered orally and reaches the colon essentially unchanged. There it is metabolized by bacteria to form low-molecular-weight acids that acidify the colonic contents, resulting in the retention of ammonia in the colon as the ammonium ion. Soft stools or diarrhea are frequently seen when high doses of lactulose are used. (10; 25:1197–98; 27:1338)

66. **C.** Ricinoleic acid is formed from hydrolysis of castor oil by intestinal lipases. This irritant substance produces a powerful laxative effect by stimulating the peristaltic motion of the small intestine. (6:982)

67. **A.** Sodium bicarbonate is considered to be a systemic antacid because it is absorbed after oral administration and is capable of producing systemic alkalosis. It is commonly administered by the IV route to treat systemic acidosis. The others listed are nonabsorbable (largely) and nonsystemic antacids. (6:960–61)

68. **B.** The initial diuretic effect of ethyl alcohol is due to inhibition of antidiuretic hormone secretion from the posterior pituitary gland. This inhibition is independent of the volume of fluid consumed as a beverage. Later, urine volume again reflects fluid intake. (6:141)

69. **D.** Triamterene appears to act on the distal tubule by blocking sodium reabsorption. Spironolactone inhibits the action of endogenous aldosterone on the distal tubule. (6:837–38)

70. **D.** Colchicine acts rapidly to relieve the pain of acute attacks of gout. It is usually administered in a regimen of one 0.5-mg tablet per hour until symptoms of the attack subside or until gastrointestinal distress ensues. A single oral course of therapy may require between 6 and 8 mg of the drug, and if a second course is indicated, it should not be given for at least 48 hours after completing the first course. Unlike other drugs used specifically for the treatment of gout (i.e., probenecid, allopurinol), colchicine has no effect on the biosynthesis, plasma level, or urinary excretion of uric acid. Rather, colchicine is believed to exert its analgesic effect in gout by inhibiting the formation of sodium urate crystals, which are responsible for the acute gout attack. (6:352)

71. **B.** Phenylbutazone should not be taken chronically because of its potential for producing a number of toxic effects, the most serious being blood dyscrasias such as aplastic anemia and agranulocytosis. (6:340)

72. **A.** Since most iron is absorbed in the duodenum, sustained release or enteric coated iron preparations may release iron in portions of the GI tract where it will not be absorbed, thereby resulting in the loss of a portion of the iron dose. (6:1310)

73. **B.** There are two mechanisms for the absorption of ferrous iron from the GI tract. Active transport, the most important physiological process, occurs in the duodenum and the adjacent jejunum. A fraction of the ferrous iron that is carried into the mucosal cell is transported into the blood. The remainder is converted to the ferric form, combines with apoferritin, and is stored in mucosal cells as ferritin. When large amounts are administered therapeutically, the active process can be partially bypassed and iron can be absorbed by diffusion. (6:1310)

74. **D.** Mites do not bite or sting. They tend to burrow beneath the stratum corneum, causing inflammation and itching. When the mite is *Sarcoptes scabiei* the condition is known as scabies. (2a:265)
A. Bedbugs are able to pierce the skin and suck blood by using their buccal stylets.
B. Fleas are known to transmit a variety of diseases, including typhus, by biting the host.
C. Lice attach themselves to the skin by use of claws while sucking blood.
E. Ticks feed on human blood by direct attachment of their mouth into the skin. If forcefully removed, part of the tick may remain embedded in the skin, causing itching and nodules.

75. **D.**
A., B., C., E. The aminoglycoside antibiotics (gentamicin and kanamycin) and tetracycline are excreted primarily by glomerular filtration. (6:1146, 1171–79)

76. **B.** Upon inhalation of amyl nitrite, the patient experiences a rapid and pronounced flush of the head, neck, and clavicular area known collectively as the blush zone. Amyl nitrite is used to treat acute attacks of angina pectoris because it can produce a transient increase in coronary blood flow. (6:729)

77. **A.** The four states through which a patient may progress when administered a general anesthetic are:
I. *Stage of Analgesia*—Patient's pain threshold is elevated but he is still conscious.
II. *Stage of Delirium*—Extends from loss of consciousness to beginning of surgical anesthesia. Breathing is irregular.
III. *Stage of Surgical Anesthesia*—Extends from the end of Stage II until spontaneous respiration ceases. Breathing is regular and muscular relaxation occurs.
IV. *Stage of Respiratory Paralysis*—Spontaneous respiration ceases, eventually leads to circulatory collapse. (6:60–61)

78. **E.** Most cells seem able to synthesize small amounts of prostaglandins rapidly when needed from the essential fatty acid precursors through the mediation of a complex of microsomal enzymes known as prostaglandin synthetase. (6:641)
D. Members of the series may show quite different pharmacological actions. For example, PGEs relax and PGFs contract bronchial musculature. (6:644)

79. **E.** Timolol maleate (Timoptic®) is a beta-adrenergic receptor blocking agent administered as an ophthalmic solution. While its precise mechanism of action in reducing intraocular pressure is unclear, some studies have suggested that its action may be related to a reduction in aqueous humor formation in the eye.

Because it does not affect pupil size, dim or blurred vision and night blindness, which are typically seen with the use of such miotics as pilocarpine, do not occur. Because of its beta-adrenergic blocking action, timolol maleate should be used with caution in patients with bronchial asthma, sinus bradycardia, or congestive heart failure and in others with a history of severe pulmonary or cardiac disease. (47:39, 40)

80. **D.** These drugs are usually prescribed only when the short-acting agents are inadequate. The patient should not expect maximum activity until approximately 24 hours after initial instillation. Effects of these drugs may persist for several days. (4:928)

81. **C.** Atropine and other anticholinergic drugs will tend to reduce the secretion of gastric fluids and are sometimes used to treat patients who suffer from gastric ulcers. Atropine is probably given more frequently than any other drug in preparation for surgical anesthesia because of its ability to minimize bronchial, nasal, and salivary secretions which could accumulate and obstruct respiratory passages. (6:518–21)

82. **C.** Antihistaminic drugs are believed to act by competing for the same receptor sites as histamine. They do not alter the rate of synthesis or inactivation of histamine. (6:595)

83. **E.** Ischemia or diminished oxygen supply to an area of the myocardium is believed to cause the pain associated with angina pectoris. Agents such as nitroglycerin, which are used to treat or prevent the occurrence of this pain, supposedly act by increasing the blood supply (and thereby the oxygen supply) to the myocardium. (6:737)

84. **D.** Sympathomimetic agents such as epinephrine and isoproterenol are useful in the symptomatic treatment of bronchial asthma because they exert beta-receptor action, which relaxes bronchial smooth muscle, and may in some cases exert alpha-receptor action, which constricts bronchial mucosal vessels, thereby reducing congestion and edema. (4:627–28)

85. **A.** Diuresis usually occurs within five minutes, with a peak action within 30 minutes. Duration of activity is approximately two hours. Furosemide inhibits sodium reabsorption in the proximal and the distal tubules and also in the loop of Henle. (6:833)

86. **B.** Acetaminophen has no anti-inflammatory action. It is ineffective in the treatment of arthritis and similar conditions. However, it is often recommended as an aspirin substitute for patients who are under anticoagulant therapy or allergic to salicylates, or have peptic ulcers. Since it is stable in water, liquid dosage forms are available for pediatric use. (1:1048)

87. **E.** Propoxyphene HCl (Darvon®) has only about half the analgesic activity of an equal dose of codeine. It exerts only an analgesic effect. The dextrorotatory isomer has the analgesic activity. The levo isomer is marketed as Novrad® and is said to have antitussive activity. (6:270)

88. **C.** A number of antineoplastic agents are produced by microorganisms and are, therefore, classed as antibiotics. They exert their cytotoxic effects by similar mechanisms, i.e., binding to polynucleotides and preventing new polynucleotide synthesis, particularly by blocking transcription of DNA or RNA. (6:1288, 1292)

89. **C.** (6:1250–51)

90. **C.** Since prostaglandins have been recovered from exudates and perfusates taken from tissue in which inflammatory conditions have been induced, it has been suggested that inflammation is at least partially mediated by prostaglandins (specifically PGE_2). Aspirin, and salicylate to a lesser degree, inhibits the synthesis of prostaglandins from arachidonic acid. This effect may be related to the anti-inflammatory action of aspirin. (6:332, 647)

91. **E.** Carbon monoxide combines chemically with the hemoglobin of the blood and renders the hemoglobin incapable of carrying oxygen to the tissues of the body. Hemoglobin has a greater affinity for carbon monoxide than for oxygen. (6:900)

92. **D.** The most serious toxic effect of hydrocarbon ingestion is the aspiration of the toxic liquid into the respiratory tract when vomiting. Such aspiration often causes pulmonary edema and pneumonitis, which are more serious than any effect the poison might have on the GI tract. For this reason, the use of emetics in

the treatment of hydrocarbon ingestions is contraindicated. (6:907–08)

93. **D.** When administered to a patient who has ingested silver nitrate, sodium chloride will cause precipitation of insoluble silver chloride and will replenish some of the chloride ions lost as a consequence of this ingestion. Secondary treatment with demulcents may aid in preventing and treating corrosion of the mucosa of the GI tract. (6:930)

94. **C.** Central nervous system depression to the extent of causing drowsiness requires warnings to avoid driving or using hazardous machinery when taking antihistamines. This same effect leads to some deliberate use of these drugs to facilitate falling asleep at bedtime. Paradoxically, CNS stimulation causing restlessness, nervousness, and insomnia is observed in some patients. The anticholinergic activity is responsible for the usefulness of some antihistamines in treating parkinsonism as well as for common side effects such as dry mouth. Because of their local anesthetic activity, some antihistamines have been incorporated into creams and lotions to relieve itching. This is a dubious use because of the relatively high incidence of hypersensitivity reactions to topically applied antihistamines. (6:603–11)

95. **D.** Acetazolamide exerts a diuretic effect by inhibiting the activity of the enzyme carbonic anhydrase in the renal tubules. This causes an increase in the excretion of sodium and bicarbonate ions, thereby drawing water out of the body and alkalinizing the urine. (6:826)

96. **C.** The thiazide diuretics are excreted in varying degrees by the same renal tubular mechanism responsible for the secretion of uric acid. Because of the limited capacity of the system, the excretion of uric acid may be reduced following thiazide administration. The resulting elevation of serum uric acid is generally of no significance in normal subjects but may precipitate or intensify gout in susceptible individuals. (6:830–31)

97. **B.** Acetazolamide is a urinary alkalinizer. The other choices would tend to acidify the urine. Another alkalinizer would be sodium bicarbonate. (6:499, 828)

98. **E.** Ethanol is metabolized in the liver to acetaldehyde, which is further oxidized to acetate or acetyl-CoA. This, in turn, enters the tricarboxylic acid cycle for further oxidation to carbon dioxide and water. Disulfiram (Antabuse®) inhibits the enzyme aldehyde dehydrogenase, which is required to oxidize acetaldehyde. The toxic symptoms ("disulfiram reaction") are extremely uncomfortable to the patient; these include weakness, dizziness, nausea, and vomiting. Metronidazole (Flagyl®) is a trichomonacide that also inhibits aldehyde dehydrogenase. Sulfonylurea antidiabetic agents may also elicit a "disulfiram reaction." (8:97, 151, 216)

99. **B.** Glutethimide (Doriden®) is an enzyme inducer. Each of the other agents is a monoamine oxidase (MAO) inhibitor. (6:180–84)

100. **D.** Many sedative and hypnotic drugs are capable of inducing the production of microsomal enzymes in the liver. Barbiturates and alcohol are included among the most potent of the enzyme inducers. (8:47)

101. **D.** In contrast with other thiazide derivatives, diazoxide produces marked salt and water retention in both normotensive and hypertensive patients. Rapid IV injection of diazoxide is used in emergencies to produce an immediate fall in blood pressure. (6:714)

102. **C.** Thiopental sodium is an ultrashort-acting barbiturate used principally as an intravenous anesthetic, usually in conjunction with inhalational agents. Amobarbital and pentobarbital are considered to be short- to intermediate-acting agents and are used as sedative-hypnotics, while phenobarbital and metharbital are long-acting barbiturates used as sedative-hypnotics as well as for their anticonvulsant action. (6:117–18)

103. **C.** Aminocaproic acid acts as a competitive antagonist to the activators of plasminogen. It therefore prevents the conversion of plasminogen (profibrinolysin) to plasmin (fibrinolysin). It also, to a lesser degree, inhibits plasmin. The drug is used in specific situations where unusually great fibrinolytic activity has been established. It is also useful in disorders such as hemophilia, where fibrin formation is so deficient that inhibition of the normal fibrinolytic process is desirable. (10; 6:1365)

104. **C.** Phenylbutazone is an anti-inflammatory compound that is rapidly absorbed following oral administration and extensively bound to plasma protein. The unbound fraction is either rapidly excreted or metabolized. The principal metabolite, oxyphenbutazone, has essentially the same anti-inflammatory action as its precursor. (6:340)

105. **E.** Phenylbutazone may aggravate the patient's peptic ulcer because of its tendency to cause irritation of the GI tract. Such irritation can be minimized by administering the drug with food or antacids. (4:369)

106. **A.** The sulfonylureas are believed to stimulate pancreatic beta cells to increase their insulin production. They do not potentiate the action of insulin and are of no value unless the pancreas is capable of producing insulin. (37:743)

107. **B.** Chlorpropamide has a half-life of approximately 36 hours. (6:1521)

108. **B.** Vidarabine has been available for several years as an ophthalmic product for the treatment of herpes simplex keratitis. It is now also available in a parenteral form for the treatment of herpes simplex en-

cephalitis, a condition which is often life-threatening. The drug is believed to act by inhibiting DNA synthesis. It has also been shown to be active in vitro against other viruses, including herpes zoster (shingles). The most common problem with its use is that the drug will help only if it is given before severe neurological deficits occur. A firm diagnosis, however, requires a brain biopsy, a procedure considered drastic for a patient without neurological problems. (25:1324–25)

109. **C.** Methenamine is absorbed orally and rapidly excreted in the urine. In an acid urine below pH 5.5 the breakdown of methenamine to form formaldehyde and ammonia occurs. Methenamine salts are contraindicated in renal insufficiency, since precipitation of organic acids (e.g., uric acid) may occur. Methenamine and sulfonamides are mutually antagonistic because methenamine may cause sulfonamide precipitation in the urine and sulfonamides may raise the pH of the urine to an alkaline or neutral level which would impair methenamine activity. (6:1006–07)

110. **A.** Pepsin activity is completely inhibited above a pH of approximately 4.0. Most commercial antacid products raise stomach pH to at least 4.0 by simple neutralization of stomach hydrochloric acid. Pepsin inactivation is due to pH alteration and not to any intrinsic antipeptic activity of the antacid. (2a:6)

111. **C.** Cyproheptadine (Periactin®) is an agent that bears a structural resemblance to the phenothiazine antihistaminic drugs. It has been shown to antagonize both histamine and 5-HT to a great extent, resulting in a high order of antipruritic activity. It is most popularly used for the treatment of a variety of pruritic dermatoses. (6:622–23)

112. **D.** Cromolyn sodium (Intal®, Aarane®) is a synthetic analogue of khellin, which was itself formerly used as a spasmolytic. Cromolyn appears to stabilize the membrane of sensitized mast cells and, thereby, to prevent the release of histamine and other mediators implicated in asthma. The drug is not effective if it is administered after these substances have been released and, therefore, is of no value in acute asthmatic attacks. (6:602)

113. **D.** The antirachitic activity of vitamin D in cod liver oil is determined by observing the calcification of the rachitic metaphyses of the radius and tibia of rats. (1:576)

114. **C.** Insulin injection and other forms of insulin are assayed by measuring the reduction in blood glucose levels in rabbits after a subcutaneous injection. (1:574)

115. **E.** The anticoagulant activity of heparin is determined by measuring the in vitro inhibition of clot formation in sheep blood. (1:575)

116. **A.** The oxytocic activity of the injection product is determined by measuring the vasodepressive activity of the drug in anesthetized chickens. (1:574)

117. **E.** Sheep blood is heparinized. Protamine is then standardized by recording the reduction of clotting time upon addition of the protamine. (1:576)

118. **D.** Ganglionic blocking agents appear to act through a competitive antagonism with acetylcholine at nerve ganglia. Because of the serious side effects of agents in the group, they are being slowly but completely replaced by safer antihypertensive agents. (6:570–73)

119. **C.** Reserpine and other rauwolfia alkaloids exert their antihypertensive effect by depleting catecholamine stores and thereby reducing sympathetic nerve discharge. These agents also have a sedating effect and may produce severe depression and suicidal tendencies. Reserpine is usually used in combination with other antihypertensive agents. (6:557)

120. **A.** Methyldopa replaces norepinephrine in nerve storage sites and is released upon stimulation of the nerve. Since this agent is not as effective a transmitter as norepinephrine, it tends to exert an antihypertensive effect. (6:707–10)

121. **B.** Hydralazine acts directly to dilate arterioles, thereby decreasing peripheral resistance and decreasing blood pressure. The most serious potential side effect of this drug is cardiac stimulation. It is, therefore, often avoided in patients who have known coronary artery disease. (6:705–07)

122. **E.** The veratrum alkaloids appear to act directly on the central nervous system to decrease peripheral vascular resistance and lower blood pressure. They also exert an emetic action, which limits the practicality of their use. (6:716–17)

123. **B.** (11:1593)

124. **D.** (11:1519)

125. **C.** (11:457)

126. **E.** (11:707)

127. **A.** (11:407)

128. **D.** (17:94)

129. **A.** (17:105)

130. **E.** (17:302)

131. **C.** (17:556)

132. **B.** (17:552)

133. **D.** (17:716)

134. **A.** (17:357)

135. **E.** (17:544)

136. **B.** (17:554)

137. **C.** (17:364)

138. **C.** (17:364)

139. **E.** (17:110)

140. **A.** (17:108)

141. **B.** (17:577)

142. **B.** (17:571)

143. **E.** (17:558)

144. **A.** (17:564)

145. **C.** (17:253)

146. **E.** (17:570)

147. **C.** (17:581)

148. **B.** (17:309)

149. **D.** (17:113)

150. **E.** (17:259)

151. **C.** (17:295)

152. **A.** (17:312)

153. **B.** (17:239)

154. **B.** (17:190)

155. **E.** (17:304)

156. **C.** (17:160)

157. **D.** (17:186)

158. **B.** (17:440)

159. **D.** (17:321)

160. **A.** (17:153)

161. **C.** (17:486)

162. **A.** (17:440)

163. **D.** (17:587)

164. **B.** (17:239)

165. **E.** (17:389)

166. **A.** (17:587)

167. **C.** (17:77)

168. **B.** (17:309)

169. **E.** (17:716)

170. **D.** (17:192)

171. **E.** (17:490)

172. **C.** (17:110)

173. **A.** (17:124)

174. **D.** (17:360)

175. **B.** (17:321)

176. **B.** (17:589)

177. **A.** (17:278)

178. **C.** (17:294)

179. **E.** (17:121)

180. **D.** (17:586)

181. **D.** (17:239)

182. **A.** (17:254)

183. **C.** (17:186)

184. **E.** (17:346)

185. **B.** (17:389)

186. **C.** Pellagra is characterized by dermatitis, inflammation of mucous membranes, diarrhea, and psychic disturbances. (11:1152)

187. **B.** Pernicious anemia is a megaloblastic anemia resulting from malabsorption of vitamin B_{12} due to failure of the gastric mucosa to secrete intrinsic factor. (11:85)

188. **A.** Scurvy is characterized by anemia, spongy gums, and induration of leg muscles. (11:1393)

189. **D.** (6:1097)

190. **E.** (6:1101)

191. **A.** (6:1103)

192. **B.** (6:1103)

193. **C.** (6:1101)

194. **D.** (6:1091)

195. **A.** (6:1091)

196. **C.** (6:1091)

197. **E.** (6:1091)

198. **B.** (6:1091)

199. **B.** (6:1091)

200. **C.** (6:1091)

201. **C.** (6:1091)

202. **E.** (6:1091)

203. **D.** (6:1091)

204. **B.** (6:1091)

205. **D.** (6:1091)

206. **E.** Bisacodyl (Dulcolax®) is a mild stimulant laxative. It acts through direct stimulation of the mucosal nerve plexus of the colon. It has been termed a "contact" cathartic because its stimulant effect on the intestine is inhibited by the topical application of local anesthetics. Oral tablets and rectal suppositories are available. (2a:41–44)

207. **A.** Magnesium Citrate Solution NF (Citrate of Magnesia) is a typical saline cathartic. Other commonly used chemicals are magnesium hydroxide and sodium sulfate. Laxative action usually occurs in two to six hours. (2a:41–44)

208. **C.** Mineral oil softens feces and eases their passage. It is useful when minimum straining during evacuation is important; for example, in patients with cardiovascular disease or hernia. (2a:41–44)

209. **D.** Poloxamer 188 is a wetting agent which lowers the surface tension of feces, thereby facilitating penetration by intestinal fluids. Poloxamer 188 is available as Polykol®. Another wetting agent is dioctyl sodium sulfosuccinate (Colace®, Doxinate®). (2a:41–44)

210. **B.** Psyllium is a hydrophilic colloid which will increase intestinal bulk by absorbing water. Its laxative action is rather slow in onset, usually 12 to 24 hours. Commercial forms of psyllium include Effersyllium®, Metamucil®, and Mucilose®. (2a:41–44)

211. **A.** Sodium biphosphate and sodium phosphate solutions are used as saline cathartics in such commercial products as Fleet® Enema, Phospho-Soda®, and Travad® Enema. These sodium salts may be contraindicated in cardiac patients with edema or evidence of congestive heart failure, or who are on low-sodium diets. (2a:41–44)

212. **E.** Oxymorphone HCl is a semisynthetic narcotic analgesic with approximately 10 times the activity of morphine. It is valuable in controlling severe postoperative pain and pain due to advanced neoplastic diseases. It is marketed as Numorphan®. (1:1041)

213. **A.** Ethylmorphine HCl is commercially available as Dionin®. Its relative strength is similar to that of codeine, which is approximately one-sixth the analgesic potency of morphine. (1:1040)

214. **A.** Ethylmorphine HCl causes hyperemia in the eye. It is useful in the treatment of indolent corneal ulcers and uveal exudates. Usually a 1 to 5% ophthalmic solution is dispensed. (1:1040)

215. **D.** Nalorphine exhibits pharmacological properties similar to those of morphine in patients not already being given opiates. However, when administered to narcotic-treated patients, nalorphine antagonizes many morphine effects. In particular, it reduces the severity of circulatory and respiratory depression of other narcotics. It will produce withdrawal symptoms in the active addict. (1:1042)

216. **B.** Hydromorphone HCl (Dilaudid®) is approximately four times stronger than morphine. The duration of analgesia from Dilaudid® is shorter than from morphine. However, Dilaudid® does not cause as much stupefaction or induction of sleep as does morphine. While oral and parenteral dosage forms are available, rectal administration is sometimes used to slow absorption. (1:1040)

217. **B.** Prazocin may cause syncope with sudden loss of consciousness, particularly within 30 to 90 minutes after the initial dose has been administered. This effect can be minimized by limiting the initial dose to 1 mg and by administering it at bedtime. (3:484)

218. **C.** When used in high doses hydralazine may produce, in some patients, a clinical picture resembling acute systemic lupus erythematosis (SLE). In such patients the drug is generally discontinued. (3:473)

219. **A.** With prolonged therapy 10 to 20% of patients on methyldopa will develop a positive direct Coomb's test, usually after six to twelve months of therapy have elapsed. On rare occasions this may be associated with hemolytic anemia, which could lead to fatal consequences. (3:469)

220. **D.** Guanethidine is a potent agent that reduces responses to sympathetic nerve activation. Although guanethidine does not directly produce impotence, inhibition of ejaculation is a common adverse effect. (10; 6:556)

221. **E.** Diazoxide is an antihypertensive agent administered rapidly by the intravenous route for the emergency reduction of blood pressure. It acts by relaxing smooth muscle in peripheral arterioles. Since diazoxide causes sodium retention, repeated injections may cause edema and congestive heart failure. (10)

CHAPTER 4

Pharmaceutical Calculations

The ability to handle the mathematics required in calculations for compounding prescriptions and formulating other products has lost much of the importance it once had for the practicing pharmacist. That is, until the occasional prescription comes in that requires a computation.

Most textbooks in pharmacy calculations have many problems to work out. We have attempted to represent the topic with relatively few, those which we believe to have the greatest currency.

Directions: Each of the questions or incomplete statements below is followed by five suggested answers or completions. Select the BEST answer in each case.

1. Both the apothecary and avoirdupois systems of weight measurement are used by the pharmacist. Units that are quantitatively identical in both systems are the
   A. drachms
   B. grains
   C. ounces
   D. pounds
   E. grains and ounces (23:70)

2. One thousand (1000) nanograms equals one
   A. centigram
   B. gram
   C. kilogram
   D. microgram
   E. milligram (41:812)

3. The Angstrom equals
   A. 0.1 nanometer
   B. 1 nanometer
   C. 10 nanometers
   D. 100 nanometers
   E. 1000 nanometers (1:79)

4. Lanoxin® Pediatric Elixir contains 0.05 mg of digoxin per ml. How many micrograms (μg) are there in 3 ml of the elixir?
   A. 0.15
   B. 0.015
   C. 1.5
   D. 0.0015
   E. none of the above (10)

5. According to USP specifications, which one of the following equivalents should be used to convert a grain measurement to milligrams when compounding prescriptions?
   A. 60 mg
   B. 62.5 mg
   C. 64.8 mg
   D. 65 mg
   E. 15.4 mg (18:794)

6. For the following prescription, what is the approximate percentage strength of the diluted solution which the patient will use as a soak?

   Rx
   Potassium Permanganate Tab. 200 mg
   Disp. # 60
   Sig: iii tab in pint of warm water.
   Use as soak.

   A. 0.06%
   B. 0.6%
   C. 0.13%
   D. 2.0%
   E. none of the above (23:135)

7. How many ml of a 0.5% gentian violet stock solution are needed to prepare one gallon of a 1:2000 solution?
   A. 47
   B. 94.5
   C. 200

D. 378
E. none of the above (23:161)

8. The adult dose of a drug is 250 mg. What would be the approximate dose for a six-year-old child? Use Young's rule.
   A. 60 mg
   B. 85 mg
   C. 100 mg
   D. 125 mg
   E. 180 mg (23:93)

9. What would be the appropriate dose for a child weighing 40 lb if the adult dose is 50 mg? Use Clark's rule.
   A. 15 mg
   B. 20 mg
   C. 25 mg
   D. 30 mg
   E. 35 mg (23:93–94)

10. The USP contains a nomograph for estimating body surface area for either children or adults. Which of the following measurements must be known in order to use this nomograph?
    A. age and height
    B. age and weight
    C. height only
    D. height and weight
    E. weight only (18:inside back cover)

11. Dopamine (Intropin®) 200 mg in 500 ml of normal saline at 5 μg/kg/min is ordered for a 155-lb patient. What is the final concentration of solution in μg/ ml?
    A. 0.4
    B. 2.5
    C. 40
    D. 400
    E. 25 (3:445; 23:321)

12. Referring to the previous question, at what rate should the solution be infused to deliver the desired dose of 5 μg/kg/min?
    A. 0.35 ml/min
    B. 0.40 ml/min
    C. 0.88 ml/min
    D. 2.0 ml/min
    E. 5.0 ml/min (23:321)

13. What is the percentage of alcohol in a mixture of 300 ml of 95% V/V alcohol, 1000 ml of 70% V/V alcohol, and 200 ml of 50% V/V alcohol?
    A. 84%
    B. 72%
    C. 8.4%
    D. 7.2%
    E. 79% (23:174)

14. A physician requests that an elixir containing 32% alcohol be prepared. How much low-alcohol elixir (10% alcohol) and high-alcohol elixir (78%) must be mixed to prepare 1 pint of the requested elixir?
    A. 148 ml of low and 325 ml of high
    B. 153 ml of low and 320 ml of high
    C. 320 ml of low and 153 ml of high
    D. 325 ml of low and 148 ml of high
    E. none of the above (23:174)

15. What would be the number of grains of pilocarpine HCl needed to fill the following prescription?

    Rx
    Pilocarpine HCl 5%
    Boric Acid 2%
    Purified Water q.s. f ℥i
    M. & Ft. Ophthalmic Sol.
    Sig: gtt ii o.u. b.i.d.

    A. 21.9
    B. 22.8
    C. 24
    D. 25
    E. none of the above (23:132)

16. What would be the correct directions to the patient for the preceding prescription?
    A. two drops in the left eye twice a day
    B. two drops in the right eye twice a day
    C. two drops in both eyes twice a day
    D. two drops in the manner prescribed twice a day
    E. two drops in the affected other eye twice a day (1:1713)

17. A physician requests one pound of bacitracin ointment containing 200 units of bacitracin per gram. How many grams of bacitracin ointment (500 units/gram) must be used to make this ointment?
    A. 182 g
    B. 200 g
    C. 227 g
    D. 362 g
    E. none of the above (23:170)

18. How many grains of benzocaine are needed for the following prescription?

Rx

Benzocaine	2% W/W
Glycerin	5%
Hydrophilic Ointment q.s.	℥ ii
Sig: Apply as needed	

A. 1.2
B. 12
C. 17.5
D. 18.2
E. 19.2 (23:138)

19. A 250-ml infusion bottle contains 5.86 g of potassium chloride. How many milliequivalents of potassium chloride are present? (molecular weight of KCl = 74.6)

A. 12.7
B. 20
C. 78.5
D. 150
E. none of the above (23:233)

20. A solution contains 1.5 mEq of calcium per 100 ml. Express the solution's strength of calcium in terms of milligrams per liter. (The atomic weight of calcium is 40.)

A. 30
B. 60
C. 150
D. 300
E. 600 (23:233)

21. Calcium chloride ($CaCl_2 \cdot 2H_2O$) has a formula weight of 147. What weight of the chemical is needed to obtain 40 meq of calcium? (Ca = 40.1; Cl = 35.5; H_2O = 18.)

A. 0.80 g
B. 2.22 g
C. 1.47 g
D. 2.94 g
E. 5.88 g (1:768; 23:233)

22. The official potassium iodide solution contains 100 g of KI in a total volume of 100 ml (dl) of solution. The density of this saturated solution is approximately 1.7 g/ ml. Express the concentration of the solution in terms of % W/W.

A. 17%
B. 59%
C. 70%
D. 100%
E. 170% (1:75)

23. From the information provided in the preceding question, determine the amount of water needed to prepare 1000 ml of saturated potassium iodide solution (SSKI).

A. 300 ml
B. 412 ml
C. 588 ml
D. 700 ml
E. 1000 ml (1:75)

24. For a Class A prescription balance rating, a balance must have a sensitivity requirement equal to or less than

A. 2 mg
B. 6 mg
C. 10 mg
D. 30 mg
E. 120 mg (1:85)

25. The minimum quantity that can be weighed on a balance with a sensitivity requirement of 6 mg if an error of 5% is permissible would be

A. 6 mg
B. 24 mg
C. 60 mg
D. 120 mg
E. 180 mg (19:1036)

26. How many ml of Hydrochloric Acid USP is needed to prepare 4 liters of Diluted Hydrochloric Acid USP? The label on the available hydrochloric acid bottle shows that the concentration of the acid is 36.8% W/W and the solution specific gravity is 1.19. The diluted acid is 10% W/V accirding to the official monograph.

A. 147
B. 400
C. 913
D. 1087
E. 1294 (1:737; 23:169)

27. How much additional sodium chloride should be added to the following prescription to maintain isotonicity? Zincfrin® is an isotonic solution.

Rx

Zincfrin	15 ml
Sodium Chloride	q.s.
Sterile Water for Injection	q.s. 60 ml

A. 0.135 g
B. 0.4 g
C. 0.54 g
D. 0.9 g
E. none (since sterile water for injection is already isotonic) (1:1407)

28. A physician places a patient on a daily dose of 48 units of U-80 insulin. How many ml should the patient inject each day?

A. 0.48
B. 0.60
C. 0.80
D. 1.0
E. 4.8 (18:253; 23:318)

29. In changing a patient from U-40 to U-100 insulin, a pharmacist would instruct him to use ____ ml of U-100 if the previous dosage was 0.8 ml of U-40 per day.

A. 0.32
B. 0.40
C. 0.50
D. 0.80
E. 2.0 (23:318)

30. A patient normally uses 60 units of NPH U-100 insulin. However, only U-80 syringes are available. To what calibration mark on the U-80 syringe should the U-100 insulin solution be drawn to obtain the correct dose?

A. 40 units
B. 48 units
C. 60 units
D. 75 units
E. impossible to measure in the U-80 syringe (23:318)

31. How many ml of glycerin would be needed to prepare 2 apothecary ounces of ointment containing 5% W/W of glycerin? The density of glycerin is 1.25 g/ml .

A. 2.3
B. 2.4
C. 2.5
D. 3.0
E. 3.9 (1:95)

32. How much sodium chloride should be added to a liter of the following formula to adjust for isotonicity? The freezing point depression or "D" values for each chemical is listed to the right of the item.

Chemical		"D" for 1% solution
Procaine Hydrochloride	1%	0.12
Benzyl Alcohol	0.5	0.09
Potassium Phosphate *(Monobasic)*	0.25	0.25
Potassium Phosphate *(Dibasic)*	0.1	0.27
Sodium Chloride	q.s.	
Water for Injection	q.s. 100%	

A. none is needed
B. 0.46 g
C. 1.7 g
D. 2.1 g
E. 4.6 g (1:1406)

33. The freezing point depression ("D" value) for a 1% solution of pilocarpine hydrochloride is 0.14. The concentration of pilocarpine hydrochloride that would be iso-osmotic with the blood is

A. 0.14%
B. 0.76%
C. 1.0%
D. 2.7%
E. 3.7% (1:1406)

34. How many grains of ammonium chloride are present in each dose of the following prescription?

Rx
Codeine gr iv
Ammonium Chloride ʒ iss
Elix. T.H. with C. q.s. f ℥ vi
Sig: ʒ i q4h p.r.n. for cough

A. 1.9
B. 2.5
C. 60
D. 90
E. 1.5 (23:91)

35. The amount of codeine per dose in the preceding prescription would be approximately

A. 1/12 gr
B. 1/9 gr
C. 5/18 gr
D. 1/3 gr
E. 5/12 gr (1:803; 23:85)

36. A formula for Magnesium Citrate Solution NF requires 27.4 g of anhydrous citric acid (mol. wt. = 192). How many grams of citric acid monohydrate could be used as a replacement?

A. 25.1 g
B. 27.4 g
C. 30.0 g
D. 34.0 g
E. 54.8 g (1:1259; 23:219)

37. How much elemental iron is present in every 300 mg of ferrous sulfate ($FeSO_4 \cdot 7H_2O$)? Atomic weights are iron = 55.9; sulfur = 32.1; oxygen = 16.0; and hydrogen = 1.0. Iron has valences of + 2 and + 3.

A. 30.2 mg
B. 60.3 mg
C. 110.3 mg
D. 120.6 mg
E. 164 mg (23:214)

38. How many 4-fluid-ounce bottles can be packaged from a 1-gallon bottle of cough syrup?
   A. 16
   B. 32
   C. 64
   D. 100
   E. 120 (23:68)

39. Hydriodic acid syrup may be prepared from the following formula:

Diluted Hydriodic Acid	140 ml
Dextrose	450 g
Purified Water	ad 1000 ml

   Diluted hydriodic acid contains 10% W/V HI. How many ml of an 18% W/W hydriodic acid solution (density = 1.18 g/ml) must be used to prepare 4000 ml of hydriodic acid syrup?
   A. 56
   B. 264
   C. 311
   D. 367
   E. 560 (23:157)

40. How many ml of Sodium Hypochlorite Solution NF will be needed to fill the following prescription? (Sodium Hypochlorite Solution NF contains 5% W/V NaOCl.)

   Rx
   Sodium Hypochlorite Sol.
   Purified Water q.s. 120 ml

   M & Ft sol. of such strength that 30 ml diluted to 1 pint contains 0.1% sodium hypo.
   A. 2.4
   B. 9.5
   C. 37.8
   D. 75.6
   E. impossible to determine since amount of sodium hypochlorite solution was not specified in the prescription (23:164)

41. A pharmacist adds 120 ml of Aluminum Acetate Solution USP containing 5% aluminum acetate to 1 liter of Sterile Water for Irrigation. What is the % W/V concentration of aluminum acetate present?
   A. 0.50%
   B. 0.53%
   C. 0.60%
   D. 1.07%
   E. 1.20% (23:166)

42. How many milliliters of a 1:50 stock solution of ephedrine sulfate would be needed to prepare 30 ml of the following prescription?

   Rx
   Ephedrine Sulfate 0.25%
   Normal Saline q.s. 10 ml
   A. 1.25
   B. 3.75
   C. 4.0
   D. 7.5
   E. 12.5 (23:163)

43. A pharmacist has 50 ml of 0.5% gentian violet solution. What will be the final ratio strength if he dilutes this solution to 1250 ml with purified water?
   A. 1:8
   B. 1:200
   C. 1:500
   D. 1:1000
   E. 1:5000 (23:160)

44. Syrup USP contains 85% W/V sucrose and has a specific gravity of 1.313. Express the concentration of sucrose in terms of % W/W.
   A. 55%
   B. 65%
   C. 75%
   D. 85%
   E. impossible to calculate with the given data (23:141)

45. Sufficient water is added to 800 ml of a liquid chemical (density = 0.8 g/ml) to make a final volume of 4000 ml. What is the % W/V concentration of the liquid chemical in the final preparation?
   A. 12.5%
   B. 16%
   C. 20%
   D. 25%
   E. 40% (23:137)

46. How many grains of potassium permanganate are needed for the following prescription?

   Rx
   Potassium permanganate 0.02%
   Pur. Water q.s. f ℥ viii
   A. 0.73 gr
   B. 0.77 gr
   C. 73 gr
   D. 77 gr
   E. 48 gr (23:134)

47. How much sodium chloride is needed to adjust the following prescription to isotonicity? (E value for zinc sulfate is 0.15.)

Rx

Zinc Sulfate	1%
Sodium Chloride	q.s.
Purified Water	q.s. 60 ml

A. 0.45 g
B. 0.54 g
C. 0.60 g
D. 0.75 g
E. 0.90 g (1:1407)

48. How many grams of ammonia water (10% W/W) can be prepared from one pound of 28% W/W Strong Ammonia Solution NF?

A. 84
B. 162
C. 280
D. 1271
E. 1400 (23:160)

49. Strong Iodine Solution USP contains 5% W/V iodine. How many mg of iodine are consumed daily if the usual dose is 0.3 ml t.i.d.?

A. 7.5 mg
B. 15 mg
C. 22.5 mg
D. 45 mg
E. 90 mg (23:97)

50. A hospital clinic requests 2 lb of 2% ammoniated mercury ointment. How many grams of 5% ammoniated mercury ointment would be diluted with white petrolatum to prepare this order?

A. 18.2 g
B. 27.5 g
C. 45.4 g
D. 363 g
E. 545 g (23:171)

Answers and Commentary

1. **B.** The grain is a measurement that is identical in both systems. The apothecary ounce (℥) contains 480 grains, while the avoirdupois ounce (oz) contains 437.5 grains. The apothecary pound is 12 ounces (5760 grains) and the avoirdupois is 16 ounces (7000 grains). The scruple and drachm measures are other units in the apothecary system. The apothecary system should be used for prescription compounding, while the avoirdupois system is employed for the purchase and selling of bulk chemicals. (23:70)

2. **D.** The prefix "nano" is a part of the S.I. (Système Internationale), which has been adopted by most countries to designate the magnitude of numbers. The system is essentially an extension of the metric decimal system. The major prefixes with the order of magnitude include:

Prefix	Magnitude	Example
kilo	1000 ×	kilogram
—	1 ×	gram
centi	0.01 ×	centigram
milli	0.001 ×	milligram
micro	$1 \times 10^{-6} \times$	microgram
nano	$1 \times 10^{-9} \times$	nanogram
pico	$1 \times 10^{-12} \times$	picogram
femto	$1 \times 10^{-15} \times$	femtogram
atto	$1 \times 10^{-18} \times$	attogram

(41:812)

3. **A.** The Angstrom is the measurement of length used mainly for wavelengths of light. This unit and the millimicron have been replaced in the scientific literature by the nanometer. The millimicron equals the nanometer; 10 Angstroms equals one nanometer. (1:79)

4. **E.** 1 mg = 1000 micrograms (μg). Therefore 0.15 mg of digoxin (contained in 3 ml of the elixir) would be equivalent to 150 μg of drug. (10)

5. **C.** The USP contains a table of equivalents of weights and measures for the metric, avoirdupois, and apothecary systems. When converting specific quantities in pharmaceutical formulas, the exact equivalents must be used. For prescription compounding, the exact equivalents may be rounded to three significant figures. The metric equivalent of 1 grain is listed as 0.06480 g, which would then be expressed as 64.8 mg. Some sources use the value of 65 mg, which does not meet USP specifications. The value of 60 mg should not be used except for rough calculations in checking doses. (18:794)

6. **C.** There are 473 ml of solution in 1 pint. Since three 200-mg tablets are dissolved in each pint:

$$\frac{0.6\ \text{g}}{473\ \text{ml}} \times 100 = 0.13\%\ \text{W/V}.$$

(23:135)

7. **D.** *Step 1.* Determine the quantity of chemical in the final solution:

1 gallon = 3785 ml therefore

$$\frac{1\ \text{g}}{2000\ \text{ml}} = \frac{x\ \text{g}}{3785\ \text{ml}}$$

$$x = 1.89\ \text{g}.$$

Step 2. Determine the amount of the available solution needed to obtain the quantity of chemical determined in Step 1: (a 0.5% solution contains 0.5 g of chemical in 100 ml (dl) of solution)

$$\frac{0.5\ \text{g}}{100\ \text{ml}} = \frac{1.89\ \text{g}}{x\ \text{ml}}$$

$$x = 378\ \text{ml}.$$

(23:161)

8. **B.** Young's rule states that:

$$\text{Child's dose} = \frac{\text{Age (yr)}}{\text{Age (yr)} + 12} \times \text{Adult dose}$$

$$\text{Child's dose} = \frac{6}{6 + 12} \times 250\ \text{mg}$$

Child's dose = 83.3 mg or 85 mg.

(23:93)

9. **A.** Clark's rule has been used to relate body weight to dosage. It states:

$$\text{Child's dose} = \frac{\text{Child's wt. (lb)}}{150} \times \text{Adult dose}$$

$$\text{Child's dose} = \frac{(40)}{(150)} \times (50\ \text{mg})$$

Child's dose = 13.3 or 15 mg.

(23:93–94)

10. **D.** The nomograph in the USP consists of three parallel, vertical lines. The left line is calibrated with height measurements in both centimeters and inches, while the right line lists weights in kilograms and pounds. Using data based upon the patient's measurements, one draws a line between the two outside parallel lines. The intercept on the middle line, which is calibrated in square meters of body surface area, allows one to estimate the patient's body surface area. (18:inside back cover)

11. **D.** $\frac{200 \text{ mg dopamine}}{500 \text{ ml solution}} = 0.4 \text{ mg/ml}$

$1 \text{ mg} = 1000\ \mu g$

$0.4 \text{ mg} = 400\ \mu g$

final concentration: $\frac{400\ \mu g}{\text{ml.}}$

(3:445; 23:321)

12. **C.**

$\frac{155 \text{ lb}}{2.2 \text{ lb/kg}} = 70.5 \text{ kg}$

$\frac{5\ \mu g/kg}{\text{minute}} \times 70.5 \text{ kg} = 352\ \mu g/\text{minute}$

concentration of solution is 400 μg/ ml

divide dosage rate by concentration of solution:

$\frac{352\ \mu g/\text{min}}{400\ \mu g/\text{ml}} = 0.88 \text{ ml/min.}$

(23:321)

13. **B.** The problem solution requires a calculation of a "weighted average." The procedure is to multiply the percentage strength of each component by its quantity, then sum up the products, then divide the sum of the products by the sum of the quantities. For this problem:

$300 \times 95 = 28{,}500$

$1000 \times 70 = 70{,}000$

$\frac{200}{1500} \times 50 = \frac{10{,}000}{108{,}500}$

$108{,}500 \div 1500 = 72.3\% = 72\%.$

(23:174)

14. **C.** This type of problem may be solved by using the technique of alligation alternate. (1) Parts of the higher concentration preparation needed = (percent desired minus the lower percent). (2) Parts of the lower concentration preparation needed = (higher percent minus the desired percent). (3) The sum of the parts gives the total parts of the final product. (4) With appropriate proportions, one can calculate the required amounts. The following diagram illustrates the general process and then further illustrates with data from this question.

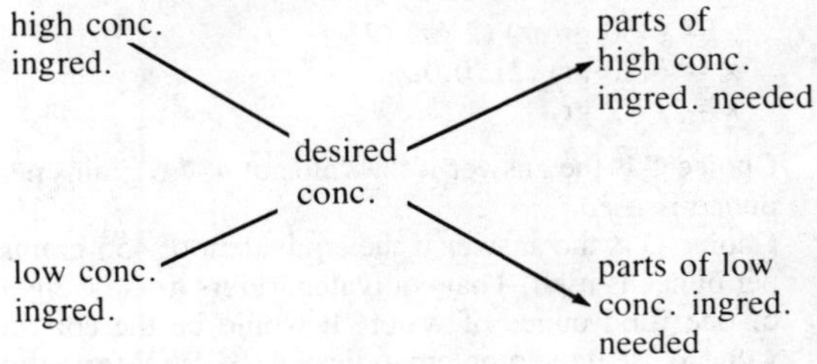

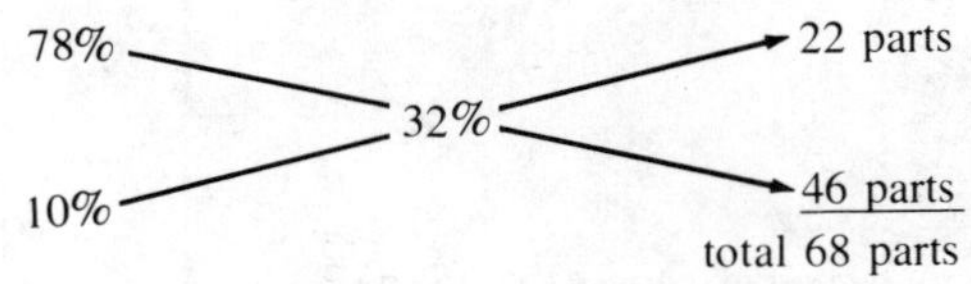

1 pint = 473 ml

low elixir needed $= 473 \text{ ml} \times \frac{46}{68} = 320 \text{ ml}$

high elixir needed $= 473 \text{ ml} \times \frac{22}{68} = 153 \text{ ml.}$

(23:174)

15. **B.** Since this is a %W/V problem, the number of grains (455) present in one fluid ounce of water is used as the fundamental equivalent.

gr needed = (455 gr/oz) (1 oz) (5%)
gr needed = (455 gr/oz) (1 oz) (0.05)
gr needed = 22.75 gr.

(23:132)

Choice C (24 gr) is obtained if the incorrect value of 480 gr per fluid ounce is used.

16. **C.** (1:1713)

17. **A.** One avoirdupois pound contains 454 grams. The total number of bacitracin units required is 200 units times 454 grams = 90,890 units. By proportion:

$\frac{500 \text{ units}}{1 \text{ g}} = \frac{90{,}800 \text{ units}}{x \text{ g}}$

$500x = 90{,}800$

$x = 181.6 \text{ g.}$

(23:170)

18. **E.** There is some potential for confusion in interpretation of the symbol ℥ although it is used only for the apothecary ounce. The avoirdupois ounce is symbolized by oz. The two are not equal weights. There are 480 gr in 1 apothecary ounce and 437.5 gr in 1 avoirdupois ounce. The grain weight is the same in the two systems. The apothecary system is always used in

prescriptions; the avoirdupois is used in commercial transactions, e.g., when the pharmacist buys or sells bulk chemicals. The usual equation used is: grains needed = (total grains in 1 ounce) × (number of ounces in final preparation × (% concentration desired).

x = (480 gr/oz) (2 oz) (2%)
x = (480 gr) (2) (0.02)
x = 19.2 gr.

Choice C is the answer if the value of 437.5 grains per ounce is used.
Choice D is the answer if the equivalent of 455 grains per ounce is used. That equivalent refers to the weight of one fluid ounce of water. It would be the correct value to use if the problem indicated a % W/V formula. (23:138)

19. **C.**

1 equivalent weight of KC1 = 74.6 g

1 milliequivalent (mEq) = 74.6 mg

$$\frac{1 \text{ mEq}}{74.6 \text{ mg}} = \frac{x \text{ mEq}}{5860 \text{ mg}}$$

74.6 x = 5860

x = 78.5 mEq.

Or by using the equation:

$$\text{mg/volume} = \frac{(\text{mEq/volume})\ (\text{Formula wt.})}{\text{Valence}}$$

$$5860 \text{ mg} = \frac{(x)\ (74.6)}{1}$$

x = 78.5 mEq.

(23:233)

20. **D.** Since the valence of calcium is +2, one mEq equals 40 mg ÷ 2 = 20 mg. Therefore, 1.5 mEq = 30 mg. If there are 30 mg per dl of solution, there will be 300 mg per liter. By use of the equation:

$$\text{mg/vol.} = \frac{(\text{mEq/vol.})\ (\text{Formula wt.})}{(\text{Valence})}$$

$$x \text{ mg/1000 ml} = \frac{(1.5 \text{ mEq/100 ml})\ (40)}{(2)}$$

$$\frac{x}{1000} = \frac{(1.5)\ (40)}{(100)\ (2)}$$

200x = 60,000

x = 300 mg.

21. **D.** $1 \text{ Equivalent} = \frac{147}{2} = 73.5 \text{ g}$

1 mEq = 73.5 mg

40 mEq = 2940 mg or 2.94 g of calcium chloride.

OR

by equation

$$\text{mg} = \frac{(\text{mEq})\ (\text{Formula wt.})}{\text{Valence}}$$

$$\text{mg} = \frac{(40)\ (147)}{2}$$

$$\text{mg} = \frac{5880}{2}$$

= 2940 mg or 2.94 g of calcium chloride.

One must remember that 40 mEq of calcium combines with 40 mEq of chloride to form 40 mEq of calcium chloride. (1:768; 23:233)
A. This answer is obtained if one multiplies the 40 mEq desired by the atomic weight of calcium and then divides by the +2 valence. The use of the atomic weight of calcium is incorrect since the official hydrated calcium chloride must be weighed to obtain the correct amount of calcium. The right answer can be obtained by this method by the additional step of:

$$\frac{0.80 \text{ g (calcium)}}{40 \text{ (Atomic Wt. Ca)}} = \frac{x \text{ g } (CaCl_2 \cdot 2\,H_2O)}{147 \text{ (Formula wt.)}}$$

$$x = 2.94 \text{ g } CaCl_2 \cdot 2\,H_2O.$$

B. The answer of 2.22 g is incorrect since it assumes that anhydrous calcium chloride (mol. wt. of 111) was used. However, the problem specified that the official form with two waters of hydration was available.
E. The answer of 5.88 g is obtained if one ignores the + 2 valence of calcium. (1:768; 23:233)

22. **B.** The solution is a 100% W/V solution since there are 100 g of solute and 100 ml of final solution volume. To express the concentration in W/W terms, one must determine the weight of 100 ml of the solution:

$$\text{Density} = \frac{W}{V}$$

$$1.7 \text{ g/ml} = \frac{W}{100 \text{ ml}}$$

W = 170 g

$$\% \text{ W/W} = \frac{100 \text{ g solute}}{170 \text{ g solution}} \times 100$$

% W/W = 58.8% or 59%.

(1:75)

23. **D.** The solution would be prepared by dissolving 1000 g KI in sufficient water to make 1000 ml of final solution. The weight of the final solution will be 1700 g since the density is 1.7. Of that 1700 g of weight, 1000 g is KI; the other 700 g must be water. Since 700 ml of water weighs 700 g, the 1000 ml of solution can be made by dissolving 1000 g of KI in 700 ml of water. (1:75)

24. **B.** To measure the sensitivity requirement, the balance rest-point is first determined. A weight is added to one pan, and the change in rest-point is observed. The magnitude of change must be such that 6 mg would alter the original rest-point by at least one index scale division. If a weight greater than 6 mg is required to bring about this change in rest-point, the balance is not sensitive enough and cannot be used in prescription compounding.
C. Ten milligrams was the sensitivity requirement specified prior to the USP XVIII.
D. Thirty milligrams is the maximum sensitivity requirement for the Class B prescription balance. This balance is not common in pharmacies but could be used for bulk manufacturing or nonprescription work. (1:85)

25. **D.** The minimum weight that may be weighed on any balance with a known sensitivity requirement (SR) with a given percent of error may be determined by the equation: SR = (minimum amount that may be weighed) × (% permissible error). In the given problem:

$$6 \text{ mg} = (x \text{ mg})\ (5\%)$$
$$6 \text{ mg} = (x \text{ mg})\ (0.05)$$
$$x = 120 \text{ mg.}$$

The NF specifies that pharmacists should not weigh quantities less than 120 mg on the Class A prescription balance in order to avoid errors of 5% or more. (19:1036)

26. **C.** *Step 1*. If pure HCl were available, how much would be needed? Since diluted HCl is 10% W/V, 4000 ml × 10% = 400 g of HCl needed.
Step 2. How much of the available 36.8% W/W solution would be needed to obtain 400 g? By definition, a 36.8% W/W solution contains 36.8 g in 100 g of solution.

$$\frac{36.8 \text{ g}}{100 \text{ g}} = \frac{400 \text{ g}}{x \text{ g}}$$

$$x = 1087 \text{ g.}$$

Step 3. What is the volume of 1087 g if the specific gravity is 1.19? 100 ml of acid weighs 119 g.

$$\frac{100 \text{ ml}}{119 \text{ g}} = \frac{x \text{ ml}}{1087 \text{ g}}$$

$$x = 913 \text{ ml.}$$

Thus 4 liters of diluted hydrochloric acid are prepared by measuring 913 ml of Hydrochloric Acid USP and diluting it with sufficient purified water to measure 4000 ml. (1:737;23:169)

27. **B.** Only 45 ml of the prescription must be adjusted to isotonicity, since the 15 ml of Zincfrin® is already isotonic. An isotonic solution of sodium chloride contains 0.9% sodium chloride: 45 ml × 0.009 = 0.4 g. (1:1407)

28. **B.** The strengths of insulin are expressed as U-40, 80, and 100. These values refer to the number of USP insulin units per ml of solution. One ml of U-80 insulin contains 80 units of insulin. This strength is no longer made in this country, but the calculation is generally illustrative. (18:253; 23:318)

$$\frac{80 \text{ units}}{1 \text{ ml of sol.}} = \frac{48 \text{ units}}{x \text{ ml of sol.}}$$

$$80\,x = 48$$

$$x = 0.60 \text{ ml.}$$

29. **A.** The number of units injected each day was:

$$\frac{40 \text{ units}}{1 \text{ ml}} = \frac{x}{0.8 \text{ ml}}$$

$$x = (40)\ (0.8)$$

$$x = 32 \text{ units.}$$

Since U-100 insulin contains 100 units per ml:

$$\frac{100 \text{ units}}{1 \text{ ml}} = \frac{32 \text{ units}}{x \text{ ml}}$$

$$100\,x = 32$$

$$x = 0.32 \text{ ml.}$$

(23:318)

30. **B.** Since the patient requires 60 units of the available U-100 insulin, 0.6 ml of solution is needed. While the volumes present in both the U-80 and U-100 insulin syringes are identical, the unit calibrations are different. Therefore,

$$\frac{1 \text{ ml volume reads}}{80 \text{ units}} = \frac{0.6 \text{ ml volume}}{x \text{ units}}$$

$$x = 48 \text{ units.}$$

(23:318)

31. **C.** Since the 5% concentration refers to a W/W strength, the problem should be solved in two steps.
Step 1. What weight of glycerin is required?
grains needed = (480 gr/℥) (2 ℥) (5%)
grains needed = (480 gr/℥) (2 ℥) (0.05)
grains needed = 48 grains
Step 2. Convert the weight to a volume measurement. At this point it is easier to convert the weight quantity from the apothecary to the metric system, which is requested for the answer.

1 grain = 64.8 mg

48 grains = 64.8 × 48 =

3110 mg or 3.11 g

Since density = $\frac{\text{Weight}}{\text{Volume}}$

1.25 g/ ml = $\frac{3.11 \text{ g}}{x}$

x = 2.5 ml.

(1:95)

It is also possible to immediately convert the prescription to the metric system:

1 apothecary ounce = 31.1 g
Amount of glycerin = (31.1) (2) (5%)
Amount of glycerin = 3.11 g.

32. **E.** Although the final answer must indicate the amount of sodium chloride to be added to 1 liter of solution, it is best to determine the percent of sodium chloride required first. Since the final isotonic solution must freeze at −0.52 degrees, the total freezing point depression caused by the formula's ingredients must be determined.
If the effect of the ingredients totals a freezing point depression of 0.255, and blood freezes at −0.52 degrees, enough sodium chloride must be added to cause a further reduction of: 0.520 − 0.255 = 0.265 degrees. Since 0.9% sodium chloride will cause a freezing point depression of 0.52 degrees, the amount of sodium chloride needed for a 0.265 depression is:

$$\frac{0.9\%}{0.52 \text{ degrees}} = \frac{x\ \%}{0.265 \text{ degrees}}$$

x = 0.46%.

Therefore, 0.46% sodium chloride must be added to the original formula. In every liter there will be 4.6 grams of sodium chloride. (1:1406)

Ingredient	"D" value if 1% solution were used	Formula concentration	Actual depression
Procaine HCl	0.12 degrees	1%	0.12 degrees
Benzyl Alcohol	0.09	0.5%	0.045
Pot. Phosphate *(Mono)*	0.25	0.25%	0.063
Pot. Phosphate *(Di)*	0.27	0.1%	0.027
		total depression =	0.255 degrees

33. **E.** A 1% solution of pilocarpine hydrochloride causes a freezing point depression of only 0.14 degrees. Thus, a greater concentration is needed to obtain a depression equal to that of blood (0.52). By simple proportion:

$$\frac{1\ \%}{0.14 \text{ degrees}} = \frac{x\ \%}{0.52 \text{ degrees}}$$

x = 3.7%.

(1:1406)

34. **B.** The directions indicate that the patient is to take one teaspoonful of the prescription every four hours. One teaspoonful is considered to be approximately 5 ml when household measures are employed. Since this prescription consists of 6 fluid ounces, which is approximately 180 ml, there are 180 ÷ 5 = 36 doses. One and one half drachms are equal to 90 grains. Therefore, the number of grains per dose would be 90 ÷ 36 = 2.5 grains. (23:91)
Choice A would be calculated if one misinterpreted ʒ i in the Sig. as meaning one fluid drachm. Since there are 8 drachms in 1 fluid ounce, the total number of doses would then be 48.
Choice D is the amount of ammonium chloride in the entire prescription, not per dose.

35. **C.** There are two sources of codeine in the prescription. Four grains are being added to the elixir, which already contains approximately 1 grain of codeine per fluid ounce. Thus the total amount of codeine will be about 10 grains.

10 ÷ 36 doses = 5/18 grains.

(1:803; 23:85)

Choice A would be based upon 48 doses rather than 36 doses. Assumption that ʒ i in the directions to the patient meant 1 fluid drachm rather than 5 ml (1 teaspoonful) would lead to this error. Also, the codeine present in the elixir was ignored.
Choice B considers only the codeine added to the prescription, thus ignoring the codeine originally present in the elixir.
Choice D: if the gr iv was read as 6 grains, the total number of grains of codeine would be 12.
Choice E is also based upon 48 doses rather than the correct 36.

36. **C.** More hydrous citric acid than anhydrous citric acid would be needed. The molecular weight of monohydrate citric acid would be 192 plus 1 water (18) = 210.

$$\frac{210}{192} \times 27.4 \text{ g} = 30.0 \text{ grams.}$$

(1:1259; 23:219)

37. **B.** The formula weight of ferrous sulfate is 278. The amount of iron present in 300 mg of the chemical will be:

$$\frac{55.9}{278} \times 300 \text{ mg} = 60.3 \text{ mg.}$$

(23:214)

Choices A and D would be obtained if the correct answer was either doubled or halved to reflect the +2 valence of iron. The valence of iron has no significance in this type of problem since only one atom of iron is present in each molecule of ferrous sulfate.
Choice C assumes that the ferrous sulfate is anhydrous, with a molecular weight of 152. This is incorrect, since the 300-mg weight is based upon a chemical formula containing 7 waters of hydration.
Choice E is the amount of anhydrous ferrous sulfate ($FeSO_4$) present in each 300 mg. The question asks for iron (Fe) only.

38. **B.** One gallon contains 128 fluid ounces.

$$128 \div 4 = 32 \text{ bottles.}$$

(23:68)

39. **B.** The amount of diluted hydriodic acid needed for this manufacturing batch is 140 ml × 4 = 560 ml. Since diluted hydriodic acid contains 10 g of HI in each 100 ml, the amount of pure hydriodic acid required is:

$$\frac{10 \text{ g}}{100 \text{ ml}} = \frac{x \text{ g}}{560 \text{ ml}}$$

$$x = 56 \text{ grams.}$$

The amount of 18% W/W hydriodic acid solution needed to obtain 56 grams of pure HI would be:

$$\frac{18 \text{ g}}{100 \text{ g}} = \frac{56 \text{ g}}{x \text{ g}}$$

$$x = 311 \text{ grams of 18\% W/W solution.}$$

The question requested that the answer be expressed in ml.

$$\text{density} = \frac{\text{weight}}{\text{volume}}$$

$$1.18 = \frac{311 \text{ g}}{x}$$

$$1.18x = 311$$

$$x = 264 \text{ ml.}$$

(23:157)

40. **C.** One pint contains 473 ml. The final solution used by the patient will contain 473 × 0.1% = 0.473 g of pure sodium hypochlorite. This amount is also present in each 30 ml of the prescription since the dilution process performed by the patient simply involves the addition of water. If each 30 ml of the prescription contains 0.473 g of pure sodium hypochlorite, the total amount is

$$0.473 \times \frac{120}{30} = 1.89 \text{ grams.}$$

The amount of Sodium Hypochlorite Solution NF required is:

$$\frac{5 \text{ g sod. hypochlorite}}{100 \text{ ml of official sol.}} = \frac{1.89 \text{ g}}{x \text{ ml}}$$

$$x = 37.8 \text{ ml.}$$

(23:164)

41. **B.** There are two methods for determining the correct answer for this question.

Method I.
a. Determine the amount of pure chemical present:
120 ml × 5% = 6.0 g of aluminum acetate.
b. Determine the new concentration.

$$\frac{6.0 \text{ g}}{1120 \text{ ml}} = 0.53\% \text{ W/V, Ans.}$$

Method II. Use of the equation:
(quantity of new solution) (strength of new sol.) = (quantity of original sol.) (strength of original sol.)

$$(1120 \text{ ml})(x\,\%) = (120 \text{ ml})(5\%)$$

$$1120x = 600$$

$$x = 0.53\%, \text{ Ans.}$$

(23:166)

C. The answer of 0.60% is incorrect since it assumes that the final volume of diluted solution is 1000 ml instead of the correct volume of 1000 + 120 ml.

42. **B.** The amount of pure ephedrine sulfate required is 30 ml × 0.25% = 0.075 gram. The stock solution contains 1 gram of ephedrine in every 50 ml of solution. Therefore:

$$\frac{1 \text{ g ephedrine sulfate}}{50 \text{ ml stock solution}} = \frac{0.075 \text{ g}}{x \text{ ml}}$$

$$x = 3.75 \text{ ml.}$$

(23:163)

43. **E.** One may solve this problem by first determining how much pure (100%) gentian violet was originally

present. The final ratio strength can then be determined by dividing the amount of chemical present by the final volume prepared.

(1) 50 ml of 0.5% contains

$$50 \times .005 = 0.25 \text{ g}$$

(2) 0.25 g is diluted to 1250 ml

$$\frac{0.25}{1250} = .0002 \text{ or } \frac{2}{10{,}000} =$$

$$\frac{1}{5000} = 1{:}5000.$$

or by equation:

$$\begin{pmatrix}\text{quantity of}\\ \text{new solution}\end{pmatrix}\begin{pmatrix}\text{strength of}\\ \text{new solution}\end{pmatrix} =$$

$$\begin{pmatrix}\text{quantity of}\\ \text{original sol.}\end{pmatrix}\begin{pmatrix}\text{strength of}\\ \text{original sol.}\end{pmatrix}$$

$$(1250 \text{ ml})(x) = (50 \text{ ml})(0.5\%)$$

$$1250\,x = 0.25$$

$$x = .0002 \text{ or } \frac{2}{10{,}000} = \frac{1}{5000}$$

$$\frac{1}{5000} = 1{:}5000.$$

(23:160)

44. **B.** A solution having a specific gravity of 1.313 is 1.313 times heavier than water. Therefore, every 100 ml of Syrup weighs 131.3 grams. Since Syrup contains 85 grams of sucrose in each 100 ml:

$$\%\ W/W = \frac{85 \text{ g}}{131.3 \text{ g}} = 64.7 \text{ or } 65\%$$

(23:141)

45. **B.** The problem requests an answer expressed as % W/V. The weight of the liquid chemical is:

$$\text{density} = \frac{\text{weight}}{\text{volume}}$$

$$0.8 = \frac{x \text{ g}}{800 \text{ ml}}$$

$$x = 640 \text{ grams (weight of 800 ml)}$$

$$\%\ W/V = \frac{640 \text{ g}}{4000 \text{ ml}} = .16 \text{ or } 16\%.$$

(23:137)

Choice C is the correct concentration for a % V/V expression.

46. **A.** One fluid ounce of water weighs 455 grains.
gr of chemical = (455 gr/f℥) (8 f℥) (.02%)
x = (455 gr/f℥) (8 f℥) (.0002)
x = .728 or .73 grains.

(23:134)

Choice B (.77 grains) occurs when the wrong equivalent for the apothecary ounce is used. The value of 480 grains is correct only when problems are expressed as % W/W.

Choices C and D are based upon 2% solutions not 0.02%.

47. **A.** If only sodium chloride were being used to render the 60 ml isotonic: 60 ml × 0.9% = 0.54 g or 540 mg would be needed. However, the zinc sulfate will contribute toward making the solution isotonic. The E value for zinc sulfate is 0.15, which indicates that 1 gram of zinc sulfate has the same effect on isotonicity as 150 mg of sodium chloride. The effect of zinc sulfate may be calculated as: (1) 60 ml × 1% = 0.60 g or 600 mg of zinc sulfate required to fill the prescription. (2) This 600 mg is equivalent to 600 × 0.15 = 90 mg of sodium chloride. Therefore, the amount of sodium chloride needed is equal to:

$$540 \text{ mg} - 90 \text{ mg} = 450 \text{ mg}.$$

(1:1407)

48. **D.** One pound of Strong Ammonia Solution NF weighs 454 grams. Since 28% of the 454 grams is pure ammonia, there is present 454 × .28 = 127.1 grams of pure ammonia. Since the new solution will contain 10 grams of pure ammonia in every 100 grams of solution, 127.1 grams of pure ammonia will be present in every 1271 grams of ammonia water.
Or by equation:

$$\begin{pmatrix}\text{quantity of}\\ \text{new solution}\end{pmatrix}\begin{pmatrix}\text{strength of}\\ \text{new solution}\end{pmatrix} =$$

$$\begin{pmatrix}\text{quantity of}\\ \text{original sol.}\end{pmatrix}\begin{pmatrix}\text{strength of}\\ \text{original sol.}\end{pmatrix}$$

$$(x \text{ gram})(10\%\ W/W) =$$

$$(454 \text{ gram})(28\%\ W/W)$$

$$10\,x = 12712$$

$$x = 1271.2 \text{ grams.}$$

(23:160)

49. **D.** The daily dose is 0.3 ml × 3 doses = 0.9 ml.
0.9 ml × 5% = .045 g or 45 mg.

(23:97)

50. **D.** Two pounds would contain 454 × 2 = 908 grams of ointment. The final preparation would contain 908 g × 2% = 18.18 grams of pure ammoniated mercury. Since the available mercury ointment is 5% strength one would use:

$$\frac{5\text{g}}{100\text{ g}} = \frac{18.16\text{ g}}{\text{x g}}$$

x = 363.2 g of the 5% ointment.

Or by equation:

$$\left(\begin{array}{c}\text{quantity of}\\ \text{new ointment}\end{array}\right)\left(\begin{array}{c}\text{strength of}\\ \text{new ointment}\end{array}\right) =$$

$$\left(\begin{array}{c}\text{quantity of}\\ \text{old ointment}\end{array}\right)\left(\begin{array}{c}\text{strength of}\\ \text{old ointment}\end{array}\right)$$

(908 g) (2% W/W) = (x g) (5% W/W)

x = 363.2 grams. (23:171)

A. This is the amount of pure ammoniated mercury needed to prepare 2 lb of 2% ointment.
Choice E is the amount of ointment diluent that would be added to the 5% ammoniated mercury ointment. (23:171)

CHAPTER 5

Pharmacy

Pharmacy has been said to require knowledge of the identification, selection, pharmacological action, preservation, combination, analysis, and standardization of drugs and medicines and to include responsibility for their proper and safe use (1:3). In practice, the pharmacist needs to know generic and trade names, dosage forms and strengths, items which compete with each other for therapeutic choice, the good and bad of OTC medications, and a host of miscellanea. These make up the areas dealt with in the test items in this chapter.

Directions: Each of the questions or incomplete statements below is followed by five suggested answers or completions. Select the BEST answer in each case.

1. The essential difference between protamine zinc insulin (PZI) and isophane insulin (NPH) is that

   A. PZI has an acetate buffer while NPH has a phosphate buffer
   B. NPH has a much longer duration of action
   C. PZI has an acid pH while NPH is neutral
   D. PZI has a large excess of protamine while NPH has essentially no excess
   E. NPH has greater stability because it is neutral (17:368)

2. Mono-component or single-component insulin

   A. is prepared from a single animal source
   B. is a highly purified form of insulin
   C. is another name for the U100 insulins
   D. can be administered on an every other day schedule
   E. has its peak activity maintained at a constant level for several hours (6:1516)

3. Which of the following is *not* true of single-peak regular insulin?

   A. can be mixed with all other insulins
   B. can only be prepared from pork insulin
   C. is more antigenic than "single-component" insulins
   D. is supplied only at neutral pH
   E. need not be refrigerated (6:1516–18)

4. Which one of the following forms of insulin has the shortest expiration dating?

   A. globin zinc insulin injection
   B. insulin injection
   C. insulin zinc suspension (lente)
   D. isophane insulin suspension (NPH)
   E. protamine zinc insulin suspension (PZI) (18:253)

5. Actifed® differs from Actidil® in that Actifed®

   A. contains an antihistamine
   B. contains aspirin
   C. contains a decongestant
   D. contains ascorbic acid
   E. contains a barbiturate (10)

6. Sterazolidin® is a combination product containing as its active ingredients

   A. phenylbutazone and prednisone
   B. oxyphenbutazone and aspirin
   C. oxyphenbutazone and hydrocortisone
   D. phenylbutazone and aspirin
   E. phenylbutazone and hydrocortisone (4:528)

7. Which of the following agents is/are available in a sublingual dosage form?

   A. isorbide dinitrate (Isordil®)
   B. nitroglycerin
   C. amyl nitrite
   D. A and B
   E. all of the above (7:812–17)

8. Pyridoxine is a component of which of the following products?
   A. Bendectin®
   B. Antivert®
   C. Dramamine®
   D. Compazine®
   E. none of the above (3:788; 4:1105)

9. Liquifilm® is a vehicle used in preparing
   A. topical gels
   B. ophthalmic solutions
   C. topical aerosols
   D. otic solutions
   E. none of the above (3:1394, 1398)

10. Micronor® differs from Ovral® in that Micronor®
   A. contains no estrogen
   B. contains no progestin
   C. is not an oral contraceptive
   D. contains a higher estrogen dose
   E. must be used for only five days each month (10)

11. Tuinal® can best be described as a combination of
   A. amobarbital and butabarbital
   B. phenobarbital and secobarbital
   C. secobarbital and pentobarbital
   D. pentobarbital and butabarbital
   E. secobarbital and amobarbital (10)

12. According to USP standards, a refrigerator may be used to store pharmaceuticals which specify storage in a
   A. cold place
   B. cool place
   C. controlled room temperature
   D. dark place
   E. both B and C (1:519; 18:8)

13. The NF describes several tests for evaluating prescription balances. These tests include all of the following *except*
   A. arm ratio
   B. rest point
   C. rider and graduated beam
   D. sensitivity requirement
   E. shift (1:85; 19:1036)

14. Weights are classified by an alphabetical system. For prescription work, the pharmacist should use what class (or better) weights?
   A. A
   B. C
   C. P
   D. Q
   E. T (19:1037)

15. According to the National Bureau of Standards (NBS), the initial calibration mark on a 100-ml graduate should be
   A. 5 ml
   B. 10 ml
   C. 15 ml
   D. 20 ml
   E. 30 ml (1:89; 22:35)

16. One example of an official saturated solution is
   A. Aluminum Acetate Solution USP XIX
   B. Acetic Acid USP XIX
   C. Iodine Solution USP XIX
   D. Strong Iodine Solution USP XIX
   E. Potassium Iodide Solution USP XIX (1:802)

17. According to the USP, a monograph's instruction of "protect from light" indicates storage in a
   A. dark place
   B. amber glass bottle
   C. light-resistant container
   D. hermetic container
   E. tight glass container (18:7, 642)

18. Solubility of a substance in a solvent may be expressed in several ways. When a quantitative statement of solubility is given in the USP and NF it is generally expressed as
   A. g of solute soluble in 1 ml of solvent
   B. g of solute soluble in 100 ml of solvent
   C. ml of solvent required to dissolve 1 g of solute
   D. ml of solvent required to dissolve 100 g of solute
   E. ml of solvent required to prepare 100 ml of saturated solution (1:230)

19. If a bottle of tablets has an expiration date of "June 1980," the pharmacist may
   A. continue to dispense the product if he has already opened the container
   B. dispense the tablets only until June 1, 1980
   C. dispense the tablets through June 15, 1980
   D. dispense the tablets through June 30, 1980
   E. dispense the tablets if he informs the patient to discard unused tablets in six months (December 1, 1980) (18 Supp.:1)

20. The expiration date on a pharmaceutical container states "Expires June, 1980." This statement means that by July 1, 1980, the product will have lost

A. 5% of its activity
B. 10% of its activity
C. 20% of its activity
D. 50% of its activity
E. sufficient activity to be outside USP or NF monograph requirements (18 Supp. 1:9)

21. The USP weight variation test for capsule dosage forms states limits for the variation of weight of individual capsules from the observed average weight of a sample of 20 capsules. None of the capsules may have net content weights varying more than ____ from the average.

A. 5%
B. 10%
C. 15%
D. 20%
E. 25% (15:137–38; 18:670)

22. Which of the following chemicals is actually a mixture of ingredients?

A. ammonium chloride
B. ferrous sulfate
C. sodium bisulfite
D. sodium bicarbonate
E. sodium thiosulfate (26:155)

23. Calamine powder is a mixture of zinc oxide and

A. aluminum oxide
B. amaranth
C. caramel
D. cochineal
E. ferric oxide (26:304)

24. The USP and NF specifies that almost all measurements and tests that are temperature-dependent must be conducted at

A. 15.6°C
B. 20°C
C. 25°C
D. 60°F
E. 98.6°F (24:25)

25. The constipating component of camphorated tincture of opium (paregoric) is

A. morphine
B. oxymorphone
C. hydrocodone
D. codeine
E. heroin (17:265)

26. The cardiac glycoside present in digitalis leaf in the largest amount is

A. digoxin
B. ouabain
C. gitalin
D. lanatoside C
E. digitoxin (33:137)

27. The official bioassay for digitalis leaf preparations utilizes which of the following animals?

A. frog
B. cat
C. pigeon
D. rabbit
E. rat (33:129)

28. The monograph for Strong Ammonia Solution NF contains a note pertaining to

A. its reaction with strong acids
B. proper dilutions for use
C. the incompatibilities of ammonia
D. the method of manufacturing
E. the manner of handling and opening of bottles (1:1257)

29. The process of grinding a substance to a very fine powder is termed

A. levigation
B. sublimation
C. trituration
D. percolation
E. maceration (14:37, 122, 173, 242)

30. The term "impalpable" refers to a substance that is

A. not tasty
B. not perceptible to the touch
C. greasy
D. nongreasy
E. tasteless (11:767; 41:659)

31. The process of wetting and smoothing zinc oxide with mineral oil in preparation for incorporation into an ointment base is

A. attrition
B. levigation
C. milling
D. pulverization by intervention
E. trituration (1:1555; 20b:160)

32. Which form of sulfur should a pharmacist use when extemporaneously preparing an ointment?

A. cake of sulfur
B. flowers of sulfur
C. precipitated sulfur
D. sublimed sulfur
E. washed sulfur (24:315)

33. Micromeritics refers to the study of

A. metric systems of measurement
B. microscopes

C. microscopic ocean life
D. dimensions of microorganisms
E. small particles (22:177)

34. Which of the following statements concerning adsorption is *not* true?
A. as the temperature increases, adsorption decreases
B. doubling the concentration of adsorbable chemical per unit adsorbent in solution will double the amount of adsorption that will occur
C. adsorption is a rapid process
D. the amount of adsorption that will occur is dependent upon the surface area of the adsorbent
E. adsorption may be either a chemical or a physical process (1:293)

35. The shrinkage that occurs when alcohol and purified water are mixed is primarily due to
A. attractive van der Waals forces
B. covalent bonding
C. hydrogen bonding
D. ionic bonding
E. temperature changes (12:67)

36. The type of flow in which the viscosity of a liquid increases with agitation is
A. plastic
B. dilatant
C. pseudoplastic
D. thixotropic
E. Newtonian (14:302–06)

37. According to the Poiseuille equation, the factor that has the relatively greatest influence on the rate of flow of liquid through a capillary tube is the
A. length of the tube
B. viscosity of the liquid
C. pressure differential on the tube
D. radius of the tube
E. temperature of the liquid (12:508)

38. Patients following low-sodium diets may resort to the use of sodium-free salt substitutes such as Co-Salt® (U.S.V.) or Neocurtasal® (Winthrop). The major ingredient in these products is
A. ammonium chloride
B. calcium chloride
C. potassium chloride
D. potassium iodide
E. none of these (3:499)

39. Potassium supplements are administered in all of the following manners *except*
A. IV infusion
B. rapid IV injection
C. elixirs, p.o.
D. effervescent tablets
E. slow-release tablets, p.o. (1:770–71)

40. Which of the following statements concerning fluorouracil is *not* true?
A. its chemical structure is a modified pyrimidine similar to uracil and thymine
B. it is effective only when administered by injection
C. anorexia or nausea and vomiting are very common side effects
D. the drug interferes with the synthesis of ribonucleic acid
E. the drug prevents the methylation of deoxyuridylic acid to thymidylic acid (3:1563; 5:527; 6:1274–77)

41. Which one of the following liquid products is *not* a source of potassium?
A. Isoclor®
B. Kaochlor®
C. Kaon®
D. Kay Ciel®
E. all of the above products are potassium supplements (3:31–33, 597)

42. Several preparations of slow-release potassium (e.g., Slow-K®) are now commercially available. Slow release of the potassium from the dosage form has been accomplished by
A. using a slowly dissolving carbonate salt of potassium
B. enteric coating of successive layers of potassium chloride
C. using a wax matrix tablet core from which the potassium slowly dissolves
D. using an outer layer of rapidly dissolving potassium chloride and an inner core of slowly dissolving potassium gluconate
E. a series of enteric coated granules of potassium chloride which have been compressed into tablet form (3:33; 10)

43. Polypropylene syringes are
A. autoclavable
B. completely transparent
C. cheaper than polyethylene syringes
D. lighter in weight than polyethylene syringes
E. unbreakable (20:652)

44. Nylon is rarely used in the manufacture of syringes because it

A. is too easily broken
B. cannot be autoclaved
C. may react with acidic drugs
D. is not flexible
E. is destroyed by dilute mineral acids (20a:701)

45. The bevel length of a hypodermic needle may vary from very short to long (regular). A short bevel is preferred for injections by which route of administration?
A. intradermal
B. intramuscular
C. intrathecal
D. intravenous
E. subcutaneous (13:342; 15:532)

46. Insulin preparations are usually administered by
A. intradermal injection
B. intramuscular injection
C. intravenous bolus
D. intravenous infusion
E. subcutaneous injection (13:159)

47. Which one of the following needles is most suited for the administration of insulin solutions?
A. 16G ⅝″
B. 21G ½″
C. 21G ⅝″
D. 25G ⅝″
E. 25G 1″ (13:344)

48. "Winged" needles are most closely associated with which type of injections?
A. intradermal
B. intramuscular
C. intrathecal
D. intravenous
E. subcutaneous (13:345)

49. Hypodermic needle sizes are expressed by gauge numbers. The gauge number refers to
A. the bevel size
B. the external diameter of the cannula
C. the internal diameter of the cannula
D. the length of the needle
E. the size of the lumen opening (15:532)

50. The Busher® Injector is
A. an automatic device for self-injecting
B. a disposable syringe and needle system
C. a device used to start an intravenous injection
D. a filled syringe unit made by Bristol mainly for the emergency administration of drugs
E. Wyeth's cartridge injection system (24:270)

51. All adjuvants used in parenteral products must be specified on the label by name *except* for
A. antimicrobial preservatives
B. antioxidants
C. pH adjustors
D. headspace gasses
E. no exemptions are allowed (18:4)

52. Which of the following commonly available large-volume dextrose solutions for intravenous use is isotonic?
A. 2.5%
B. 5.0%
C. 10%
D. 20%
E. 50% (13:123)

53. An injectable drug product whose literature specifically contraindicates reconstitution with vehicles containing parabens, phenol, or cresol is
A. chlordiazepoxide hydrochloride (Librium®)
B. mithramycin (Mithracin®)
C. nitrofurantoin sodium (Furadantin®)
D. oxacillin sodium (Prostaphlin®)
E. tetracycline hydrochloride (Achromycin® HC1) (21:249)

54. Which one of the following injectable solutions should *not* be added to any infusion bottles?
A. diazepam (Valium®)
B. folic acid (Folvite®)
C. furosemide (Lasix®)
D. gentamicin sulfate (Garamycin®)
E. succinylcholine chloride (Anectine®) (21:121)

55. Becton Dickinson supplies packages of insulin syringes and needles. Which one of the following statements concerning these products is *not* true?
A. syringes are available for U40 and U100 insulins
B. syringes are color coded and calibrated according to the insulin strengths available
C. the syringes are available either individually wrapped or in bags of 10 each

D. the syringes have 26-gauge needles
E. the smallest volume syringe available is 1.0 ml (10)

56. The method of preparation must be indicated on labels for
A. Bacteriostatic Water for Injection USP
B. Milk of Magnesia USP
C. Purified Water USP
D. Stronger Rose Water NF
E. Water for Injection USP (18:540)

57. Of the following vehicles, which is the most appropriate for an IV admixture of ampicillin (500 mg per 50 ml)?
A. dextrose 5% injection
B. dextrose 5% and sodium chloride 0.9% injection
C. dextrose 2.5% and sodium chloride 0.45% injection
D. sodium chloride 0.9% injection
E. all of the above (21:29)

58. A parenteral solution that is preferably administered by hypodermoclysis is
A. dextrose 50% injection
B. lactated potassic saline injection
C. lactated Ringer's injection
D. Ringer's injection
E. sodium lactate injection (1:771)

59. The storage directions on a parenteral solution specify "store in a cool place." This solution may be stored in
A. an air-conditioned area at 68°F
B. a refrigerator
C. a cooler set at 59°F
D. both A and C
E. both B and C (1:519)

60. Water for Injection USP may be prepared from tap water by
A. chemical treatment with $KMnO_4$
B. deionization followed by filtration through pyrogen-retaining filters
C. simple distillation
D. reflux distillation
E. sterilization by autoclaving (18:716)

61. Product literature often suggests that sterile water for injection be used as the reconstituting solvent for injectable antibiotic powders. However, sodium chloride injection (normal saline) is frequently used. Normal saline would *not* be used to reconstitute
A. ampicillin sodium
B. erythromycin lactobionate
C. methicillin sodium
D. penicillin G potassium
E. polymyxin B sulfate (21:143)

62. Although isotonicity is desirable for almost all parenterals, it is particularly critical for which injections?
A. intra-articular
B. intradermal
C. intramuscular
D. intravenous
E. subcutaneous (1:1461)

63. The osmotic pressure of a 0.1 molar dextrose solution will be approximately how many times that of a 0.1 molar sodium chloride solution?
A. 0.5
B. 1
C. 2
D. 3
E. 4 (1:245–47)

64. Parenteral solutions that are isotonic with human red blood cells have an osmolality of approximately how many mOsm/l?
A. 20
B. 40
C. 50
D. 150
E. 300 (13:262)

65. The form of water most commonly used as a solvent during the manufacture of parenterals is
A. Bacteriostatic Water for Injection USP
B. deionized water
C. distilled water
D. Sterile Water for Injection USP
E. Water for Injection USP (1:1240, 1241, 1464)

66. A suspension is *not* a suitable dosage for what type of injection?
A. intra-articular
B. intradermal
C. intramuscular
D. intravenous
E. subcutaneous (1:1461)

67. Which one of the following parenteral solutions is considered to most closely approximate the extracellular fluid of the human body?
A. dextrose 2½% and sodium chloride 0.45% injection

B. lactated Ringer's injection
C. Ringer's injection
D. sodium chloride injection
E. sodium lactate injection (1:758)

68. Storage conditions for Normal Human Serum Albumin USP are

A. below 2°C
B. 2 to 4°C
C. 5 to 8°C
D. 8 to 15°C
E. room temperature (1:756)

69. Ringer's solution is an aqueous solution containing

A. sodium, potassium, and magnesium cations
B. dextrose and sodium chloride
C. sodium, potassium, and calcium chloride
D. fructose and sodium chloride
E. dextrose and sodium bicarbonate (1:758)

70. The quantities of all ingredients present in parenteral solutions must be specified on the label *except* for

A. antimicrobial preservatives
B. chelating agents
C. isotonicity adjustors
D. pH adjustors
E. there are no exceptions (18:253)

71. Which one of the following statements concerning Sodium Chloride Irrigation USP is *not* true? The Solution

A. may contain an antimicrobial preservative
B. is intended for either topical or rectal administration
C. may be packaged in bottles as large as three liters
D. contains the same concentration of sodium chloride as present in Sodium Chloride Injection USP
E. is sterile (18:457)

72. The manufacturing formula for Ascorbic Acid Injection USP may include

A. acetic acid
B. hydrochloric acid
C. propylene glycol
D. sodium hydroxide
E. tetracycline hydrochloride (18:37)

73. The IV fluid systems which utilize glass bottles may be divided into two types according to the

A. presence or absence of a vacuum in the bottle
B. presence or absence of an airway tube in the bottle
C. type of closure utilized (i.e., screw cap versus rubber plug)
D. size (volume) of the available solutions
E. presence or absence of pressure in the bottle (30:134)

74. In 1971, Travenol introduced large-volume IV solutions in flexible plastic containers (Viaflex®). Which of the following is *not* an advantage of this system over the glass bottle system?

A. danger of air embolism is reduced since no air enters the system
B. lightweight containers save storage space and are easier to handle
C. easier to dispose of the empty container
D. easier visual check for particulate matter
E. plastic bags are essentially unbreakable (30:136)

75. Which one of the following parenteral antibiotics is the most stable in aqueous solution?

A. gentamicin sulfate
B. methicillin sodium
C. oxacillin sodium
D. tetracycline hydrochloride
E. vancomycin hydrochloride (21:156)

76. Which of the following drug products is a combination of two different antimicrobial drugs?

A. Mysteclin-F®
B. Polycillin-PRB®
C. Tetrex bid-Caps®
D. V-Cillin K®
E. Bicillin® (4:751; 25:713, 1654)

77. Which of the following sulfisoxazole salts or derivatives would most likely be the best choice in formulating a flavored liquid dosage form of the drug?

A. sulfisoxazole diethanolamine
B. sulfisoxazole sodium
C. acetylsulfisoxazole
D. sulfisoxazole potassium
E. none of the above (6:1118)

78. Naturally occurring vitamin K_1 is also called

A. menadione
B. phytonadione
C. tocopherol
D. dihydrotachysterol
E. biotin (17:172)

79. The aromatic waters are generally outdated as dosage forms. One that is still often used is

Hamamelis Water NF XI, which is also known as

A. bay rum
B. camphorated water
C. neroli water
D. peppermint water
E. witch hazel (24:371)

80. All of the following are reasons why aromatic waters are *not* commonly used *except*

A. most are saturated solutions
B. preparation requires 12 to 24 hours
C. poor solvent properties
D. unpleasant taste
E. susceptibility to mold growth (1:1439)

81. The USP has established limits on dissolved solids in the official waters, assuming that such values should reflect the relative purity of the waters. Which of the following has the lowest permissible level of dissolved solids?

A. Bacteriostatic Water for Injection USP
B. Purified Water USP
C. Sterile Water for Injection USP (in 30-ml vials)
D. Sterile Water for Injection USP (in 1-liter bottles)
E. potable water (18:540)

82. Blood taken from volunteer donors is usually prevented from clotting by

A. freezing
B. addition of heparin
C. the removal of calcium ions from the blood by adding citrate salts
D. separating the formed elements (cells) from the plasma
E. maintaining the blood at 4 to 10°F (36:110)

83. Biologicals can be used to obtain either active or passive immunity. Which one of the following pairs is *not* correct?

A. antiserum, passive immunity
B. antitoxin, passive immunity
C. human immune serum, active immunity
D. toxoid, active immunity
E. vaccine, active immunity (24:278)

84. All of the following biologicals may be administered to humans. Which one is the most dangerous in respect to body response and potential toxicity?

A. antiserums
B. antitoxins
C. toxins
D. toxoids
E. vaccines (1:1324)

85. The Schick test is used to determine susceptibility to

A. diphtheria
B. measles
C. polio
D. TB
E. typhoid fever (1:1341)

86. All of the following biologicals are used for active immunization *except*

A. bacterial vaccines
B. bacterial antigens
C. multiple antigen preparations
D. toxoids
E. toxins (1:1328)

87. Which one of the following statements concerning Immune Serum Globulin is true?

A. Immune Serum Globulin contains approximately 50% gamma globulin
B. serum hepatitis is one of the most often reported adverse reactions
C. skin tests should not be performed before injecting any of the globulins
D. virus infections attenuated by gamma globulin are noninfectious
E. all of the above statements are true (3:1279–80)

88. Special forms of gamma globulin such as tetanus or pertussis differ from immune gamma globulin in that they are

A. obtained from humans hyperimmunized with either tetanus toxoid or pertussis vaccine
B. effective after the onset of the disease symptoms
C. administered by slow infusion
D. prepared from foreign (animal) serum
E. unsuitable for administration to children (1:1340; 3:1279–82)

89. Immune serum globulin (gamma globulin) is usually administered by what type of injection?

A. intradermal
B. intramuscular
C. intravenous
D. subcutaneous
E. any of the usual methods of injection (1:760, 1339–40; 3:1279–83)

90. Which statement concerning mumps immune globulin is *not* true?

A. globulin is obtained from humans
B. the intramuscular route of administration is used
C. globulin provides passive immunity for the patient
D. the globulin may also be used in larger doses to prevent complications of mumps such as orchitis
E. the biological product is commercially available as immune serum globulin (3:1281)

91. The Sabin poliomyelitis vaccine is

A. administered orally as a live attenuated vaccine
B. available only in a monovalent form
C. available only in a trivalent form
D. a killed vaccine
E. similar to the Salk vaccine (1:1333)

92. The Mantoux test uses

A. diagnostic diphtheria toxin
B. DPT toxin
C. mumps skin test antigen
D. old tuberculin
E. scarlet fever streptococcus toxin (1:1342)

93. The intermediate tuberculin skin test (intermediate strength PPD) contains

A. 2 tuberculin units
B. 5 tuberculin units
C. 25 tuberculin units
D. 250 tuberculin units
E. 500 tuberculin units (3:1335; 37:132)

94. All of the following are used for the prophylaxis or treatment of diseases *except*

A. antitoxins
B. antivenins
C. globulins
D. serums
E. serum albumin (1:756)

95. The usual storage condition specified for biologicals is

A. below 2°C
B. 2 to 8°C
C. cool place
D. 8 to 15°C
E. room temperature (24:277)

96. All of the following statements concerning toxoids are true *except*

A. toxoids are detoxified toxins
B. toxoids are antigens
C. toxoids produce permanent immunity
D. toxoids are often available in a precipitated or adsorbed form
E. toxoids produce artificial active immunity (1:1330)

97. Several vaccines and toxoids are precipitated and adsorbed onto aluminum hydroxide, aluminum phosphate, or other suitable media. This process results in a dosage form that, in comparison to fluid products, is

A. more effective orally
B. more slowly absorbed
C. more stable
D. less irritating upon injection
E. less likely to cause abscesses (1:1330)

98. All of the following are viral infections *except*

A. influenza
B. measles
C. mumps
D. poliomyelitis
E. typhoid fever (1:1330–33)

99. All of the following are bacterial infections *except*

A. cholera
B. plague
C. rabies
D. pertussis
E. tuberculosis (1:1333)

100. Most vaccines are administered in two or more doses separated by a time interval of several weeks. The exception to this statement is in the administration of

A. BCG vaccine
B. cholera vaccine
C. pertussis vaccine
D. plague vaccine
E. typhoid vaccine (1:1329–30)

101. The route of administration for antitoxins in the prophylactic treatment of tetanus would be

A. intramuscular
B. intravenous
C. intradermal
D. subcutaneous
E. either subcutaneous or intramuscular (1:1336–37)

102. Which of the following preparations will induce passive (rather than active) immunity?

A. tetanus toxoid
B. botulism antitoxin
C. typhoid vaccine

D. mumps virus vaccine, attenuated
E. cholera vaccine (26:582–89)

103. Bactrim® and Septra® are trade names for a synergistic combination of

A. sulfamethoxazole and trimethoprim
B. sulfamethizole and trimethizole
C. sulfamethoxazole and trimethadione
D. sulfadiazine and phenazopyridine
E. sulfisoxazole and methenamine (3:1239)

104. Atropine sulfate is included in the Lomotil® formulation in order to

A. enhance the laxative action of diphenoxylate
B. diminish the unpleasant side effects of diphenoxylate
C. enhance the antidiarrheal action of diphenoxylate
D. minimize the abuse potential for Lomotil®
E. diminish the output of gastric secretions (6:266)

105. Which one of the following statements concerning propoxyphene napsylate is *not* true?

A. the drug is water soluble
B. the drug is claimed to have better stability than propoxyphene hydrochloride
C. the drug is available as Darvon N®
D. both solid and liquid dosage forms are available
E. the drug has analgesic activity (24:149)

106. Acetone salts have been prepared to improve the solubility characteristics of the active drug. Which of the following is available as the acetonide salt?

A. dexamethasone (Decadron®)
B. hydroxyzine (Vistaril®)
C. procainamide (Pronestyl®)
D. prochlorperazine (Compazine®)
E. triamcinolone (Kenalog®) (1:897)

107. The most hygroscopic of the following liquids is

A. acetone
B. alcohol
C. glycerin
D. mineral oil
E. PEG 400 (1:1255; 22:255, 330)

108. Glass used to make pharmaceutical containers is designated as Types I, II, III, and NP. All of these glasses are composed of soda-lime *except*

A. Type I
B. Type II
C. Type III
D. Type NP
E. Types II and III (19:879)

109. Type II glass is prepared from Type III glass by surface treatment with

A. lime
B. nitrogen
C. oxygen
D. silicone
E. sulfur dioxide (1:1468)

110. The water resistance of glass containers is tested by measuring

A. amount of alkali released into water
B. amount of acid released into water
C. changes in pH
D. determination of silicate levels
E. turbidity of an aqueous solution after autoclaving (1:1468)

111. The containers used to package drugs may consist of several components and/or be composed of several materials. The release of an ingredient from packaging components into the actual product is best described by the term

A. adsorption
B. diffusion
C. leaching
D. permeation
E. porosity (24:49)

112. Flexible collodion contains

A. camphor and castor oil
B. menthol and castor oil
C. camphor and salicylic acid
D. salicylic acid and ether
E. menthol and salicylic acid (5:338)

113. Which of the following statements concerning Coal Tar Solution USP is *not* true?

A. alcohol is used as the solvent
B. L.C.D. is another name for the solution
C. the solution is used only externally
D. sand is used during its manufacture
E. the final solution contains only coal tar and a volatile solvent (1:721; 24:323)

114. Which of the following descriptors concerning sodium bicarbonate is *not* true?

A. acid pH in aqueous solution
B. antacid
C. poor alcohol solubility
D. known as baking soda
E. solutions unstable when heated (1:736)

115. Acetic Acid USP contains approximately what percentage W/W of acetic acid ($C_2H_4O_2$)?

A. 36%
B. 50%
C. 70%
D. 92%
E. 100% (1:737, 1256, 1261, 1262)

116. Iodine Solution USP contains iodine and

A. alcohol
B. isopropanol
C. potassium iodide
D. sodium iodide
E. PVP (1:392, 1093)

117. Iodine Tincture USP differs from Iodine Solution USP in that the tincture contains

A. Alcohol USP as the vehicle
B. Diluted Alcohol USP as the vehicle
C. potassium iodide as the hydrotropic agent
D. more iodine
E. less iodine (1:1093)

118. All of the following statements concerning Sodium Hypochlorite Solution NF are true *except*

A. the solution has an alkaline pH
B. a major use of the solution is as an antiseptic
C. the solution contains 4 to 6% NaOCl
D. a common name for the solution is Dakin's solution
E. the solution is similar to commercial household bleach such as Clorox (26:319)

119. Ipecac fluid extract was deleted from the official compendia because it

A. had poor chemical stability
B. tended to evaporate
C. was sometimes confused with ipecac syrup
D. was too weak to be therapeutically useful
E. could not be assayed accurately (1:800; 18:268)

120. The official Hydrogen Peroxide Solution USP is also known as

A. bleaching peroxide
B. diluted peroxide
C. 10-volume peroxide
D. 20-volume peroxide
E. 30-volume peroxide (26:314)

121. The antiseptic action of hydrogen peroxide solution is dependent upon the presence of

A. an acidic pH
B. an alkaline pH
C. blood
D. the enzyme catalase
E. a body temperature of 37°C (26:314)

122. All of the following topical products contain benzoyl peroxide as the active ingredient *except*

A. Benisone® Gel (Warner-Chilcott)
B. Benzagel® (Dermik)
C. Desquam® X (Westwood Pharmaceuticals)
D. Persa-Gel® (Texas Pharmacal Co.)
E. all contain benzoyl peroxide (3:1434–35, 1484; 10)

123. Which of the following statements concerning wild cherry syrup is *not* true?

A. contains both glycerin and sucrose
B. manufacturing procedure includes percolation
C. tannins are present in the final preparation
D. has some expectorant activity
E. has a pleasant cherry flavor (24:128)

124. The HLB system is most applicable for the classification of which surfactants?

A. anionic
B. ampholytic
C. cationic
D. nonionic
E. either anionic or cationic (1:335)

125. An example of a nonionic surfactant would be

A. ammonium laurate
B. cetylpyridinium chloride
C. dioctyl sodium sulfosuccinate
D. sorbitan monopalmitate
E. triethanolamine stearate (1:332)

126. A vehicle for nasal medication should possess all of the following properties *except*

A. an acid pH
B. isotonicity
C. high buffer capacity
D. ability to resist growth of microorganisms
E. all of the above are important properties; no exceptions (20b:248)

127. An antimicrobial preservative commonly used for nasal solutions is

A. benzalkonium chloride
B. benzyl alcohol
C. phenylmercuric acetate
D. sorbic acid
E. thimerosal (20a:917)

128. All of the following laxatives contain mineral oil *except*

A. Agoral®
B. Kondremul®
C. Neoloid®
D. Petrogalar®
E. Neo-Cultol® (3:1042, 1053)

129. Which one of the following statements concerning bisacodyl is *not* true?

A. laxative action occurs within six hours after oral administration
B. action of suppositories occurs within one hour of insertion
C. suppositories may cause rectal irritation with continued administration
D. tablets should be swallowed whole
E. tablets should be administered with milk to avoid gastric irritation (4:1074)

130. Which of the following products does *not* contain an anionic surfactant as the active ingredient?

A. Dorbantyl®
B. Gentlax®-S
C. Peri-Colace®
D. Senokot®
E. Surfak® (2b:40, 53)

131. Iron salts are usually administered orally. A commercially available parenteral product is

A. Chel-Iron®
B. Feosol®
C. Ferronord®
D. Imferon®
E. Troph-Iron® (1:777; 4:101)

132. Which one of the following chemicals is believed to be the most effective and safe drug in the treatment of diarrhea?

A. activated charcoal
B. bismuth salts
C. kaolin
D. attapulgite
E. polycarbophil (1:752; 2a:31)

133. All of the following OTC laxative products contain phenolphthalein except

A. Agoral® (Warner-Chilcott)
B. Alophen® (Parke-Davis)
C. Carter's Little Pills® (Carter)
D. Correctol® (Plough)
E. Phenolax® (Upjohn) (2a:42)

134. Not only are the insoluble bismuth salts adsorbent, but they also possess useful astringent and protective properties. A commercial product containing a bismuth compound is

A. BiSoDol® (Whitehall)
B. Donnagel® (Robins)
C. Pargel® (Parke-Davis)
D. Pepto-Bismol® (Norwich)
E. Quintess® (Lilly) (2a:31)

135. Which of the following antidiarrheal products contains the adsorbent clay, attapulgite?

A. Donnagel®
B. Kaopectate®
C. Parelixir®
D. Parepectolin®
E. Quintess® (2a:35; 2b:36; 4:1068)

136. In 1972 the FDA established expert panels to study the efficacy and safety of OTC products. These advisory panels classified drugs using three categories. Category III contains those drugs

A. evaluated as being safe and effective for the intended use
B. evaluated as being unsafe for the intended use
C. evaluated as being ineffective for the intended use
D. for which insufficient data were available to judge efficacy
E. which should be immediately removed from OTC status (2a:310; 2b:xvi)

137. Which of the following statements is *not* true? Vitamin E

A. appears to be compatible with mineral supplements such as calcium and iron
B. can be taken in large doses without toxic effects
C. consists mainly of alpha tocopherol
D. deficiency is not common in the general population
E. is an antioxidant (2a:142; 2b:150)

138. Sympathomimetics are often included in nasal decongestant sprays as vasoconstrictors. The agent found in most OTC nasal sprays is

A. ephedrine
B. naphazoline
C. phenylephrine
D. pseudoephedrine
E. phenylpropanolamine (2a:87; 2b:85; 4:648–51)

139. A sympathomimetic often present in OTC appetite suppressants is

A. ephedrine
B. phenylephrine
C. phenylpropanolamine

D. pseudoephedrine
E. caffeine (2a:179)

140. The active ingredient in Bacid® is best described as a/an

A. antacid
B. astringent
C. clay
D. demulcent
E. microorganism (2a:33; 2b:35; 4:1059)

141. All of the following products contain buffered aspirin *except*

A. Ascriptin®
B. Arthritis Pain Formula®
C. Cope®
D. Excedrin®
E. Vanquish® (2a:131; 2b:138)

142. The dose of codeine present in 5 ml of terpin hydrate and codeine elixir is approximately

A. 5 mg
B. 10 mg
C. 30 mg
D. 65 mg
E. 100 mg (1:803)

143. Which of the following statements concerning terpin hydrate elixir is *not* true?

A. the elixir has a high level of alcohol (40%)
B. a prescription is needed for dispensing the product
C. the amount of terpin hydrate per teaspoonful dose is too low to be effective as an expectorant
D. terpin hydrate may precipitate from the elixir if water is added
E. all of the above statements are true (1:803)

144. All of the following expectorants are found in OTC cough formulas. Which one is believed to be the *most* effective?

A. ammonium chloride
B. guaifenesin
C. ipecac
D. potassium iodide
E. terpin hydrate (2a:88; 4:658)

145. An OTC cough syrup that contains ipecac as the expectorant is

A. Cerose DM®
B. Novahistine®
C. Robitussin®
D. Triaminic®
E. Trind® (2a:97; 2b:99)

146. Advantages of dextromethorphan as a cough suppressant include all of the following *except*

A. as effective as codeine on a weight/weight basis
B. does not cause respiratory depression
C. is nonaddicting
D. doses of 10 to 15 mg suppress coughing for at least four hours
E. doses of 30 mg are effective for cough suppression for up to 12 hours (2a:18; 2b:89)

147. The main ingredient in Absorbable Dusting Powder USP is

A. cornstarch
B. magnesium oxide
C. magnesium stearate
D. pumice
E. talc (15:506; 18:162)

148. Which of the following statements when completed is *not* true? The liquid product Emetrol®

A. is effective in both the prevention and treatment of motion sickness
B. contains both levulose and dextrose
C. is manufactured by Rorer
D. may be dispensed without a prescription
E. should be either diluted or administered with water ot other fluids (3:787)

149. Disadvantages of calcium carbonate as an antacid include all of the following *except*

A. some patients may develop hypercalcemia
B. capacity for acid neutralization is poor
C. may cause constipation
D. may induce gastric hypersecretion
E. prolonged use may induce renal calculi and decreased renal function (2a:7)

150. Magaldrate is a chemical combination of aluminum and magnesium hydroxides. It is commercially available in

A. Aludrox®
B. Creamalin®
C. Maalox®
D. Riopan®
E. WinGel® (1:734)

151. Which one of the following antacids is *contraindicated* for individuals on a low-sodium diet?

A. Chooz® tablets
B. Digel® tablets
C. Mylanta® tablets

D. milk of magnesia tablets
E. Rolaids® tablets (1:734; 2b:17)

152. Fleet's Enema® differs from Fleet's Pediatric Enema® in that
A. Fleet's Enema® contains magnesium sulfate while the pediatric form does not
B. Fleet's Enema® is twice as concentrated as the pediatric form
C. a bottle of Fleet's Enema® contains twice as much enema solution as a bottle of the pediatric form
D. Fleet's Pediatric Enema® contains magnesium sulfate while Fleet's Enema® does not
E. none of the above statements are true (10)

153. Which one of the following products is *not* an example of a soft gelatin capsule?
A. Atromid-S® (Ayerst)
B. Declomycin® (Lederle)
C. Placidyl® (Abbott)
D. Tace® (Merrell)
E. Trinsicon® (Lilly) (24:187, 189)

154. The Wurster process can be used to
A. coat tablets
B. determine the disintegration time for tablets
C. gas-sterilize parenteral solutions
D. directly compress tablets
E. automatically fill capsules (24:212)

155. Poorly manufactured tablets may have small pinholes on the surface. This phenomenon is known as
A. capping
B. cracking
C. impacting
D. mottling
E. picking (15:131)

156. Picking of tablets may be caused by all of the following *except*
A. excessive compression pressure
B. a granulation which is too damp
C. scratch punches
D. static charges on the powder
E. unsatisfactory lubricant (15:131)

157. Which of the following is *not* used primarily as a diluent in tablet formulations?
A. calcium stearate
B. dicalcium phosphate
C. lactose
D. mannitol
E. starch (20b:125)

158. Which of the following is *not* a function of the lubricant in a tablet formulation?
A. improving flow properties of granules
B. reducing powder adhesion onto the dies and punches
C. improving tablet wetting in the stomach
D. reducing punch and die wear
E. facilitating tablet ejection from the die (1:1579; 20b:125)

159. The splitting of the top of a tablet is known as capping. Reasons for capping include all of the following *except*
A. excessive lubricant
B. excessive pressure of compression
C. excessive fine powder
D. insufficient binder
E. too dry a granulation (15:131)

160. A water-insoluble shellac coating is sometimes applied to tablets as a/an
A. enteric coat
B. film coat
C. subcoat for sugar coating
D. final coat
E. ingredient in the polishing coat (15:142)

161. All of the following ingredients have been commonly used as the coating agents for film coating *except*
A. carnauba wax
B. cellulose acetate phthalate
C. hydroxyethylcellulose
D. sodium carboxymethylcellulose
E. zein (15:144)

162. Which of the following trade-marked dosage forms is enteric coated?
A. Enduret®
B. Enseal®
C. Extentab®
D. Filmtab®
E. all of the above (15:144, 150)

163. A sweetener that is widely employed in chewable tablet formulas is
A. cyclamate sodium
B. glucose
C. lactose
D. mannitol
E. sucrose (24:213)

Directions: Each set of the following questions consists of several numbered items followed by a list of five lettered words or phrases. MATCH the lettered words or phrases most closely associated with the numbered item. Use each letter once only unless otherwise indicated.

Questions 164 to 168
Select the lettered formulation design that best describes the mechanism of release for each of the following numbered drug products.

164. Triaminic® Tablets
165. Donnatal® Extentabs
166. Pro-Banthine® PA Tablets
167. Rynatan® Tablets
168. Tenuate® Dospan

A. complexation
B. pellets in a tablet
C. repeat action
D. slow erosion core
E. slow erosion core with an initial dose (34:149–56)

Questions 169 to 172
MATCH the numbered sustained-action principle with the corresponding lettered drug product.

169. enteric-coated pellets in capsules
170. ion-exchange resin
171. microencapsulated drug
172. pellet form in capsule

A. Ornade® (SKF)
B. Ionamin® (Pennwalt)
C. Medrol® Medules (Upjohn)
D. Pavabid® (Marion)
E. Theracombex® HP (Parke-Davis) (34:153–56)

Directions: Each of the questions or incomplete statements below is followed by five suggested answers or completions. Select the BEST answer in each case.

173. Which one of the following OTC asthmatic products does *not* contain ephedrine as an active ingredient?

A. Bronkaid® Mist
B. Bronkaid® Tablets
C. Bronkotabs®
D. Tedral® Tablets
E. all contain ephedrine (2b:118)

174. Which of the following comments concerning dextran is *not* true?

A. available in two types—Dextran 40 and 75
B. administered by intravenous injection
C. useful in emergency treatment of shock
D. used as a blood substitute
E. may be used in relieving edema of nephrosis (1:757)

175. Labels for liotrix (Thyrolar®) tablets bear a number designation such as ½, 1 or 3. This number refers to the

A. level of sodium liothyronine (T_3) present
B. level of sodium levothyroxine (T_4) present
C. combined total of liothyronine and levothyroxine present
D. equivalence in terms of thyroid
E. μg of bound iodine present (1:910; 10)

176. Which of the following commercially available thyroid preparations contains both of the thyroid hormones (T_4 and T_3) in roughly the same ratio in which they are secreted by the thyroid gland?

A. Proloid®
B. Synthroid®
C. Thyrolar®
D. Levothroid®
E. Cytomel® (17:346)

177. Which of the following narcotics may *not* be used for medicinal purposes in this country?

A. diacetylmorphine
B. ethylmorphine
C. dihydrocodeinone
D. methylmorphine
E. all are permitted (1:1039)

178. Sodium heparin is obtained from

A. adrenal medulla
B. beef lung
C. human plasma
D. liver
E. whole blood (1:568, 766)

179. Burns are classified according to relative severity. Characteristics of a first degree burn are

A. erythema, pain, no blistering
B. erythema, pain, blistering
C. blisters, pain, skin will regenerate
D. no blisters, leathery appearance to skin, skin grafting necessary
E. blackened skin, danger of deep infection (2a:272; 2b:336)

180. The local anesthetic most commonly used in OTC burn remedies is

A. benzocaine
B. butamben picrate
C. lidocaine

D. phenol
E. tetracaine
(1:1263; 2a:274; 2b:336; 4:269)

181. Which one of the following statements concerning dextranomer (Debrisan® by Pharmacia) is *not* correct? The product

A. aids in the removal of wound exudates
B. can be used to treat decubitus ulcers
C. consists of spherical hydrophilic beads
D. is effective in the healing of both secreting and nonsecreting wounds
E. must be physically removed after treatment (3:1525)

182. For effectiv[...]

A. merbromin
B. Mercresin®
C. Metaphen®
D. Phemerol®
E. thimerosal (3:1391, 1532)

185. Rectal clinical thermometers differ from oral thermometers in

A. bulb shape
B. stem length
C. distance between graduation marks on the stem
D. standards for accuracy
E. stem shape (1:1806; 15:481)

186. A basal thermometer is

A. a rectal thermometer
B. used to estimate time of ovulation
C. used to determine basal metabolic rate
D. graduated only in Celsius degrees
E. used vaginally (15:484, 485)

187. What length crutch would usually be correct for a person who is 5′11″ tall?

A. 42 inches
B. 48 inches
C. 54 inches
D. 58 inches
E. 71 inches (15:556)

188. The scale most commonly used in this country for denoting catheter sizes is the

A. American
B. English
C. French
D. Stubbs
E. Foley (15:502, 504)

[...]gham clamp is a device used to
[...]ow of solutions through an enema

[...]ack the edges of incisions made
[...] surgery
[...] sutures for closing wounds
[...]ine flow in an incontinent male
[...]os stoma during irrigation (15:496)

[...]f the following is *not* suitable for
[...]in around the ostomy opening?
[...]nd tincture of benzoin
[...]eal®
[...]gum
[...]esive®
[...] of benzoin (24:72)

[...] the following statements concern-
[...]actions to insect bites and stings is
not true?

A. cross-sensitization to bites of different insects (ants, wasps, bees, etc.) can be expected
B. death may occur due to anaphylactic shock
C. the initial systemic reaction will usually occur within 20 minutes of the time of the bite
D. the toxicity of the venom is the prime cause of the severe reaction or death
E. subsequent sting episodes usually cause more severe reactions than the earlier ones do (2a:266, 2b:328)

192. Lanolin differs from wool fat in that lanolin

A. contains more water
B. contains less water
C. has been further purified
D. is obtained from natural sources
E. contains a greater quantity of cholesterol
(1:1249)

193. Lanolin has been reported to be a sensitizing agent. The component(s) of lanolin believed to be allergenic is/are the

A. wool wax alcohols
B. aliphatic fraction of the lanolin acids
C. aromatic alcohols
D. low-molecular-weight esters
E. minor impurities that may be present (1:1531)

194. The ointment base Eucerin® is most similar to

A. Aquaphor®
B. cold cream
C. Jelene®
D. polyethylene glycols
E. Unibase® (product label)

195. Plastibase® (Jelene) is a common ointment vehicle. It is a/an

A. mixture of mineral oils and hydrocarbon waxes
B. oil in water emulsion base
C. polyethylene glycol type base
D. polyethylene-gelled mineral oil
E. undisclosed patented formula (1:1530)

196. Which one of the following procedures would *not* improve the absorption of a drug into the skin?

A. application of the ointment and covering the area with an occlusive bandage or Saran wrap
B. incorporating an oil-soluble drug in polyethylene glycol ointment rather than white ointment
C. applying the medicated ointment on the back of the hand rather than on the palms
D. increasing the concentration of the active drug in the ointment base
E. using an ointment base in which the active drug has excellent solubility (1:1524–29; 22:239–44)

197. All of the following substances have been shown to increase the permeability of the skin *except*

A. benzene
B. chloroform
C. dimethyl sulfoxide
D. propylene glycol
E. sodium lauryl sulfate (22:243)

198. Aqueous solutions may be incorporated into all of the following ointment bases *except*

A. Aquaphor®
B. lanolin
C. Polysorb®
D. Unibase®
E. white ointment (1:1533; 20b:152)

199. Silicones are useful in ointment formulas since they are good

A. humectants
B. nonpolar solvents
C. preservatives
D. surfactants
E. water repellents (1:1530)

200. Aluminum paste is prepared by levigating 10% powdered aluminum into

A. hydrophilic ointment
B. hydrophilic petrolatum
C. petrolatum
D. white petrolatum
E. zinc oxide ointment (20a:822)

201. Lassar's Paste is

A. benzoic and salicylic acid ointment
B. zinc oxide ointment
C. zinc oxide paste
D. zinc oxide paste with salicylic acid
E. none of these (24:316)

202. Hydrophilic petrolatum contains what as an emulsifier?

A. cholesterol
B. glyceryl monostearate, self-emulsifying
C. sodium lauryl sulfate
D. Span 80®
E. Tween 80® (1:1243, 1249)

203. Most commercial emulsion bases are O/W emulsion systems. An exception, which is a W/O emulsion, is

A. Allercreme® Skin Lotion
B. Cetaphil®
C. Keri® Lotion
D. Neobase®
E. Polysorb® Hydrate (20b:198)

204. Tarbonis® cream contains allantoin which is present as a/an

A. antibacterial agent
B. antifungal agent
C. antipruritic
D. emollient
E. healing agent (1:729; 3:1511)

205. A synonym for Cold Cream USP is

A. Galen's cerate
B. petrolatum rose water ointment
C. rose water ointment

D. wool fat emulsion
E. vanishing cream (1:1250)

206. Rectal suppositories are suitable for the treatment of many diseases or symptoms. For which one of the following is a commercial suppository dosage form *not* available?
A. asthma
B. fever
C. epilepsy
D. insomnia
E. migraine (3:528, 698, 734, 865, 902–38)

207. Characteristics of rectal drug administration include all of the following *except*
A. neutral pH of colon fluids lessens possible drug inactivation by stomach acidity
B. drugs may avoid first-pass hepatic inactivation
C. drugs intended for systemic activity can be administered
D. the release and absorption of drugs is predictable
E. irritating drugs have less effect on the rectum than on the stomach (24:351–52)

208. Most commercial vaginal suppositories use a base of
A. beeswax
B. cocoa butter
C. glycerin
D. glycerinated gelatin
E. polyethylene glycols (24:363)

209. A prescription order for "Triple Sulfa Cream" may be filled with
A. Gantrisin® Vaginal Cream
B. Mycostatin®
C. Sporostacin®
D. Sultrin®
E. Trimo-San® (3:1415, 1420, 1422, 1424)

210. A vaginal product whose main purpose is to restore normal vaginal acidity is
A. Delfen® Cream
B. AVC® Cream
C. Betadine® Cream
D. Nylmerate® Jelly
E. Vagitrol® Cream (3:1424)

211. An excellent choice of diluent for a compressed vaginal tablet formulation would be
A. lactose
B. starch
C. sucrose
D. talc
E. all are equally effective (24:364)

212. Norforms® suppositories may be used as a/an
A. antitrichomonal agent
B. contraceptive
C. deodorant
D. mild laxative
E. tampon (10)

213. Certain vaginal products must be refrigerated for greater stability. The pharmacist should attach a "store in the refrigerator" label on which one of the following products?
A. Betadine® Vaginal Gel
B. Monistat® Cream
C. Sultrin® Cream
D. Sporostacin® Cream
E. Vanobid® Ointment (10)

214. All of the following properties are classified as colligative properties *except*
A. elevation of boiling point
B. osmotic pressure
C. increase in conductivity
D. lowering of freezing point
E. lowering of vapor pressure (1:245–50, 256; 14:190–95)

215. The colligative properties of a solution are related to the
A. total number of solute particles
B. pH
C. number of ions
D. number of unionized molecules
E. the ratio of the number of ions to the number of molecules (1:245)

216. Colligative properties are useful in determining
A. tonicity
B. pH
C. solubility
D. sterility
E. stability (1:245–50; 14:196–99)

217. The vapor pressure of a liquid
A. decreases with increases in temperature
B. equals atmospheric pressure at the liquid's boiling point
C. is independent of temperature
D. increases when a solute is added to the liquid
E. none of the above (12:75)

218. An isotonic solution has the same
   A. salt content as blood
   B. pH as blood
   C. fluid pressure as blood
   D. osmotic pressure as blood
   E. specific gravity as blood (12:251)

219. All of the following substances readily permeate the red blood cell, causing hemolysis, *except*
   A. boric acid
   B. glucose
   C. glycerin
   D. propylene glycol
   E. urea (1:1408)

220. Mixing a hypertonic solution with red blood cells will cause ____ of the red blood cells.
   A. bursting
   B. chelating
   C. crenation
   D. hemolysis
   E. hydrolysis (1:247)

221. Sodium chloride equivalents are used to estimate the amount of sodium chloride needed to render a solution isotonic. The sodium chloride equivalent or "E" value may be defined as the
   A. amount of sodium chloride that is theoretically equivalent to one gram of a specified chemical
   B. amount of a specified chemical theoretically equivalent to one gram of sodium chloride
   C. milliequivalents of sodium chloride needed to render a solution isotonic
   D. weight of a specified chemical that will render a solution isotonic
   E. percent sodium chloride needed to make a solution isotonic (1:1407)

222. A second method for adjusting solution to isotonicity is based upon
   A. boiling point elevations
   B. blood coagulation times
   C. freezing point depressions
   D. milliequivalent calculations
   E. refractive indexes (1:1406)

223. All aqueous solutions that freeze at $-0.52°C$ are isotonic with red blood cells. They are also iso-osmotic with each other. Which of the following apply?
   A. both statements are true
   B. both statements are false
   C. the first statement is true but the second is false
   D. the second statement is true but the first is false
   E. there is no correlation between freezing points and osmotic pressures of solutions (1:247)

224. One disadvantage in calculating isotonicity adjustments using either the sodium chloride equivalent or freezing point depression methods is
   A. D values are not accurate
   B. E values are not accurate
   C. it is difficult to locate the values in the literature
   D. only sodium chloride can be used for tonicity adjustments
   E. the adjusted solution will be iso-osmotic but may not be isotonic (1:247, 1405, 1408–12)

225. An ophthalmic solution that is highly hypertonic is
   A. atropine sulfate solution 1%
   B. Pilocar® 2% Solution
   C. Stoxil® Solution
   D. Sodium Sulamyd® 30%
   E. zinc sulfate solution 0.25% (20:884)

226. Methylcellulose and similar agents are used in ophthalmic solutions to
   A. increase drop size
   B. increase ocular contact time
   C. reduce inflammation to the eye
   D. reduce tearing during instillation of the drops
   E. reduce drop size (20b:236)

227. The presence of *Pseudomonas aeruginosa* would be of particular danger in an ophthalmic solution of
   A. atropine sulfate
   B. fluorescein sodium
   C. pilocarpine hydrochloride
   D. silver nitrate
   E. zinc sulfate (1:1218)

228. An antimicrobial preservative for ophthalmics is considered adequately effective if it will
   A. kill all microorganisms within five minutes
   B. reduce microbial counts to 1% of original count within one hour
   C. reduce microbial counts to not more than

10 microorganisms per ml within one hour
D. resterilize the solution within one hour
E. resterilize the solution within 24 hours (1:1500)

229. The most popular commercial combination of perservatives that appears to be effective for ophthalmic use is
A. benzalkonium chloride and EDTA
B. benzalkonium chloride and chlorobutanol
C. chlorobutanol and EDTA
D. methyl and propyl paraben
E. phenylmercuric nitrate and phenylethyl alcohol (1:1501, 1502; 20b:237)

230. Which one of the following ophthalmic solutions does *not* require storage in the refrigerator?
A. Chloroptic®
B. Eppy®
C. Ophthochlor®
D. Sulamyd Sodium®
E. all require refrigeration (10)

231. Which one of the following anesthetics is available as an ophthalmic solution?
A. dibucaine hydrochloride
B. hexylcaine hydrochloride
C. lidocaine hydrochloride
D. procaine hydrochloride
E. tetracaine hydrochloride (4:982)

232. All of the following viscosity builders have been used in ophthalmic solutions *except*
A. polyethylene glycols
B. polyvinyl alcohol
C. polyvinylpyrrolidone
D. methylcellulose
E. veegum (20:236)

233. The function of papain in a soft contact lens product is to
A. remove grease
B. disinfect
C. keep the lens soft
D. remove proteinaceous residues
E. prevent dehydration of the lens (3:1401)

234. Which of the following would be most irritating to the eye?
A. purified water
B. 0.7% sodium chloride solution
C. 0.9% sodium chloride solution
D. 1.2% sodium chloride solution
E. both B and D (20:236)

235. pH is mathematically
A. the log of the $(OH)^-$ ion concentration
B. the negative log of the $(OH)^-$ concentration
C. the log of the H^+ ion concentration
D. the negative log of the H^+ ion concentration
E. none of the above (12:202)

236. The pH of a buffer system can be calculated by using the
A. pH partition theory
B. Noyes-Whitney Law
C. Henderson-Hasselbalch equation
D. Michaelis-Menten equation
E. none of the above (12:237)

237. pH is equal to pK_a at
A. pH1
B. pH7
C. the neutralization point
D. the end point
E. the half-neutralization point (32:16)

238. Radium (^{226}Ra) is never used as an unsealed internal source of radiation or tracer because
A. of its extremely long half-life and retention time in the body
B. it accumulates in brain tissue
C. radium is not a naturally occurring endogenous element that can be utilized by the body
D. of its extremely short half-life
E. it emits only high-energy gamma rays (1:493)

239. Which of the following radioisotopes is used in therapeutic doses to treat polycythemia vera?
A. gold (^{198}Au)
B. iridium (^{192}Ir)
C. yttrium (^{90}Y)
D. sodium phosphate (^{32}P)
E. sodium iodide (^{131}I) (1:493)

240. A radioisotope generator is a/an
A. pharmaceutical product which has been labeled with a radioactive substance
B. ion-exchange column upon which a nuclide has been absorbed
C. ionization chamber
D. high-energy-yielding radioactive isotope that produces one or more isotopes that emit low energy radiation
E. apparatus in which radioactive isotopes are incorporated into biological molecules (1:478)

241. Which of the following widely used radioisotopes is considered to be an almost ideal isotope for medical applications and is commercially available as a radioisotope generator?

A. ^{131}I (iodine)
B. ^{99m}Tc (technetium)
C. ^{32}P (phosphorus)
C. ^{59}Fe (iron)
E. ^{198}Au (gold) (1:478, 515)

242. Isotopes are atomic species having the same number of

A. protons and neutrons
B. protons and electrons
C. protons but a different number of electrons
D. neutrons but a different number of protons
E. protons but a different number of neutrons (1:474–75)

243. The decay of radioactive atoms occurs

A. at a constant rate
B. as a first-order reaction
C. as a zero-order reaction
D. as a second-order reaction
E. at constantly increasing rates (1:481)

244. Which of the following forms of radiation has the least penetrating power?

A. alpha radiation
B. beta radiation
C. gamma radiation
D. x-rays
E. ultraviolet radiation (1:474)

245. When using a technetium-99m generator (Technetope®), which of the following would be a possible chemical impurity in the eluate?

A. molybdenum (^{99}Mo)
B. alumina
C. sodium pertechnetate ($NaTcO_4$)
D. sodium chloride
E. sodium perchlorate (15:645–46)

246. The dose rate (roentgens/hour) from a point source of a gamma-emitter varies

A. directly in linear relationship to distance
B. inversely in linear relationship to distance
C. directly with the square of distance
D. inversely with the square of distance
E. by a constant factor as distance is increased (15:629)

247. Which of the following commonly used radiopharmaceuticals is used for both diagnostic and therapeutic purposes?

A. sodium iodide ^{131}I
B. cyanocobalamin ^{57}Co
C. iodinated ^{125}I serum albumin
D. sodium chromate ^{51}Cr
E. sodium iodide ^{125}I (22:439, 440)

248. A specially formulated sodium iodide crystal is a major component in

A. ionization chamber detectors
B. proportional detectors
C. Geiger-Müller counters
D. scintillation counters
E. photographic detectors (22:446)

249. The diluent used in Sodium Iodide ^{131}I Capsules USP is

A. lactose
B. starch
C. potassium perchlorate
D. nonradioactive sodium iodide
E. no diluent is used (22:439)

250. Which of the following terms refers to the amount of radiation energy that has been absorbed by living tissue?

A. roentgen (r)
B. curie (Ci)
C. rem
D. rad
E. electron volt (22:426, 427)

251. The agency in the United States responsible for selecting appropriate nonproprietary names for drugs is the

A. AMA
B. APhA
C. FDA
D. USAN
E. USP (1:447)

252. The product inserts for many drug products contain cautionary statements. Which one of the following sequences lists the three types of cautions in the order of least serious to most serious?

A. contraindication, precaution, warning
B. precaution, warning, contraindication
C. warning, contraindication, precaution
D. warning, precaution, contraindication
E. contraindication, warning, precaution (24:38)

Directions: Each set of the following questions consists of several numbered items followed by a list of five lettered words or phrases. MATCH the lettered words or phrases most closely associated with the numbered item. Use each letter once only unless otherwise indicated.

Questions 253 to 268
MATCH the lettered manufacturer with the associated numbered trademarked dosage form.

253. Filmtab®
254. Kapseal®
255. Extentab®
256. Spacetab®

A. Robbins
B. Abbott
C. Parke-Davis
D. Schering
E. Sandoz (25:1–40)

257. Chronotab®
258. Caplet®
259. Wyseal®
260. Enseal®

A. Wyeth
B. Lilly
C. Schering
D. Winthrop
E. Abbott (25:1–40)

261. Filmseal®
262. Repetab®
263. Spansule®
264. Supprette®

A. Smith Kline & French
B. Wyeth
C. Webcon
D. Parke-Davis
E. Schering (25:1–40)

265. Gradumet®
266. Infatab®
267. Medilet®
268. Glosset®

A. Schering
B. Abbott
C. Sandoz
D. Winthrop
E. Parke-Davis (25:1–40)

Questions 269 to 283
MATCH the lettered manufacturer to the numbered brand name for its drug product.

269. Phenergan®
270. Librium®
271. Feosol®
272. Colace®
273. Flagyl®

A. Roche
B. SKF
C. Searle
D. Wyeth
E. Mead-Johnson (10)

274. Hydrodiuril®
275. Aristocort®
276. Polycillin®
277. Coumadin®
278. Pro-Banthine®

A. Bristol
B. Lederle
C. Searle
D. MSD
E. Endo (10)

279. Indocin®
280. Orinase®
281. Actifed®
282. Ovral®
283. Premarin®

A. Upjohn
B. Wyeth
C. Ayerst
D. MSD
E. Burroughs Wellcome (10)

Questions 284 to 298
MATCH the lettered dosage strength most closely corresponding to the numbered drug brand name.

284. Lasix®
285. Miltown®
286. Cleocin®
287. Pro-Banthine®
288. Indocin®

A. 400 mg
B. 15 mg
C. 40 mg
D. 25 mg
E. 150 mg (10)

289. Lanoxin®
290. Tetrex®
291. Hygroton®
292. Valium®
293. Premarin®

A. 250 mg
B. 50 mg
C. 0.25 mg
D. 5 mg
E. 1.25 mg

294. Aldomet®
295. Pyribenzamine®
296. Chlor-Trimeton®
297. Darvon-N®
298. Sudafed®

A. 4 mg
B. 100 mg
C. 50 mg
D. 60 mg
E. 250 mg (10)

Questions 299 to 313
MATCH the lettered generic name most closely corresponding to the numbered drug brand name.

299. Inderal®
300. Talwin®
301. Dyrenium®
302. Tofranil®
303. Flagyl®

A. pentazocine
B. imipramine
C. metronidazole
D. propranolol
E. triamterene (10)

304. Benadryl®
305. Valium®
306. Tofranil®
307. Dilantin®
308. Aldomet®

A. diazepam
B. diphenhydramine
C. methyldopa
D. imipramine
E. phenytoin (10)

309. Lomotil®
310. Lasix®
311. Equanil®
312. Atromid-S®
313. Tandearil®

A. furosemide
B. oxyphenbutazone
C. diphenoxalate
D. clofibrate
E. meprobamate (10)

Directions: The incomplete statement below is followed by five suggested completions. Select the BEST one.

314. Some states now allow or even require the substitution of bioequivalent drug products. A product with the same active ingredient as Tylenol® No. 3 is

A. Darvocet® 100
B. Darvocet N® 100
C. Empracet® No. 3
D. Empirin Comp® No. 3
E. none are equivalent (3:702–25)

Directions: Each set of the following questions consists of several numbered items followed by a list of five lettered words or phrases. MATCH the lettered words or phrases most closely associated with the numbered item. Use each letter once only unless otherwise indicated.

Questions 315 to 323
MATCH the lettered drug brand name having the same active therapeutic ingredient as the numbered drug brand name.

315. Penbritin®
316. Hydrodiuril®
317. Isordil®
318. Milpath®
319. Meltrol®

A. Alpen®
B. DBI®
C. Esidrix®
D. Sorbitrate®
E. Pathibamate® (10)

320. Pediamycin®
321. Eskalith®
322. E-Mycin®
323. Mycostatin®

A. Ilotycin®
B. Nilstat®
C. Sumycin®
D. Erythrocin®
E. Lithane® (10)

Questions 324 to 328
MATCH the lettered trade name with the related numbered nonproprietary name.

324. phenylephrine
325. phenylpropanolamine
326. oxymetazoline
327. naphazoline
328. tetrahydrozoline

A. Afrin®
B. Privine®
C. Neo-Synephrine®
D. Propadrine®
E. Tyzine®

Questions 329 to 332
MATCH each lettered nonproprietary name with the corresponding numbered trade name for an ophthalmic solution.

329. Floropryl® (3:519, 544–46)
330. Humorsol®
331. Isopto Eserine®
332. Phospholine®

A. demecarium bromide
B. echothiophate iodide
C. isoflurophate
D. neostigmine bromide
E. physostigmine salicylate (4:927–29)

Questions 333 to 337
MATCH the lettered brand name with the numbered nonproprietary name most closely related to it.

333. lidocaine
334. hexylcaine
335. dibucaine
336. tetracaine
337. procaine

A. Pontocaine®
B. Cyclaine®
C. Novocaine®
D. Xylocaine®
E. Nupercaine® (6:388–90)

Questions 338 to 342
MATCH the lettered antacid ingredients with the corresponding numbered commercial antacid product.

338. Amphojel®
339. Gelusil®
340. Mylanta®
341. Pepto-Bismol®
342. Robalate®

A. aluminum hydroxide
B. mixture of aluminum and magnesium hydroxides
C. mixture of aluminum hydroxide and magnesium trisilicate
D. calcium carbonate
E. dihydroxy-aluminum aminoacetate (2:13; 4:1036, 1040)

Questions 343 to 349
MATCH the lettered manufacturer with the associated numbered disposable syringe system.

343. Unimatic®
344. Isoject®
345. Carpuject®
346. Tubex®

A. Wyeth
B. Roche
C. Squibb
D. Winthrop
E. Pfizer (13:309)

347. Steri-Dose®
348. Tel-E-Ject®
349. Hyporet®

A. Lily
B. Parke-Davis
C. Bristol
D. Upjohn
E. Roche (13:309)

Questions 350 to 353
MATCH the lettered nonproprietary name with the associated numbered B complex vitamin.

350. B_1
351. B_2
352. B_6
353. B_{12}

A. cyanocobalamin
B. pyridoxine
C. thiamine
D. riboflavin
E. pantothenic acid (1:951–56)

Questions 354 to 356
Alcohol has many pharmaceutical uses and is available in several concentrations. MATCH the lettered concentration (% V/V) with the associated numbered official product.

354. Alcohol NF
355. Diluted Alcohol USP
356. Rubbing Alcohol NF

A. 49%
B. 70%
C. 92%
D. 95%
E. 100% (1:1088, 1252, 1254)

Questions 357 to 361
For many drugs in the USP and NF, exact solubility limits are not listed. Instead descriptive terminology is employed. MATCH the lettered solubility limits with the correct numbered solubility expression.

357. freely soluble
358. slightly soluble
359. soluble
360. sparingly soluble
361. very soluble

Parts of solvent required for 1 part of solute

A. less than 1
B. 1 to 10
C. 10 to 30
D. 30 to 100
E. 100 to 1000 (18:6)

Questions 362 to 365
MATCH the lettered term concerning hypodermic needles with the associated numbered description.

362. extension of needle that fits onto the syringe
363. portion of needle that is ground for sharpness
364. shaft portion of the needle
365. the needle hole

A. bevel
B. cannula
C. hub

D. heel of bevel
E. lumen (15:531–33)

Questions 366 to 369
MATCH the lettered ingredients with the numbered official product of which they are constituents.

366. Cherry Syrup NF 14
367. Ipecac Syrup USP 19
368. Tolu Balsam Syrup NF 14
369. Wild Cherry Syrup USP 18

A. benzoic and cinnamic acids
B. emetine and cephaeline
C. amodin and aloe emodin
D. malic and citric acids
E. prunase and emulsin
(1:800, 1236, 1237; 18:268; 19:788, 839; 24:130–32)

Questions 370 to 372
MATCH the lettered ointment base with the numbered ointment in which it is used.

370. coal tar ointment
371. compound undecylenic acid ointment
372. simple ointment

A. hydrophilic ointment
B. PEG ointment
C. white petrolatum
D. zinc oxide ointment
E. zinc oxide paste (1:1247, 1261, 1533)

Questions 373 to 376
As a pharmacist you may be asked for advice in selecting a suitable product for a skin condition. MATCH the lettered OTC ointment with the most appropriate numbered request.

373. a drawing salve for a localized infection
374. a protective to prevent further infection to the skin
375. to treat a mild case of scabies
376. to treat a mild eczematic condition

A. calamine
B. Butesin®
C. coal tar
D. ichthammol
E. sulfur (1:718, 721, 1180)

Questions 377 to 387
MATCH the lettered category of ointment base with the numbered ointment base which it describes. Letters may be used once, more than once, or not at all.

377. Aquaphor®
378. cold cream
379. hydrophilic petrolatum
380. Jelene®
381. lanolin
382. petrolatum
383. polyethylene glycol
384. white ointment
385. wool fat
386. hydrophilic ointment
387. Unibase®

A. oleaginous
B. absorption (anhydrous)
C. absorption (hydrous)
D. emulsion
E. water-soluble (1:1529)

Questions 388 to 391
MATCH the lettered ointment base with the most appropriate numbered use. Letters may be used once, more than once, or not at all.

388. for an ophthalmic drug
389. for an antibiotic with limited stability
390. for application to a seeping infection
391. for absorbing a large quantity of water

A. cold cream
B. hydrophilic ointment
C. hydrophilic petrolatum
D. PEG ointment
E. white petrolatum (24:328)

Questions 392 to 394
It is often desirable to formulate a dosage form so that its pH approximates that of the area to which it is administered. MATCH the lettered pH value that is nearest to the pH usually found in the numbered body areas. Answers may be used once, more than once, or not at all.

392. blood
393. eye
394. skin

A. 4.6
B. 5.5
C. 6.4
D. 7.0
E. 7.4 (1:596, 1495, 1524)

Questions 395 to 400
MATCH the lettered route(s) of administration with the numbered anesthetic. Letters may be used once, more than once, or not at all.

395. cocaine
396. dimethisoquin
397. lidocaine
398. mepivacaine
399. procaine
400. tetracaine

A. intravenous and local injection
B. local injection
C. topical
D. topical and local injection
E. topical, local injection, and intravenous injection (4:273–83)

Answers and Commentary

1. **D.** Before NPH insulin was developed to meet the need, it was common practice to extemporaneously prepare 2:1 mixtures of regular insulin and PBZ insulin to get an intermediate duration of action. The proportion of protamine in the 2:1 mixture is about 0.5 mg per 100 units of insulin which is about the same as in NPH insulin. PZI has 1.0 to 1.5 mg of protamine per 100 units. (17:368)

2. **A.** Prior to 1973, commercially available insulins contained significant amounts of proinsulin and its incompletely converted products. Since that time two highly purified forms of insulin, "single-peak" and "single-component" insulin, have been prepared. While both of these insulins are chromatographically prepared, the purity of single-component insulin is greater than 99%. The purity of commercially available insulin is now that of single-peak insulin (i.e., 99%). In spite of this degree of purity, these insulins still appear to contain antigenic components. Single-component insulin (purity greater than 99%) appears to be markedly less antigenic. While this product is not commercially available, it may be obtained from the manufacturer if needed. (6:1516)

3. **B.** Virtually all commercially available insulins in the U.S. may be prepared from beef or pork sources and are usually combinations of both. Pure beef or pork insulins are also available. Single-peak insulin is a purified form of insulin that exhibits only a single protein peak when a chromatographic analysis is performed. (6:1516–18)

4. **A.** All insulin products are refrigerated for stability and have expiration dates that start from the time the immediate container is filled. All but one of the official forms of insulin have 24-month expiration dates. The exception is globin zinc insulin injection, which has an 18-month dating. (18:253)

5. **C.** Both Actifed® and Actidil® contain equal quantities of triprolidine HCl per dosage unit. In addition to this antihistamine, Actifed® also contains the decongestant pseudoephedrine HCl. (10)

6. **A.** This combination is used for patients requiring anti-inflammatory activity but who require as low a corticosteroid dose as possible. Some authorities feel that fixed combinations of antirheumatic agents do not represent a rational approach to treatment since dosage flexibility is important for the maximum effectiveness of treatment. (4:528)

7. **D.** Both nitroglycerin and Isordil® are available in a sublingual dosage form. Amyl nitrite is administered by inhalation. All of these agents are used as coronary vasodilators in the treatment and (or) prevention of anginal attacks. (7:812–17)

8. **A.** Bendectin® is a product containing a combination of doxylamine succinate, pyridoxine HCl, and dicyclomine HCl. It is used in the treatment of nausea and vomiting of pregnancy. Some authorities have claimed that fixed combinations of antiemetics and pyridoxine have no proven advantage over the use of the antiemetic drug alone. (3:788; 4:1105)

9. **B.** Liquifilm® is a name used for an ophthalmic vehicle containing polyvinyl alcohol. The polyvinyl alcohol increases the viscosity of the ophthalmic solutions, thereby prolonging the contact with the corneal surface. (3:1394, 1398)

10. **A.** Micronor® is a progestin-only contraceptive product which is administered on a continuous daily dosage regimen starting on the first day of menstruation (i.e., one tablet each day, every day of the year). Ovral® is a combination product containing estrogen and progestin and is administered on a cyclical regimen for 21 days, each cycle beginning on day 5. (10)

11. **E.** Tuinal® (Lilly) is a rapidly effective, moderately long-acting hypnotic combination which currently is classified in Schedule II by the Federal government. (10)

12. **A.** A cold place indicates a temperature not exceeding 8°C (46°F). A refrigerator is a cold place in which the temperature is maintained between 2° and 8°C (36 to 46°F.
B. A cool place indicates temperatures between 8° and 15° (46 to 59°F).
C. Controlled room temperature is 15 to 30°C (59 to 86°F). (1:519; 18:8)

13. **B.** The rest point is simply the point at which the balance indicator point stops. It may be easily shifted by adjusting the leveling screws of the balance.
A. This test confirms that the two arms of the balance are equal in length.
C. The rider test confirms the accuracy of the calibrated beam or dial at both the 500 mg and 1 g position.
D. The sensitivity is reflected by the minimum weight that will shift the indicator point one unit or mark on the indicator plate. This shift is considered

the smallest change that an operator can consistently observe. Therefore it is the smallest discernible weighing error. The sensitivity requirement (S.R.) for the Class A prescription balance is 6 mg. For the less precise Class B prescription balance, the S.R. is 30 mg. (1:85, 19:1036)
E. The shift tests check the balance construction, especially the arm and lever components. (1:85; 19:1036)

14. **D.** The accuracy of weights is expressed in tolerances which are + or − deviations from the stated weight. The Class Q weights have tolerances smaller than the sensitivity requirement of the Class A prescription balance. (19:1037)
C. The Class P weights are more accurate than Class Q and are suggested for performance of the balance tests and to check other weights. (19:1037)

15. **D.** The NBS specifications state that a graduate shall have an initial interval of not less than one fifth nor more than one fourth of the capacity of the graduate. Therefore, a 100-ml graduate would probably have either a 20- a 25-ml calibration mark as the initial calibration. This regulation is intended to discourage small-volume measurements in large graduates when a smaller size graduate should be utilized. For some measurements, the conical graduate is less accurate than the cylindrical graduate. NBS specifications state that graduates holding 10 ml or less must be cylindrical. Whatever the shape and size of the graduate, one should not attempt to measure volumes less than one fourth to one fifth of the total capacity. (1:89; 22:35)

16. **E.** Potassium Iodide Solution USP is referred to as Saturated Potassium Iodide Solution (SSKI). It contains 97 to 103% W/V of potassium iodide. (1:802)

17. **C.** A container that reduces light transmission in the range between 290 and 450 nanometers to the level specified in the USP may be considered light-resistant and suitable protection from light. The container may be constructed of glass or plastic. Although amber units are most common, other colored or opaque containers could meet the official requirements. (18:7, 642)

18. **C.** For example, boric acid 1:18 in water indicates that 1 g of boric acid is soluble in 18 ml of water. In extemporaneous compounding, it is advisable to use excess solvent since saturated solutions are difficult to prepare and their concentrations are usually temperature dependent. (1:230)

19. **D.** When expiration dates are expressed only in terms of month and year, the intended expiration date is the last day of the stated month. (18 Sup. 1:1)

20. **E.** The expiration date for a pharmaceutical is based on the length of time for which the product should continue to meet the specified monograph requirements. Requirements are stated in terms of amount of active ingredient that is present as determined by suitable assay. Most drug products are considered usable until approximately 10% loss of drug or drug activity has occurred. However, some monographs specify other ranges. For example, digoxin tablets must assay between 92 and 108% of label claim. (18 Supp. 1:9)

21. **E.** Twenty intact capsules are weighed individually and the average weight is calculated. The requirement is met if each of the individual weights is within 90% to 110% of the average. However, the test allows for instances in which one or more capsules may be outside the limits. In these cases, the powder from the individual capsules is weighed and the difference between each individual net content and the average net content is determined. The requirements are met if (a) not more than two of the differences are greater than 10% of the average net content and (b) in no case is the difference greater than 25%. (15:137–38; 18:670)

22. **C.** Sodium bisulfite is theoretically $NaHSO_3$. However, the official salt is a mixture of sodium bisulfite and sodium metabisulfite ($Na_2S_2O_5$). When dissolved in water, the sodium metabisulfite converts to sodium bisulfite. The busulfites are strong reducing agents. They are preferentially oxidized, thereby protecting an oxygen-sensitive drug from oxidation. (26:155)

23. **E.** Calamine consists of 98% zinc oxide and 2% ferric oxide. The ferric oxide imparts a pink color to the mixture which is more cosmetically acceptable than the white zinc oxide. (26:304)

24. **C.** Unless otherwise specified, 25°C is the "official" temperature.
B. The National Bureau of Standards usually uses 20°C as a standard temperature.
A. A temperature of 15.56°C (60°F) is used for determining alcohol volumes. (24:25)

25. **A.** Camphorated tincture of opium (paregoric) is one of the traditional preparations for the treatment of diarrhea. (17:265)

26. **E.** Digitoxin is the primary active glycosidal constituent of digitalis and consequently its absorption, cumulative properties, duration of action, and therapeutic effects are very comparable to digitalis itself. (33:137)

27. **C.** The various bioassay methods that have been used depend on the fact that a continuous infusion of a dilute tincture of digitalis will lead to cardiac arrest in systole or in ventricular fibrillation. Frogs and cats were formerly used in the official assay but pigeons are currently used. (33:129)

28. **E.** The NF warning statement (caution) emphasizes the caustic nature of the solution and the irritating properties of its vapor. Bottles of the solution must be cooled before opening and the closure covered with a cloth while opening. Do not taste the solution or inhale the vapor. (1:1257)

29. **C.** (14:37)
A. Levigation is the process of reducing the particle size of solids by the addition of a small amount of a liquid or ointment base to make a paste which is then rubbed with a spatula against a tile. (14:37)
B. Sublimation is the conversion of a solid to a vapor without passing through a liquid phase. (14:122)
D. Percolation is the extraction process in which the desired constituents are dissolved from a granulated or powdered drug by the descent of a suitable solvent at a controlled rate through a column of the drug. (14:173)
E. Maceration is an extraction process in which the ground drug is soaked in the solvent until the cellular structure is penetrated and the soluble constituents have been dissolved. (14:242)

30. **B.** Powders that are either directly applied to the skin or are incorporated into topical products should be extremely fine, or impalpable. Trituration is often needed to reduce particles to an extremely fine size so that the patient will not discern individual particles when the product is rubbed on the skin. Usually a particle size of 50 microns or smaller is desired. (11:767; 41:659)

31. **B.** Incorporating powders into ointment bases may be aided by first wetting the powders with a small amount of a nonsolvent liquid, then rubbing the paste so formed on an ointment slab with a spatula. Usually mineral oil is employed when the vehicle is oleaginous. Glycerin may be used for more hydrophilic vehicles. (1:1555)

32. **C.** Precipitated sulfur has a finer particle size and greater surface area than the other listed forms. A smoother ointment will be formed. (24:315)
A., B., D. These are all forms of sulfur purified by sublimation.

33. **E.** Micromeritics is a study of all aspects of small particles including particle size, separation of particles, comminution, and behavior of particles in pharmaceutical systems. (22:177)

34. **B.** The amount of chemical adsorbed per unit of adsorbent is a logarithmic function. Therefore doubling the concentration of chemical will increase the amount that is adsorbed but will not double it. (1:293)

35. **C.** Hydrogen bonding is an attractive force between hydrogen atoms and electronegative atoms such as oxygen, fluorine, and nitrogen. Although weak, hydrogen bonds can bring about the miscibility of certain solvents or the solubility of certain chemicals. Hydrogen bonding is also responsible for the shrinkage phenomenon that occurs when mixing certain liquids. For example, when equal volumes of Alcohol USP and purified water are mixed, there is approximately 3% shrinkage from the theoretical volume. If one wishes to prepare 100 ml of Diluted Alcohol USP containing 49% V/V ethanol and purified water, equal volumes of each are used. However, one must also remember to use an excess of at least 3% of each to assure obtaining the required volume. (12:67)

36. **B.** Starch suspension and zinc oxide paste show dilatancy. (14:306)
A. A plastic liquid does not flow until a certain minimum shearing stress is applied. After plastic flow begins, the apparent viscosity decreases with increasing rates of shear. (14:304)
C. A pseudoplastic liquid does not require a certain minimum shearing stress before it begins to flow. Flow begins as soon as force is applied and viscosity decreases with increasing rates of shear. (14:305)
D. Thixotrophy is a property that certain plastic materials may exhibit. While standing, many plastic systems form a gel, which will break down to form a sol if mechanical agitation is applied. This reversible isothermal gel-sol transformation is known as thixotrophy. (14:305)
E. Newtonian flow is characterized by constant viscosity at varying rates of shear. (14:302, 303)

37. **D.** The equation may be expressed as:

$$V = \frac{\pi r^4 t \Delta P}{8 \, l n}$$

The volume of liquid (V) passing during a unit of time (t) is directly proportional to the radius of the tube (r) and the pressure differential (ΔP) at each end of the tube and inversely proportional to the length of the tube (l) and the viscosity of the liquid (n). Since the radius is raised to the fourth power, doubling the radius would cause a 16-fold change in the flow provided all other factors remained constant. The capillary can be envisioned as a simple glass tube or a human blood vessel. (12:508)

38. **C.** Potassium chloride is an obvious substitute for sodium chloride since it has a similar salty taste, is crystalline, and is an electrolyte already present in the body. However, the use of these salt substitutes is contraindicated in patients with severe kidney disease or oliguria.
Symptoms such as weakness, nausea, and muscle cramps indicate excessive sodium depletion. Increased sodium intake is warranted. (3:499)

39. **B.** IV injection of high concentrations of potassium may cause cardiac arrest. Intravenous administration must be by slow infusion to allow dilution of the potassium to occur. When plasma potassium levels are above 2.5 mEq per liter, rates up to 10 mEq per hour (total of 100 to 200 mEq per day) may be set. In more serious conditions, with plasma levels below 2 mEq per liter, rates of 40 mEq per hour (total of 400 mEq per day) have been employed. Available injection forms contain 10 to 80 mEq per vial. IV admixtures are prepared by diluting these solutions to 250 to 1000 ml. Oral dosage forms include Kay Ciel® elixir, Kaon® tablets, K-Lor® and K-Lyte® packets. A recently marketed timed-release tablet (Slow-K®) has a wax matrix from which the KCl is slowly dissolved in the GI tract. (1:770–71)

40. **B.** Topical dosage forms are used. For example, both creams and solutions are available under the trade names of Efudex® and Fluoroplex®. In fact, however, fluorouracil is usually administered by intravenous injection. It is not given orally because of irregular absorption from the gastrointestinal tract. (3:1563–64; 5:527; 6:1274–77)

41. **A.** Isoclor® Liquid (Arnar-Stone Labs) is a preparation containing 2 mg of chlorpheniramine maleate and 12.5 mg of pseudoephedrine HC1 per teaspoonful. It is used for the relief of upper respiratory and bronchial congestion. (3:31-33, 597)

42. **C.** Potassium chloride is embedded in a wax matrix core to provide slow release as the salt is leached from the core. Slow release of the potassium in this manner is believed to minimize high local concentration of potassium ion near the gastrointestinal wall. These preparations have advantages over liquid potassium supplements since they are tasteless and are easier to take. It should be pointed out, however, that there have been some reports of small bowel ulceration associated with the use of these slow-release preparations. Although it appears that the incidence of this adverse effect is considerably less than that associated with oral liquid potassium preparations, the clinical significance of these reports remains to be determined. (3:33; 10)

43. **A.** Polypropylene syringes can withstand autoclaving while most of the other plastics used for syringes must be gas-sterilized. (20:652)

44. **C.** Because of the polyamide nature of nylon, acidic drugs such as benzoic acid will be adsorbed onto the plastic. (20:701)

45. **D.** A short bevel needle reduces the possibility of perforating the back wall of the vein.
A. A very short bevel is preferred. (13:342; 15:532)

46. **E.** Insulin is usually administered by subcutaneous injection into the arm or thigh. Absorption of the insulin is good, and this route is both convenient and safe for self-administration of the drug. (13:159)

47. **D.** Insulin solutions have low viscosities, and only small volumes are injected. Therefore, small-bore needles (25G or 26G) may be used. Short (½'' to ⅝'') needles are adequate for the usual subcutaneous route of insulin administration. (13:344)

48. **D.** The winged (scalp-vein, scalp, or butterfly) needle consists of a stainless steel needle with two flexible plastic, wing-like projections. The wings serve two purposes—they ease manipulation of the needle during insertion into the vein and then allow the needle to be anchored with tape to the skin. (13:345)

49. **B.** Hypodermic needle sizes are expressed by a gauge system based upon the external diameter of the cannula; the larger the number, the smaller the diameter of the needle. For example, the 21-gauge needle is smaller in diameter than the 19-gauge needle. Generally, the length of the cannula is specified also. This measurement, expressed in inches, usually represents the distance from the needle tip to the junction with the hub. (15:532)

50. **A.** The Busher® Automatic Injector is a metal device into which the patient places a filled hypodermic syringe and needle. By releasing a spring on the unit, the patient administers the injection automatically. This unit is used mainly by patients using insulin. (24:270)
D. The Bristol unit is called the Bristoject®.
E. Wyeth's cartridge and metal syringe system is known as the Tubex® system.

51. **D.** Inert gases are sometimes introduced into parenteral containers during the manufacturing procedure to improve the product's stability by displacing oxygen. Unless otherwise specified in the individual monograph, the use of an inert gas does not have to be indicated on the label. (18:4)

52. **B.** (13:263)

53. **C.** Nitrofurantoin is precipitated by certain commonly used antimicrobial preservatives. Suitable vehicles include sterile water for injection and 5% dextrose injection. (21:249)

54. **A.** There have been reports that diazepam will precipitate even when added to normal saline or 5% dextrose solution. (21:121)

55. **E.** While the most widely used syringe size is 1-ml syringe, Becton Dickinson markets a Lo-Dose® 0.5-ml disposable insulin syringe. This size is particularly useful for administering small volumes (0.1 or 0.2 ml) of insulin. (10)
A. The U-80 insulin is no longer being made, and syringes calibrated for delivering that form are obsolete.

56. **C.** Purified Water USP may be prepared by distillation, ion-exchange treatment, reverse osmosis, or other suitable processes provided that assay requirements are met. Labels must indicate the method of preparation. One possible disadvantage of ion-exchange is the higher microbial count which occurs in deionized water because the resin beds generally become contaminated. (18:540)

57. **D.** Although there is some disagreement concerning the shelf life of ampicillin solutions, it is generally agreed that sodium chloride solutions are more stable (approximately eight hours at room temperature) than dextrose solutions (less than four hours at room temperature). (21:29)

58. **B.** Except for emergencies, slow administration by hypodermoclysis is preferred to avoid potassium overdosage which would result in heart cessation in diastole. Potassium blood levels should be monitored during therapy. (1:771)

59. **E.** Since the USP specifications for a "cool place" include a temperature range of 8° to 15°C (46° to 59°F) both a refrigerator and the cooler set at 59°F are appropriate. It should also be noted that articles specifying cool-place storage may be stored in a refrigerator unless otherwise specified in the monograph. (1:519)

60. **C.** Careful handling of freshly prepared distilled water will result in nonsterile but pyrogen-free water (Water for Injection).
A. Chemical treatment of water with $KMnO_4$ will result in the oxidation of microorganisms. However, the water would have to be distilled to remove remnants of the micro-organisms.
B. Although pyrogen-retaining filters are available, deionized water is too contaminated to be used.
E. Sterilization will destroy microorganisms but will not destroy pyrogens. (18:716)

61. **B.** Sterile water for injection is recommended as the reconstituting solvent for erythromycin lactobionate since a precipitate develops in solutions made with normal saline and others containing inorganic salts. However, once reconstituted, the solution can be diluted with normal saline or lactated Ringer's solution provided the pH remains in the range of 6.0 to 7.5. (21:143)

62. **E.** A subcutaneous injection will come into contact with a large number of nerve endings and extreme pain will be felt if the solution is other than isotonic. The potential isotonicity effects of hypotonic or hypertonic intravenous solutions are offset by dilution in the large volume of blood into which they are injected, provided (1) the volume injected is not excessive and (2) the rate of injection is slow. (1:1461)

63. **A.** The osmotic pressure of the dextrose solution will be approximately one-half that of an equimolar sodium chloride solution. The osmotic pressure of a substance in a solution is an example of a colligative property. Equimolar concentrations of nonelectrolytes will have similar osmotic pressures. However, electrolytes ionize to form particles which quantitatively increase the magnitude of the colligative property. Since sodium chloride ionizes into two particles, a 0.1 molar solution has twice the osmotic pressure of a 0.1 molar solution of a nonelectrolyte such as dextrose. Deviations from this simple theory arise from interionic attractions, solvation, and other factors. (1:245–47)

64. **E.** Osmolarity, expressed as mOsm/l, is included on the labels of many large-volume parenteral bottles. Those injections with a value of approximately 300 mOsm/l will be iso-osmotic and presumably isotonic with the blood. For example, 5% dextrose injection has a value of 280 mOsm/l, whereas 0.9% sodium chloride injection has a value of 308 mOsm/l. One calculates the osmolarity of a solution by first determining the millimoles of chemical present, then multiplying by the number of ions formed from one molecule. One liter of 0.9% sodium chloride solution contains 9 g of sodium chloride (MW = 58.4). The millimole concentration will be:

$$\frac{9\text{g}}{58.4} = 0.154 \text{ moles or } 154 \text{ millimoles.}$$

The milliosmole (mOsm) concentration will be:
154 mM × 2 (ions present in NaCl) = 308. (13:262)

65. **E.** Water for Injection (W.F.I.) is pyrogen-free water that is freshly prepared by careful treatment of distilled water. If not used within 24 hours, it is discarded since it may have contained microorganisms. The parenteral prepared with W.F.I. must be sterilized near the end of the manufacturing process. Bacteriostatic Water for Injection USP and Sterile Water for Injection USP are also used for parenterals. (1:1240, 1241, 1464)

66. **D.** There is the potential danger of blockage of a blood vessel by suspension particles. (1:1461)

67. **B.** Except for the lactate concentration and the absence of sodium bicarbonate, lactated Ringer's (Hartmann's solution) closely approximates the extracellular fluid. Although the injection has a pH of 6 to 7.5, it has an alkalinizing effect since the lactate is metabolized to bicarbonate. (1:758)

68. **E.** Normal human serum albumin is stable to heat and does not require special storage. (1:756)

69. **C.** Ringer's solution is an electrolyte solution which consists of an isotonic solution of sodium, potassium, and calcium cations and chloride anion in a balanced physiological proportion. (1:758)

70. **D.** The pH of solutions is often adjusted during the manufacturing procedure by addition of either acid (hydrochloric acid) or alkali (sodium hydroxide). The amount needed may vary from batch to batch. Therefore, the label cannot specify an exact quantity. (18:253)

71. **A.** Products such as Sodium Chloride Irrigation USP and Sodium Chloride Injection USP are intended for unit dose administration, and unused portions must be discarded. Antimicrobial preservatives are not used in solutions when large volumes are being administered and absorption into the body is possible since the relatively large amount of preservative may be toxic.
B. Sodium Chloride Irrigation USP is intended for topical application to wounds and for irrigation of body cavities when there is little possibility of absorption into the blood. It is also used as an enema.
C.,D., E. Sodium Chloride Irrigation USP is similar to Sodium Chloride Injection USP in respect to sterility requirements, concentration (0.9% sodium chloride), and vehicle (water for injection). While the maximum container size for large volume parenterals is one liter, irrigation solutions may be packaged in larger containers. (18:457)

72. **D.** A simple solution of ascorbic acid would be too acidic for injection purposes. Therefore an alkali such

as sodium hydroxide, sodium bicarbonate, or sodium carbonate is used to adjust the pH to between 5.5 and 7.0. (18:37)

73. **B.** The Baxter and McGraw systems utilize a plastic airway tube that extends from the rubber stopper to above the fluid surface when the bottle is inverted for administration. The Abbott and Cutter systems utilize a filtered airway that is an integral part of the administration set. (30:134)

74. **D.** Because the plastic bags are not completely transparent, it is almost impossible to examine the solutions for particulate matter. However, in-line filters can be attached to the administration sets to remove any particulate matter that may be present in the solution. (30:136)

75. **A.** Gentamicin sulfate (Garamycin®) is stable for two years at room temperature. Of the five antibiotics listed, it is the only one manufactured in solution form, ready for injection. The others are packaged as powders for reconstitution. (21:156)

76. **A.** Mysteclin-F® is a combination of tetracycline and amphotericin B. The former is used for its antibacterial activity while the latter is used for its antifungal activity against candidal suprainfections which occur in some patients taking broad-spectrum antibiotics. During the FDA-sponsored drug efficacy review, the panel of experts stated the Mysteclin-F® is ineffective as a fixed combination in the prevention of disease due to monilial organisms. In the panel's opinion, it is preferable to prescribe antifungal drugs when clinically indicated rather than to use them indiscriminately as prophylaxis against an uncommon clinical entity. (4:751; 25:1654)
B. Polycillin-PRB is ampicillin-probenecid for oral suspension. (25:713)

77. **C.** Actylsulfisoxazole, being virtually water insoluble and therefore tasteless, would be the best choice in formulating a flavored liquid dosage form. The sodium, potassium, and diethanolamine salts of this drug are water soluble and would be more capable of imparting an unpleasant taste to such a formulation. (6:1118)

78. **B.** Vitamin K occurs naturally in two forms, vitamin K_1 and K_2. Phytonadione (Mephyton®) is a naturally occurring vitamin K_1. Menadione is an inactive synthetic derivative that is transformed by the liver into active vitamin K_2. (17:172)

79. **E.** Witch hazel is prepared by distillation. It differs from the other aromatic waters in that it contains alcohol (as a preservative). It is used as an astringent.
C. Neroli water is orange flower water. (24:371)

80. **B.** Although there is a method of manufacture that requires 24 hours for preparation (known as simple solution method), the waters could be prepared by the alternate solution method using talc. This method requires less than one hour.
A. Since the aromatic waters are usually saturated, it is often difficult to obtain stable solutions when chemicals are added. Electrolytes will often "salt out" the volatile oil.
D. Since there is no sweetener present, the solutions are bitter.
E. The absence of any preservative in most of the waters results in susceptibility to microbial growth. (1:1439)

81. **B.** Freshly prepared distilled water has very low limits (10 ppm). Autoclaving and storing the waters in glass will cause leaching of soluble solids from the container walls. The limits for Sterile Water for Injection tighten with increased container size (40 ppm for 30-ml vials versus 20 ppm for 1-liter bottle) because of the relatively smaller surface area compared to volume. (18:540)

82. **C.** Extravascular blood can be prevented from clotting by removing calcium ions from the liquid. The addition of a mixture of citrate salts (sodium, potassium, and ammonium) results in the formation of calcium citrate, a soluble but almost totally unionized compound. Upon slow administration of the blood to a recipient, the citrate is rapidly destroyed by the liver and the blood again becomes capable of clotting normally. (36:110)

83. **C.** Human immune serum is obtained from human blood. It contains specific antibodies reflecting the diseases contracted by the donor. The immunity is passive since the recipient's body does not actively develop either antibodies or sensitized lymphocytes in response to a foreign antigen. Passive immunity does not last long; usually not more than two or three weeks of protection are achieved. Active immunity implies that the recipient of the biological will develop specific immunity due to an active response to the introduction of antigenic substances. (24:278)

84. **C.** Toxins are unattenuated poisonous bacterial products that act as antigens, stimulating the body to develop antibodies. The main use of toxins is to discover whether or not an individual is susceptible to a specific disease. The amount administered is small. Schick test toxin is an example. All of the other choices are used to obtain immunity or to attenuate the severity of a disease.
A. Antiserums consist of antibody-rich blood serum obtained from animals previously injected with bacteria or viruses.
B. Antitoxins are prepared using blood from animals previously injected with specific bacterial toxins.
D. Toxoids are modified, detoxified toxins which retain antigenic properties.
E. Vaccines contain either live, attenuated, or killed microorganisms. (1:1324)

85. **A.** A sterile solution of the diluted, standardized toxic products of growth of the diphtheria bacillus (Diphtheria Toxin for Schick Test USP) is injected intradermally (0.1 ml) into the forearm. A positive

reaction denotes susceptibility to diphtheria and consists of redness and infiltration which appear at the injection site in 24 to 36 hours and persist four or five days. (1:1341)

86. **E.** Toxins are primarily used as diagnostic aids for determining the state of immunity. (1:1328)

87. **C.** Intradermal skin tests with gamma globulin will cause a localized inflammation which may be incorrectly interpreted as a positive reaction. It is best to have epinephrine available to combat the occasional sensitivity reaction. (3:1279–80)
A. Approximately 16 to 17% gamma globulin is present.
B. Serum hepatitis has very seldom been reported.

88. **A.** (1:1340; 3:1279–82)

89. **B.** The immune gamma globulin is used to prevent or modify several diseases including measles, infectious hepatitis, German measles, and chickenpox. The immunity is passive, lasting for one to two months. There are also special forms for individuals exposed to mumps, pertussis, tetanus, vaccinia, and rabies. (1:760, 1339–40; 3:1279–83)

90. **E.** Immune Serum Globulin (Gamma Globulin) is the general immune serum used to prevent or modify several diseases, including measles, hepatitis A, poliomyelitis, and chickenpox. It is available under the generic title from Hyland and Wyeth. Trade name products include Gamastan® (Cutter), Gammagee® (MSD), Gammar® (Armour) and Immu-G® (Parke-Davis). Mumps Immune Globulin (Human) is specific for the prevention or attenuation of mumps. It is commercially available as Hyparotin® (Cutter). (3:1281)

91. **A.** Poliomyelitis is caused by Poliovirus Types 1, 2, and 3. Some vaccines consist of only one type (monovalent) while others combine all three (trivalent). Sabin's vaccine is available in both forms. Salk's vaccine contains killed virus and is given by IM or SC injection. (1:1333)

92. **D.** Another intradermal test for detecting tuberculin sensitivity is the tuberculin tine test, which utilizes a disposable stainless steel unit with prongs (tines) tipped with old tuberculin. It has been standardized to conform to the Mantoux test. (1:1342)

93. **B.** The tuberculin skin test is based on skin hypersensitivity to a specific bacterial protein antigen. Tuberculin can be administered intracutaneously (Mantoux Test) or by the multiple puncture method (tine test). The intracutaneous method using purified protein derivative (PPD) is more reliable. Generally the intermediate strength (5 U/0.1 ml) is used. The first strength (1 U) is generally used for individuals suspected of being highly sensitive, and the second strength (250 U) is exclusively for those who do not react to previous injections of either one or five units. (3:1335; 37:132)

94. **E.** Serum albumin is the protein in the plasma which controls blood volume through its water-containing capacity. Normal Human Serum Albumin USP which is used in the treatment of shock or hemorrhage may be either a 5 or 25% sterile solution. (1:756)

95. **B.** The labeling on biologicals is required to specify the recommended storage temperature. With few exceptions, biologicals are stored in a refrigerator at 2° to 8°C. (24:277)

96. **C.** Booster doses of the common toxoids are required to sustain immunity. For example, a 0.5- ml dose of tetanus toxoid may be administered as a routine booster about every 10 years or, as a booster in the management of minor clean wounds, not more often than every five years. (1:1330)

97. **B.** The depot site slowly releases the immunizing agent and yields higher levels of immunity, probably because of the prolongation of the presence of the antigen. (1:1330)

98. **E.** Typhoid fever is a bacterial infection. (1:1330–33)

99. **C.** Rabies is a viral infection. (1:1333)

100. **A.** BCG vaccine is given as a single dose. It also differs from the other vaccines in being administered intradermally or placed on the skin followed by multiple skin puncturing. The other vaccines are administered SC or IM. (1:1329–30)

101. **E.** For therapeutic effects, antitoxins are usually administered by the IM or IV routes. While the more slowly absorbed subcutaneous injection is generally preferred for prophylactic effects, the intramuscular route is also used. (1:1336–37)

102. **B.** Passive immunizations are usually accomplished by the administration of purified and concentrated antibody solutions (antitoxins) derived from humans or animals that have been actively immunized against a live antigen. Active immunizations are usually accomplished by the administration of one of the following: (1) toxoids (e.g. Choice A) (2) inactivated (killed) vaccines (e.g. Choices C and E) (3) live attenuated vaccines (e.g. Choice D). (26:582–89)

103. **A.** Sulfamethoxazole inhibits the conversion of para-aminobenzoic acid to dihydrofolic acid and trimethoprim inhibits the subsequent conversion to tetrahydrofolic acid. (3:1239)

104. **D.** Each dose of Lomotil® tablets and liquid contains 2.5 mg of diphenoxylate HCl and 0.025 mg of atropine sulfate. The diphenoxylate HCl exerts a constipating effect. The atropine sulfate is added to minimize the abuse potential of the product. While the dose of atropine sulfate in this formulation is much too low to exert any significant therapeutic effect, an excessive dose of Lomotil® will give rise to unpleasant effects of atropine overdosage (6:266)

105. **A.** The water insolubility of propoxyphene napsylate is an advantage since a stable oral suspension of propoxyphene napsylate can be formulated. Propoxyphene hydrochloride (Darvon®) is water soluble, but aqueous solutions are too unstable to be marketed commercially. (24:149)

106. **E.** Triamcinolone (Kenalog®) is available as the acetonide salt. Squibb uses this salt in Kenalog® cream, lotion, ointment, and aerosol spray. Syntex uses fluocinolone acetonide in its Synalar® line of products. (1:897)

107. **C.** Hygroscopicity is the ability of a substance to attract and retain moisture. Because glycerin will absorb water even in low relative humidities, it is used as a humectant to keep creams and other semi-solid formulations from drying out. (1:1255; 22:255, 330)

108. **A.** Type I glass consists of borosilicate. This is the best material as it is more resistant to water attack. Type II is a specially treated soda-lime glass. Type III is the typical soda-lime glass. NP (Nonparenteral) glass is unsuitable for injection purposes. (19:879)

109. **E.** Dealkalizing the surface of Type III glass with sulfur dioxide will improve the glass resistance to surface breakdown and migration of alkali into the parenteral product. This internal coating will be weakened by repeated sterilization or exposure to alkaline detergents. (1:1468)

110. **A.** Migration of alkali into a parenteral product will elevate the pH and may decrease the stability of the product. The amount of alkali released into water is measured by titration with a standard solution of sulfuric acid after an autoclaving cycle. (1:1468)

111. **C.** The term *leaching* is used specifically to designate the release of a container ingredient into the product. For example, zinc and accelerators may be leached from a rubber closure into a parenteral vial solution. (24:49)
A. Adsorption would refer to the binding of a substance onto the surface of the container wall.
B. Diffusion is the passage of a substance through a second substance. For example, volatile oil or dye may diffuse from a solution through the walls of a plastic container.
D. Permeation would denote the solution of a substance in the cell wall followed by passage through the wall.
E. Porosity indicates small holes or passages through which a substance could pass.

112. **A.** Flexible collodion is prepared by dissolving 2% camphor and 3% castor oil in collodion. Both ingredients act as plasticizers thereby forming a more flexible film. Collodion consists of pyroxylin in a solvent system of ether and alcohol. Salicylic acid collodion is prepared by dissolving salicylic acid in flexible collodion. (5:338)

113. **E.** The solution also contains Polysorbate 80. This nonionic surfactant is included to disperse the water-insoluble components of coal tar which will precipitate when the highly alcoholic solution is mixed with an aqueous preparation.
B. The Latin name of coal tar solution is Liquor Carbonis Detergens (L.C.D.).
C. The solution is diluted (1:9 usually) before external use.
D. Sand is mixed with the coal tar during the maceration process to enlarge the surface area of coal tar, thereby increasing its dissolution rate in alcohol. (1:721; 24:323)

114. **A.** Sodium bicarbonate hydrolyzes in water to yield alkaline solutions. Admixture with acidic solutions will result in evolution of carbon dioxide gas. In hot water, sodium bicarbonate is converted to the more alkaline carbonate. (1:736)

115. **A.** Three forms of acetic acid are official. Acetic Acid USP refers to a 36 to 37% W/W solution. There is a Diluted Acetic Acid NF of 6% W/V strength and a Glacial Acetic Acid USP which is 100% W/W. Several other acids are official in varying concentrations. Hydrochloric Acid USP is 35 to 38% W/W. Diluted Hydrochloric Acid is 10% W/V. Phosphoric Acid NF contains 85 to 88% W/W of acid. Diluted Phosphoric Acid is 10% W/V. (1:737, 1256, 1261, 1262)

116. **D.** Iodine and sodium iodide react to form KI_3, which is readily soluble in water. There is no loss of bacterial activity since the iodine is readily available from the complex. This phenomenon of forming a more water-soluble complex without loss of activity is known as hydrotropy. (1:392, 1093)

117. **B.** Iodine tincture and solution each contain 2% iodine and 2.4% sodium iodide. The products differ in their vehicles. The solution uses Purified Water USP while the tincture uses Diluted Alcohol USP. Diluted Alcohol USP contains 49% alcohol. Since iodine is soluble in alcohol, sodium iodide is included in the formula, not as a hydrotropic agent as needed in iodine solution, but rather to allow the tincture to be diluted with water without precipitation. (1:1093)

118. **B.** The National Formulary classifies Sodium Hypochlorite Solution as a disinfectant. It also states "Caution: this solution is not suitable for application to wounds." The alkalinity and oxidizing action are too strong for application to tissue. Diluted Sodium Hypochlorite Solution NF is a 10x dilution of Sodium Hypochlorite Solution. It is known as modified Dakin's solution and is used as a germicide and disinfectant. (26:319)

119. **C.** Ipecac fluidextract was used for the manufacture of ipecac syrup. Its strength was approximately 14 times that of the syrup. Because of several mixups in which the more potent fluid extract was dispensed rather than the syrup, the preparation of the fluid

extract is now part of the manufacturing directions for the syrup. (1:800; 18:268)

120. **C.** Hydrogen Peroxide Solution USP is a 3% solution. It is known as a 10-volume solution since 1 ml of solution liberates 10 ml of oxygen. (26:314)
A., D. A 6% hydrogen peroxide solution (20 volume peroxide) is commercially available for use as a hair and fabric bleach. It is too strong for medicinal use. (26:314)

121. **D.** The enzyme catalase is believed to catalyze the decomposition of hydrogen peroxide to water and oxygen, which then oxidizes bacteria. Undiluted, the hydrogen peroxide solution is used as a mild antiseptic and as a cleanser for wounds. A 1:1 dilution with water is used as a mouthwash for treating Vincent's angina. (26:314)

122. **A.** Benisone® Gel contains a steroid, betamethasone benzoate, which has anti-inflammatory, antipruritic, and vasoconstrictive activity for the relief of inflammatory dermatosis. All of the other products are available with either 5 or 10% benzoyl peroxide. These products are used in the treatment of acne vulgaris. The mode of action appears to be a drying and desquamation action plus an antiseptic effect of hydrogen peroxide against *Propionibacterium acnes*. (3:1434–35, 1484; 10)

123. **E.** Wild cherry syrup has a somewhat bitter taste mainly because of the tannins present. It is manufactured by percolation of the bark of a tree that is a member of the plum family. The chief objection to wild cherry syrup as a vehicle is its incompatibility with commonly used prescription ingredients. The tannins will form insoluble salts with alkaloids such as codeine. Also discoloration will occur if other drugs such as iron salts are added. When a cough syrup vehicle is needed, cherry syrup is often a better choice.
A. Sucrose is added to the syrup as a sweetener. Glycerin is included to prevent precipitation of the tannins. (24:128)

124. **D.** The HLB system was originally designed by using combinations of nonionic surfactants in the preparation of a standard emulsion. Although some anionic and cationic emulsifiers have been assigned HLB values, the system's prime use is to classify the thousands of nonionics that are commercially available. In the HLB system, emulsifiers are given numerical designations between 1 and 20, depending on the relative strength of the hydrophilic and hydrophobic portions of the molecule. Emulsifiers with low HLB values are hydrophilic, whereas emulsifiers with high HLB values are hydrophilic. Generally an emulsifier with an HLB of less than nine will produce water in oil (W/O) emulsions, those with values of greater than 11 will produce oil in water (O/W) emulsions, and those with intermediate values (nine to 11) are susceptible to other factors which influence the type of emulsion that is formed. (1:335)

125. **D.** Sorbitan monopalmitate is a sorbitan fatty acid ester, commercially available as Span® 40 (Atlas). It is classified as nonionic since the molecules would not have the tendency to migrate to either pole in an electric field. (1:332)
A., C., E. These compounds are anionic surfactants. This designation implies that the large, active portion of the surfactant molecule would bear a negative charge and, therefore, would migrate to the anode in an electric field. For example, the stearate portion of triethanolamine stearate is considered the active ion.
B. Cetylpyridinium chloride is a cationic surfactant. The active surfactant portion, cetylpyridinium, has a positive charge and migrates to the cathode.

126. **C.** Both ophthalmic and nasal preparations should have only mild buffer capacity so that the organ's natural buffer system can overcome any pH differences. Otherwise irritation might result.
A. Nasal preparations usually have pH's in the range of 5.5 to 7.5. Often phosphate buffers are used.
B. Rendering the nasal solution isotonic will decrease potential for damage to the local tissue.
D. The presence of an antimicrobial preservative is important because there may be accidental contamination of the dropper or nasal spray tip. (20b:248)

127. **A.** (20a:917)

128. **C.** Neoloid® is an aqueous emulsion containing 36% castor oil as the active ingredient.
A. Agoral® contains mineral oil and phenolphthalein.
B. Kondremul® contains mineral oil and the suspending agent Irish moss.
D. Petrogalar® is an aqueous suspension of mineral oil.
E. Neo-Cultol® is a chocolate-flavored, refined mineral oil jelly. (3:1042, 1053)

129. **E.** The tablets are enteric coated to avoid gastric irritation. They should not be taken within one hour of ingestion of milk or antacids since the enteric coating may be dissolved prematurely. (4:1074)

130. **D.** Senokot® contains a senna concentrate as the active laxative. All of the other choices contain either calcium or sodium dioctyl sulfosuccinate. Besides Senokot®, Purdue Frederick markets Senokot-S®, which contains both a senna concentrate and dioctyl sodium sulfosuccinate. (2b:40, 53)

131. **D.** Imferon® is Iron Dextran Injection USP, a colloidal solution of ferric hydroxide complexed with partially hydrolyzed dextran. It is intended for treatment of iron-deficiency anemias, particularly in those patients who cannot tolerate or who fail to respond to oral administration. (1:777; 4:101)

132. **E.** The FDA OTC panel on laxatives, antidiarrheals, antiemetics, and emetics reported that only the opiates and polycarbophil were recognized as safe and effective as antidiarrheal agents. Polycarbophil absorbs large quantities of water, allowing the formation of stools. There does not appear to be any effect on the digestive enzymes or nutrients. The drug itself is not absorbed systemically. Polycarbophil is present in Schering's Sorboquel®. (1:752; 2a:31)
A. Activated charcoal possesses good adsorption properties but is seldom used as an antidiarrheal. (2a:31)
C., D. Kaolin and attapulgite are typical examples of adsorbent clays. Attapulgite is a colloidal hydrated magnesium aluminum silicate clay. Studies have indicated that it is an effective adsorbent for alkaloids, toxins, bacteria, and strains of human enteroviruses. However, attapulgite and kaolin are not selective and will also adsorb nutrients and digestive enzymes. Probably their greatest efficacy will be in the treatment of mild, functional diarrhea. (2a:31; 4:1059)

133. **C.** Carter's Little Pills® contain two stimulant laxatives, aloe and podophyllin, but do not contain phenolphthalein.
Persons sensitive to phenolphthalein may develop a polychromatic rash. Phenolphthalein-induced rashes vary greatly in size and color. Usually the rash itches or causes a burning sensation. Among the other commercial products containing phenolphthalein are Ex-Lax®, Feen-A-Mint®, and Espotabs®. (2a:42)

134. **D.** Pepto-Bismol® contains bismuth subsalicylate and calcium carbonate. The subsalicylate salt is the preferred insoluble form since the subnitrate may form the nitrite ion in the gut. Absorption of this ion could cause hypotension and possibly methemoglobinemia. The FDA panel concluded that the bismuth salts are safe when taken orally, but data establishing effectiveness of bismuth in diarrhea are questionable.
A. BiSoDol® is an antacid product containing calcium carbonate, magnesium oxide, and sodium bicarbonate.
B. The major ingredients in Donnagel® are the adsorbents kaolin and pectin, and several belladonna alkaloids.
C. Pargel® contains kaolin and pectin.
D. The adsorbent in Quintess® is attapulgite. (2a:31)

135. **E.** Quintess® is a suspension containing activated attapulgite. Another product containing this agent is Polymagma®. (2a:35; 2b:36)
A. Donnagel® contains kaolin as the adsorbent clay. Another component is pectin, a purified carbohydrate extracted from citrus fruit rinds. Pectin is classified as an intestinal adsorbent, absorbent, and protective. Several belladonna alkaloids are included for antispasmodic activity, but the effectiveness is questionable because of the low dosage used (2a:31, 34; 2b:35; 4:1068)
B. Kaopectate® contains kaolin and pectin. (2a:34; 2b:35)
C. Parelixir® is a clear liquid containing pectin and opium tincture. (2a:34; 2b:36)
D. Parepectolin® is a suspension containing kaolin, pectin, and paregoric. (2a:34; 2b:36)

136. **D.** Some manufacturers of OTC products did not have or did not submit sufficient data for a complete evaluation of their products or ingredients. In some cases the panels recommended that a time period be allowed in which more data could be generated for submission. (2a:310; 2b:xvi)

137. **A.** Iron should not be consumed simultaneously with vitamin E since the iron appears to prevent the absorption of the vitamin.
B. Large doses of vitamin E have been administered without toxicity. It is interesting to note that the RDA for the adult is only 15 international units (IU), yet vitamin E capsules containing 400 and 1000 IU are marketed.
D. Deficiencies of vitamin E are rare. The vitamin is readily available in vegetable oils, nuts, cereals, etc.
E. Because of its antioxidant properties, vitamin E has been suggested for slowing the aging process. This activity has not be proved or disproved. (2a:142; 2b:150)

138. **C.** The action of phenylephrine is similar to that of epinephrine, but the duration of action is longer. While most of the side effects common to epinephrine and ephedrine occur with phenylephrine, there is little or no central nervous system stimulation. All of the adrenergic nasal decongestants appear to act by stimulating the alpha adrenergic receptors of vascular smooth muscles. Constricting the dilated arterioles locally decreases blood flow to the inflamed edematous area. (2a:87; 2b:87; 4:650)
A. Ephedrine is effective topically but causes secondary turgescence of nasal mucosa and tachyphylaxis. (4:648)
B. Naphazoline is also effective topically but may cause rebound congestion and other more serious side effects. (4:649)
D. In oral dosage forms, pseudoephedrine is used as a decongestant because of its nasal vasoconstrictor activity. It causes little CNS stimulation and is safe and effective for administration to children. (2b:87)
E. Phenylpropanolamine is available in oral dosage forms as a nasal decongestant. (4:651)

139. **C.** Phenylpropanolamine appears to suppress the appetite center in a manner similar to that of the amphetamines. While phenylpropanolamine appears to have anorexigenic properties, the dose present in most OTC products (25 mg) is too low. However, higher doses increase the incidence of side effects such as nervousness, insomnia, hypertension, nausea, and tachycardia. (2a:179)

140. **E.** Bacid® is used in the treatment of diarrhea. It contains the microorganism *Lactobacillus acidophilus* which aids in the rebalancing of intestinal flora. Usually normal bowel function is established

within 24 to 48 hours after the start of therapy. A similar product is Lactinex® which contains both *Lactobacillus acidophilus* and *bulgaricus*. (2a:33; 2b:35; 4:1059)

141. **D.** Excedrin® contains aspirin, caffeine, salicylamide, and acetaminophen but no buffering agents. All of the other preparations contain aluminum hydroxide, magnesium hydroxide, magnesium carbonate, or some combination of these antacids. (2a:131; 2b:138)

142. **B.** Terpin hydrate and codeine elixir contains approximately one grain of codeine per fluid ounce of solution. One grain, or 64.8 mg, divided by 6 doses per fluid ounce yields approximately 10 mg per dose. (1:803)

143. **B.** The "plain" terpin hydrate elixir may be dispensed without a prescription. It is sometimes used as a vehicle for other medications. However, the low water solubility of the terpin hydrate and the high alcohol level limit its usefulness.
C. The usual teaspoonful dose contains 85 mg of terpin hydrate; the expectorant dose is 125 to 300 mg. (1:803)

144. **C.** Ipecac appears to increase bronchial secretions by reflex stimulation of gastric mucosa. Although all of the other agents are used as expectorants, their effectiveness is doubtful particularly at the low dosage being employed. (2:18; 4:475)

145. **A.** Cerose DM® contains ipecac and potassium guaiacolsulfonate; the other products contain glyceryl guaiacolate (guaifenesin) as the expectorant. A second product containing ipecac is Quelidrine®. (2b:99)

146. **A.** While increasing the dosage of dextromethorphan may increase the duration of antitussive activity, it does not increase the intensity of the action. (2a:18, 2b:89)

147. **A.** While the main ingredient in Absorbable Dusting Powder USP is cornstarch, small amounts (not more than 2%) of magnesium oxide may also be present. The powder is categorized as a surgical aid (glove lubricant). Even absorbable powder can cause granulomatous lesions and adhesions in the abdominal tract. (15:506; 18:162)

148. **E.** Emetrol® is a phosphorated carbohydrate solution containing levulose, dextrose, and orthophosphoric acid with a controlled pH. It is believed to relieve nausea and vomiting by a local action on the gastrointestinal wall and by reducing smooth muscle contraction. The Emetrol® label states that the oral solution should *not* be diluted with or accompanied by other fluids. (3:787)

149. **B.** Calcium carbonate is a rapid, prolonged, potent neutralizer of gastric acid. Some scientists and consumer groups have advocated its use because of its high effectiveness and low cost. However, the listed side effects should warrant curtailment of its use, particularly for chronic therapy. (2a:7)
A. Some of the insoluble calcium carbonate is converted to soluble calcium chloride which is absorbed. Significant amounts of calcium may be absorbed after a few days of antacid therapy.
D. Gastric hypersecretion is believed to be caused by the local effect of calcium on the gastrin-producing cells.

150. **D.** Riopan® is considered to be a more effective antacid than aluminum hydroxide. Prolonged use of magaldrate may cause constipation and hypermagnesemia in patients with impaired renal function. All of the other preparations contain mixtures of aluminum and magnesium hydroxides. (1:734: 4:789)

151. **E.** Rolaids® contains dihydroxyaluminum sodium carbonate which combines the antacid properties of aluminum hydroxide and sodium bicarbonate. The approximate sodium level is 53 mg per tablet. (1:734; 2b:17)

152. **C.** Fleet's Enema® and Fleet's Pediatric Enema® are both aqueous solutions containing 6 g of sodium phosphate and 16 g of sodium biphosphate per 100 ml. A container of Fleet's Enema® contains 4½ oz while Fleet's Pediatric Enema® contains 2¼ oz of solution. (10)

153. **E.** Trinsicon® is a hard gelatin capsule with the usual two portions (head and body). Soft gelatin capsules consist of medication enclosed by a soft, elastic shell made of gelatin plus glycerin, sorbitol, or other polyhydric alcohol. These capsules are quite easy to swallow. They are capable of containing liquid formulations. The Schering Corporation manufactures an automatic machine for production of soft gelatin capsules. Two ribbons are formed from the liquid gelatin, a pocket is formed by dies, the medication is placed between the ribbons, and the capsule is sealed by heat. (24:187, 189)

154. **A.** Granules, powders, and tablets can be rapidly coated by suspending them in a column of air and spraying with a coating solution. The rotating motion of the solids and the introduction of hot air will result in rapid drying and uniform coating. This coating technique bears the inventor's name. (24:212)

155. **E.** Picking occurs when the tablet powder sticks to the punch face.
D. Mottling is uneven color distribution, probably due to poor mixing of the tablet granulation. (15:131)

156. **A.** Excessive compression would result in hard tablets that would not stick to the punches and would not be picked. However, excessively hard tablets may not disintegrate in the body fluids. (15:131)

157. **A.** Calcium stearate (as well as other stearates) is included in tablet formulations as a lubricant. (20b:125)

158. **C.** Tablet lubricants are characterized by lubricity and are usually water insoluble and difficult to wet. The waterproofing property might retard disintegration and dissolution. (1:1579; 20b:125)

159. **A.** Capping implies that the compressed powder is not cohesive. A tablet lubricant insures uniform feeding of granules into the dies and prevents sticking of powder to the dies and punches. Excessive lubricant may render the granulation too slippery, preventing cohesiveness, but will not cause capping. (15:131)

160. **C.** Shellac is sometimes included in a sealing subcoat in the production of sugar-coated tablets. It will prevent the tablet from absorbing water from the subsequent coating solutions. (15:142)

161. **A.** Carnauba wax and beeswax combinations are commonly used as a polishing coat for sugar coating, but not for film coating.
B., C., D., E. In film coating, a thin film of coating material is applied or sprayed on tablets. Alcohol solutions of cellulosic polymers are commonly used. The thin film does not change the shape of the tablet and designs imprinted on the tablet are easily seen through it. (15:144)

162. **B.** Products such as Potassium Chloride Enseals® are enteric coated to protect the stomach from irritating substances or to prevent drug decomposition in the stomach. (15:150)
A. Endurets® are sustained-release tablets. Preludin® is an example. (15:150)
C. Extentabs® are prolonged-action tablets, for example, Dimetane® Extentabs. (15:150)
D. Filmtabs® are tablets coated with a transparent protective coating, for example, Eutron® Filmtabs. (15:144)

163. **D.** Mannitol possesses characteristics that make it an almost ideal sweetener for chewable tablets. While not as sweet as sucrose, it leaves a cool taste in the mouth and is nonhygroscopic. Mannitol is also easily compressed by wet granulation. (24:213)

164. **C.** Triaminic® tablets are designed to release an initial dose followed by a second dose at a later time. This type of product reduces the number of doses the patient must take during the day. Similarly designed products are Butisol® RA (McNeil), and Schering's repetabs (Chlortrimeton® , Polaramine®, and Demazin®).

165. **E.** This type of product is formulated by mixing the drug with an insoluble material and compressing into a tablet. The tablet does not disintegrate. Instead, it maintains its geometric shape and releases drug as erosion takes place at the surface of the tablet. Other product examples of this principle are Preludin® Endurets, Obedrin® LA, and Novahistine® Singlets. (34:149)

166. **B.** This dosage form is prepared by compressing medicated pellets into tablets. Release can be designed for one or more time spans. Product examples include Bellergan® Spacetabs and Isordil® Tembids. (34:155)

167. **A.** The Durabond principle consists of complexing amine drugs with tannic acid to form the corresponding tannates. These relatively insoluble drug forms are slowly released over a 12-hour period. (34:156)

168. **D.** For this type of drug, an initial dose is not as important as a prolonged blood level. Therefore, the equivalent of three normal doses are formulated into a core that slowly releases the drug by surface erosion. Unlike Extentabs, no initial dose is released. Other examples of slow erosion-core include Tepanil® Ten-Tab and Roniacol® Timespan. (34:153)

169. **C.** Upjohn's Medrol® Medules are formulated by incorporating the drug in acid-resistant styrene-maleic acid copolymer pellets. These pellets release drug in the intestinal tract over a period of time, thereby giving a sustained-release effect.

170. **B.** The active drug (phentermine) in Ionamin® capsules is combined with a polystyrene sulfonic acid resin. As the capsule passes through the GI tract, the resin exchanges active drug for ions such as sodium and potassium. Biphetamine® capsules are similarly formulated. (34:155)

171. **D.** Drug particles can be coated by encapsulation with a thin film that acts as a dialysis membrane. GI fluids slowly diffuse into the coated powder and dissolve the drug, which then diffuses out of the microcapsule. (34:156)

172. **A.** SKF's spansule formulation consists of medicated pellets in a capsule dosage form. Some pellets are uncoated to give almost immediate release, and other pellets have lipid coatings of various thicknesses. Thus, the initial dose is reinforced with additional drug release over a period of time. Another group of products based upon medicated pellets are Lederle's Sequels (e.g. Diamox® Sequels). (34:153)

173. **A.** Bronkaid® Mist contains epinephrine; all of the other products contain ephedrine. Ephedrine has been widely used in asthma therapy. Its slow onset of action (30 to 60 minutes) precludes its use for acute attacks. Instead, it has been used alone (two to three hours' duration of action) or in combination with theophylline to prevent attacks in patients with milder forms of asthma. For acute asthmatic attacks, epinephrine offers relief within a few minutes of administered by inhalation or injection. A major difficulty with epinephrine inhalation products is that tolerance quickly builds up. If patients do not obtain the necessary relief after several inhalations, they should consult their physician for a more effective prescription product. (2b:118)

174. **D.** The dextrans are plasma extenders which will restore blood volume. However, since they have no

oxygen-carrying functions, they are not substitutes for blood. Therefore, plasma or blood should be administered as soon as possible after the use of dextrans in emergency situations. Dextran 40 is used to prevent aggregation of erythrocytes during surgery and as a plasma expander during hypovolemic shock. Dextran 75 is mainly used in the treatment of hypovolemic shock, especially for toxemia of pregnancy and for nephrosis. (1:757)

175. **D.** Liotrix has been successfully used in place of thyroid. Some authorities believe that the 4:1 ratio of levothyroxine and liothyronine in liotrix closely approaches the composition of the normal physiological hormone. Expressing the tablet effectiveness in terms of equivalence in grains of thyroid is a convenience for the prescriber. (1:910; 10)

176. **C.** Thyrolar® (sodium levothyroxine with sodium liothyronine in a ratio of 4:1) is a combination product designed to mimic the natural secretion of the thyroid gland.
A. Proloid® is thyroglobulin extracted from animal thyroid glands and contains T_4 and T_3 in the ratio of 2:1.
B., D. Synthroid® and Levothroid® are products containing pure sodium levothyroxine (T_4).
E. Cytomel® contains pure sodium liothyronine (T_3). (17:346)

177. **A.** Diacetylmorphine is commonly known as heroin. It is a Class I controlled substance; this means that it may be used only for experimental work by special permit. (1:1039)

178. **B.** Heparin is also obtained from mammalian intestinal mucosa or other suitable tissues. The USP requires that heparin sodium contain not less than 120 USP Heparin Units when derived from lungs and not less than 140 when obtained from other tissues. (1:568, 766)

179. **A.** The first degree burn is the mildest injury since only the epidermis is affected.
C. These are characteristics of a second degree burn, which affects the epidermis and portions of the dermis.
D. A third degree burn penetrates through the entire skin. Damage may be permanent.
E. These are characteristics of the fourth degree or char burn. Both the skin and underlying tissues are affected. (2a:272; 2b:336)

180. **A.** Benzocaine is widely used for surface anesthesia of the skin and mucous membranes. It remains on the skin for a long time since it has poor water solubility and is poorly absorbed. Systemic toxicity is rare. While the possibility of local sensitization should be considered, the incidence is low considering the frequent use of benzocaine. (2a:274; 2b:336; 4:269)
B. Butamben picrate is available only in Butesin Picrate with Metaphen® ointment. (2a:277; 2b:341)
C. Lidocaine is present in Medi-Quick® Aerosol, Unguentine® First Aid Spray, and Unguentine Plus®. (2a:278; 2b:341)
D. Although phenol possesses both antiseptic and local anesthetic effects, there is the possibility that it may accentuate tissue damage because of its caustic properties. (1:1263)
E. Tetracaine is present in Pontocaine® Cream and Ointment. (2a:278; 2b:342)

181. **D.** Debrisan® is *not* useful in the treatment of *nonsecreting* wounds. Its action appears to be to absorb fluids and particles that impede tissue repair. The product is available as 0.1- to 0.3-mm spherical beads (4-g packets) which are sprinkled on secreting wounds. The hydrophilic nature of the beads creates a strong suction force; each gram absorbs about 4 ml of fluid. The beads become grayish yellow when they are saturated with fluid; they should then be washed away by irrigating with sterile water or saline. (3:1525)

182. **E.** A topical preparation should contain a minimum of 5% benzocaine. Some studies have indicated that 20% of the drug is needed. (2a:274; 2b:336; 4:269)

183. **A.** Butamben is *n*-butyl *p*-aminobenzoate, while benzocaine is the ethyl ester. (1:987, 988)

184. **D.** Phemerol® is benzethonium chloride, a quaternary ammonium compound. Since the mercury present in the other products is tightly bound in the molecule, there is little possibility of sensitization. (3:1391, 1532)

185. **A.** The rectal thermometer bulb has a strong, blunt shape which facilitates insertion into the rectum and retention by sphincter muscles. The oral bulb is cylindrical, elongated, and thin-walled for quick registration of temperature. Rectal thermometers can be used orally. The oral bulb is too easily broken and is not suitable for rectal use. The short, sturdy security bulb represents a compromise intermediate shape. (1:1806; 15:481)

186. **B.** Since fertilization can occur only within a few hours (perhaps 24) after ovulation, accurate knowledge of this event could permit timing of intercourse to either increase or decrease the possibility of conception. Basal temperature (the lowest temperature of the body during waking hours) typically passes through a biphasic cycle over the course of the menstrual cycle. From an initially low temperature, a mid-cycle thermal shift occurs to a high level, where it remains until it again becomes low premenstrually. The temperature rise roughly corresponds with the time of ovulation. (15:485)
A. The thermometer is used orally or rectally, once daily, immediately upon awakening in the morning, and before getting out of bed. (15:484)
D. The scale may be either Fahrenheit or Celsius. The temperature rise is only about 0.5°F, which would be hard to measure on the usual clinical thermometer. The basal thermometer scale ranges only

from 96°F to 100°F and is graduated to 0.1°F. (15:484)

187. **C.** If the height in inches is an odd number, subtract 17 to get the crutch length; if even, subtract 16. The crutch length selected should be tried out by the patient so that necessary adjustment can be made. (15:556)

188. **C.** One French unit equals 1 mm in outside circumference. A catheter with an outside circumference of 20 mm is identified as a 20F or 20Fr. size. Sizes range from 10F to 34F. (15:502, 504)
D. Catheters are less commonly sized by the American or English scales. (15:502)
E. The Foley catheter is a type of self-retaining or indwelling catheter. (15:504)

189. **D.** An incontinent male may use a penile clamp to mechanically compress the urethral wall in order to stop the involuntary flow of urine. The Cunningham clamp has a small, lightweight, rubber-covered, malleable metal frame that can be bent by hand to adjust the size. It is clamped over the penile shaft by forcing the two wings together with a snap-button or a spring-ratchet closure. An inverted V in the lower half of the clamp exerts pressure directly on the urethra along the underside of the penis. (15:496)

190. **A.** In addition to benzoin, compound tincture of benzoin contains tolu balsam and storax, ingredients which may irritate the sensitive skin surrounding the stoma. (24:72)
B. Colly-Seal® is an adhesive seal containing karaya. It is claimed to have a longer duration of adhesiveness than plain karaya powder.
C. Karaya gum is a resin. It is placed around ostomies for both its adhesive and healing properties. The powder can be used after wetting either with water or aluminum hydroxide gel. Karaya rings consisting of hardened karaya and glycerin are also commercially available. These rings are also wetted before use.
D. Stomahesive® is used as an adhesive seal. Wafers containing gelatin, pectin, CMC, and polyisobutylene are available.
E. Benzoin tincture may be placed on the skin before application of an adhesive cement. It is claimed that the tincture makes the skin more adhesive and reduces skin irritation.

191. **D.** While the venoms of some insects are potent, the amounts injected are too small to be toxic. The severity of the sting reaction in some individuals is due to hypersensitivity to certain proteins in the venom. This results in the anaphylactic shock. (2a:266; 2b:328)

192. **A.** Lanolin (hydrous wool fat) is a W/O emulsion containing 25 to 30% water. It is a hydrous absorption base into which more water can be incorporated if desired. Wool fat (anhydrous lanolin) contains no water; it is classified as an anhydrous absorption base. (1:1249)

193. **A.** Although the reported incidence of allergies to lanolin is relatively small, those individuals with histories of allergies should be advised to avoid lanolin-containing products. The exact chemical composition of the allergens has not been determined, but the greatest allergenicity is in the fraction containing the wool wax alcohols. The fraction is valuable for patch testing since the incidence of positive reaction is much higher than when lanolin is used. (1:1531)

194. **A.** Eucerin® consists of equal parts of Aquaphor® and water. (product label)

195. **A.** This jelly-like base maintains a good consistency over a wide temperature range. It appears to be compatibile with many active ingredients. (1:1530)

196. **E.** Diffusion of a drug from a vehicle into the skin is often related to the solubility of the drug in the vehicle relative to the solubility in the skin, i.e., the partition coefficient. Drugs that are very soluble in a vehicle will tend to remain in the vehicle and will show slower rates of penetration than less soluble drugs.
A. Covering the area to which a topical drug has been applied will often enhance the rate of absorption. Sweat accumulation at the skin-vehicle interface induces hydration of the skin, a condition which facilitates penetration of drugs.
B. Poorer solubility of the drug in PEG ointment than in white ointment may lead to faster diffusion. This is the converse of choice E.
C. The thicker epidermis of the palms will result in slower drug penetration than that which will occur on the back of the hands.
D. Higher drug concentrations will increase the rate of diffusion and penetration. (1:1524–29; 22:239–44)

197. **D.** Propylene glycol is usually included in topical formulations as a solvent and/or a humectant.
A., B. Several nonpolar solvents such as benzene and chloroform appear to increase skin permeability by removal of lipids from the stratum corneum.
C. Dimethyl sulfoxide (DMSO) has been used experimentally as a penetration enhancer for a variety of drugs. It may solvate the stratum corneum and also cause swelling of the cells, thereby opening channels for drug penetration.
E. Certain surfactants, such as sodium lauryl sulfate, appear to cause a reversible denaturation of skin protein, thereby interrupting the barrier nature of the stratum corneum. (22:243)

198. **E.** White ointment is composed of white wax and white petrolatum, both consisting of aliphatic hydrocarbons which are hydrophobic. This ointment base has a very low "water number." The water number is defined as the largest amount of water that 100g of an ointment base will hold at 20°C. (1:1533; 20b:152)

199. **E.** Silicones will form a thin occlusive film on the skin, producing an emollient effect because water loss by evaporation from the skin surface is reduced. The film also can protect the skin from irritants.

A. A humectant is an ingredient that will either absorb water from the air or retain water in a formula. Glycerin and propylene glycol are often included in aqueous ointments and creams to prevent drying out of the product.
B. Although the silicones are nonpolar, they have not been used as pharmaceutical solvents because of poor solvent characteristics and relatively high cost. They are entirely unsuitable for parenteral solutions since they would not be assimilated from tissue. (1:1530)

200. **E.** Because of the incorporation of a higher proportion of powdered ingredients, pastes are stiffer, less greasy, and more absorptive than ointments. Aluminum paste is used as a skin protective. Ostomates sometimes apply it around the stoma to protect the skin from the digestive action of the intestinal content. (20:822; 24:338)

201. **D.** Zinc oxide paste with salicylic acid contains 2% salicylic acid. It is used as an astringent and protective. (24:316)

202. **A.** Cholesterol is a steroid alcohol which is available from several sources, including wool fat. Usually W/O emulsions are formed when cholesterol is the emulsifier. (1:1243, 1249)

203. **E.** Polysorb® Hydrate contains the lipophilic sorbitan sesquioleate as an emulsifier. Two other W/O emulsion bases are Eucerin® and Nivea® Cream, both of which contain wool wax alcohols as emulsifiers. (20b:198)

204. **E.** Allantoin is included in many topical formulations as a healing agent. Presumably, it stimulates cell proliferation. (1:729; 3:1511)

205. **B.** The official Cold Cream USP contains a borate/fatty acid surfactant system and mineral oil. Rose Water Ointment NF (cold cream, Galen's cerate) contains a similar surfactant system but with almond oil rather than mineral oil. (1:1250)

206. **C.** None of the several drugs used by the epileptic patient are available as rectal suppositories. (3:902–38)
A. Asthma may be treated with aminophylline, which is available in several strengths of suppositories. (3:528)
B. Aspirin suppositories are available in both adult and pediatric dosage strengths. (3:698)
D. An example of a sedative/hypnotic drug available as rectal suppositories is chloral hydrate. (3:865)
E. Migraine may be relieved with ergotamine tartrate. A commercial form is Cafergot® Suppositories (Sandoz), a combination of 2 mg Gynergen® (ergotamine tartrate) and 100 mg caffeine. (3:734)

207. **D.** The extent of drug release and absorption will vary depending upon the properties of the drug, the suppository base, and the condition of the colon. Oil-soluble drugs will be poorly released from a cocoa butter base because of the high lipid/water solubility. (24:351–52)
A. The rectal fluids are essentially neutral and have a low buffer capacity. Therefore, drugs that can be destroyed by the acidity of the stomach may be successfully administered rectally. (24:352)
B. Drugs that are absorbed through the colon pass into the lower hemorrhoidal veins and into the general systemic circulation. Avoidance of first-pass exposure to the liver may enhance the effect of drugs that the liver inactivates. Drugs that are absorbed from the upper intestinal tract pass directly through the portal vein into the liver, where metabolism to inactive products can occur. (24:352)
E. The lesser dose frequency and lower propensity for irritation explains why certain drugs can be administered rectally but not orally. (24:351)

208. **E.** Selected combinations of the polyethylene glycols (PEGs) can be formulated into water-miscible suppositories with a range of consistence. They are easy to insert and do not require refrigeration. (24:363)

209. **D.** Sultrin® Cream (Ortho) contains the triple sulfa combination of sulfathiazole, sulfacetamide, and sulfabenzamide. It is indicated in the treatment of *Hemophilus vaginals* vaginitis. (3:1420)
A. Gantrisin® is Roche's sulfisoxazole. (3:1420)
B. Mycostatin® (Squibb) contains the antifungal agent nystatin. (3:1415)
C. Sporostacin® (Ortho) contains 1% chlordantoin and is used to treat mixed vaginal infections. (3:1422)
E. Trimo San® (Milex) is a product similar to Nylmerate®. (3:1424)

210. **D.** Nylmerate® Jelly (Holland-Rantos) contains 0.02% phenylmercuric acetate as a mild anti-infective, and boric and acetic acids for pH adjustment. It is intended for administration twice a day for a 10-day period to return the vaginal pH to normal. (3:1424)

211. **A.** Lactose is a readily compressible, water-soluble, and inert ingredient. It will also encourage the growth of Doderlein's bacilli, a microorganism present in the healthy vagina. (24:364)

212. **C.** The active ingredient in Norforms® vaginal suppositories is the quaternary ammonium germicide, methylbenzethonium chloride, which will have the tendency to decrease odor-producing microorganisms. (10)

213. **E.** Vanobid® Ointment contains the antibiotic candicidin which is unstable at elevated temperatures. (10)

214. **C.** An electric current is conducted in an electrolytic solution by the movement of ions. Conductivity (the ability to conduct current) depends upon the number and kinds of ions present. It is the reciprocal of the resistance of the solution. (1:256)

A., B., D., E. Properties of a solution that depend on the number of particles of the solute and are independent of the chemical nature of the solute are termed colligative properties. The magnitude of vapor pressure and freezing point reduction, boiling point elevation, and osmotic pressure are all related to the number of particles in solution. (1:245–50; 14:190–95)

215. **A.** Colligative properties are a series of properties possessed by solutions. The magnitude of the properties is determined by the total number of solute particles regardless of whether the particles are ions, molecules, or of dissimilar species. (1:245)

216. **A.** Solutions which have equal osmotic pressure are iso-osmotic and also are isotonic if separated by a membrane permeable to the solvent but impermeable to the solute. Any of the colligative properties can be used to determine tonicity of solutions. Freezing point depression is most frequently used. The freezing point of a 0.9% aqueous solution of sodium chloride is −0.52°C, the same as that of human blood and tears. Saline solutions of this concentration are isotonic with these body fluids. More concentrated solutions are hypertonic; less concentrated are hypotonic. (1:245–50; 14:196–99)

217. **B.** When the vapor pressure of a liquid approaches atmospheric pressure (760 mm Hg), the escape tendency of the molecules increases and the liquid begins to boil.
A. Temperature increases cause greater molecular motion, thereby increasing the vapor pressure.
D. Addition of solutes to the liquid causes a depression of the vapor pressure, thereby increasing the boiling point. (12:75)

218. **D.** Solutions that have the same osmotic pressure as blood are isotonic with blood. Solutions that have a high osmotic pressure (i.e. are hypertonic) will cause water to pass out of the red blood cells to compensate for the pressure difference. Because of the loss of volume, the red cells will shrink and take on a wrinkled appearance (crenation). Solutions that have a lower osomotic pressure (i.e., are hypotonic) will allow water to pass into the cells. This causes them to swell and rupture with a release of hemoglobin (hemolysis). (12:251)

219. **B.** Appendix A in *Remington's Pharmaceutical Sciences* lists sodium chloride equivalents, freezing-point depressions, and the hemolytic effects of many chemicals in aqueous solutions. Even when boric acid, glycerin, propylene glycol, and urea solutions are iso-osmotic, hemolysis occurs when red blood cells are added. Glucose does not cause hemolysis. If it did, it could not be used in large-volume parenterals for infusion into the bloodstream. (1:1408)

220. **C.** A hypertonic solution will draw water from within the cell until an equilibrium is reached with equal pressure on each side of the cell membrane. The shrinkage of the cell as a result of fluid loss is known as crenation. (1:247)

221. **A.** A sodium chloride equivalent is the weight of sodium chloride that will produce the same osmotic effect as one gram of the specified chemical. For example, morphine hydrochloride has an E value of 0.15. This indicates that 1 g of morphine hydrochloride produces the same osmotic pressure (and depression of freezing point) in solutions as 0.15 g of sodium chloride. (1:1407)

222. **C.** Any two solutions that have the same freezing points will have the same osmotic pressure and should be isotonic. Since blood freezes at −0.52°C, any solution that freezes at this temperature will be iso-osmotic. The use of freezing point data for isotonicity adjustment for both ophthalmic and parenteral solutions is common in the pharmaceutical industry because freezing points can be easily measured. (1:1406)

223. **D.** Aqueous solutions that have the same freezing or boiling point will have the same osmotic pressure, since these are all colligative properties. Blood freezes at −0.52°C; other aqueous solutions that freeze at this point are considered to be iso-osmotic with blood and with each other. The term *isotonic* further qualifies the relationship by indicating that the solutions have the same "tone" as the red blood cells in the blood and will not cause changes in the cell size. Since some chemicals will readily pass through the red blood cell wall, equalized pressure on both sides of the cell wall is not possible without changes in the cell volume. Such solutions may be described as being iso-osmotic but not isotonic with red blood cells. (1:247)

224. **E.** Although it is possible to experimentally determine whether a solution is iso-osmotic with a 0.9% sodium chloride solution or blood, one cannot assume that the solution is also isotonic. To be isotonic, a solution must maintain a certain pressure or "tone" in the red blood cells. If the chemical in a solution freely passes through the red blood cell membrane, it will not maintain a tone and therefore will not be truly isotonic. The pharmacist in product development will adjust a solution to the correct iso-osmotic pressure, then mix the solution with red blood cells to observe if hemolysis occurs. (1:247, 1405)
C. *Remington's Pharmaceutical Sciences* presents extensive tables of values. (1:1408–12)
D. Other chemicals may be used as tonicity adjustors. Concentrations of chemicals that are iso-osmotic are listed in the Remington or can be calculated by simple proportions. (1:1408)

225. **D.** Sodium sulfacetamide solution (30%) is equivalent to a 9% solution of sodium chloride in tonicity. Any solution of sodium sulfacetamide stronger than 12% will sting when instilled into the eyes. The patient should be warned to expect this. (20:884)

226. **B.** Increasing the contact time between a drug and the cornea will often increase the amount of drug absorption that will occur. (20b:236)

227. **B.** Sodium fluorescein is an ophthalmic diagnostic agent. It is instilled into the eye to delineate scratches and corneal lesions. It would be very dangerous to place a contaminated solution on a damaged cornea, through which microorganisms may easily pass. Pharmacists should not extemporaneously prepare sodium fluorescein solutions unless sterility can be guaranteed. Pharmaceutical manufacturers supply fluorescein as unit dose solutions or individual paper strips. (1:1218)

228. **D.** The effectiveness of an antimicrobial preservative depends upon several factors including the concentration of preservative, strains of microorganisms present, degree of contamination, and length of contact time. The higher the concentration of preservative, the greater its effectiveness. However, too high a concentration may cause irritation and tearing. Rapid action is desirable, of course. Realistically, the ability to resterilize a solution in less than one hour is considered satisfactory since the solution would be decontaminated before the next dose would be administered. (1:1500)

229. **A.** The combination of benzalkonium chloride and EDTA (0.01% of each) is effective against most common microorganisms, including strains of *Pseudomonas* that are resistant to benzalkonium chloride. (1:1501, 1502; 20b:237)

230. **D.** Sodium Sulamyd® is a brand of sulfacetamide sodium manufactured by Schering. The label specifies storage in a "cool place," which according to the USP has a temperature range between 8° and 15°. However, storage of Sulamyd® Ophthalmic Solution in the refrigerator (2° to 8°) will not damage the product. (10)
A. Chloroptic® is Allergan's brand of chloramphenicol 0.5% solution.
B. Barnes-Hind's Eppy® is a borate complex containing the equivalent of 1% 1-epinephrine.
C. Parke-Davis markets Ophthochlor®, which is also a 0.5% solution of chloramphenicol.

231. **E.** Tetracaine hydrochloride is useful for topical eye anethesia since it is five to eight times more potent than cocaine and does not produce mydriasis, cycloplegia, or intraocular hypertension. (4:982)

232. **E.** In spite of its name, veegum is not an organic gum but is an inorganic clay. It is water insoluble and would probably be unsuitable for ophthalmic administration since insoluble particles could be deposited in the ocular areas. (20b:236)

233. **D.** Papain is a proteolytic enzyme which will aid in the removal of proteinaceous residues that slowly build up on soft lenses. Allergan markets Soflens® Enzymatic Contact Lens Cleaner as tablets containing papain. Once weekly the soft lenses are soaked overnight in a solution prepared from the tablets. (3:1401)

234. **A.** Investigators have shown that solutions with a range of sodium chloride concentrations from 0.5 to 2.0% can be put into either normal or inflamed eyes without causing pain or detectable tissue change. Purified water will sting because it has such a low tonicity. (20b:236)

235. **D.** By definition. (12:202)

236. **C.** The Henderson-Hasselbalch equation, or buffer equation for a weak acid and its salt, is represented by:

$$pH = pK_a + \log \frac{salt}{acid}$$

where pK_a is the negative log of the dissociation constant for the weak acid and salt/acid is the ratio of the molar concentration of salt and acid in the system. (12:237)

237. **E.** According to the Henderson-Hasselbalch equation, pH will equal pK_a when the expression

$$\log \frac{[salt]}{[acid]} \text{ is equal to zero.}$$

This can occur only when the ratio

$$\frac{[salt]}{[acid]} = 1 \text{ since the log of } 1 = 0.$$

The point where the salt concentration equals the acid concentration is the half-neutralization point. (32:16)

238. **A.** When radioisotopes are used in medicine, the radiation dose delivered to the patient is maintained at as low a level as possible. This is accomplished through judicious choice of isotope for the best combination of minimum half-life, minimum retention in the body, and minimum quantity of isotope which will permit its detection and accurate measurement. Accordingly, certain isotopes, such as ^{90}Sr and ^{226}Ra, are never used as unsealed internal sources or tracers. (1:493)

239. **D.** Since ^{32}P is metabolized in a manner similar to naturally occurring phosphorus, the isotope is readily distributed to all tissues and is concentrated in those tissues where proliferation is most rapid. A therapeutic dose of ^{32}P (1.5 to 5 mCi) will concentrate in bone marrow and partially suppress erythrogenesis. (1:493)

240. **B.** Although it is desirable to use isotopes with short half-lives to minimize the radiation dose received by the patient, it is evident that the shorter the half-life, the greater will be the problem of supply. Radioisotope generators, or "cows," have been developed to deal with this problem. A radioisotope generator, or "cow," is an ion-exchange column

containing a resin of alumina upon which a long-lived parent nuclide is absorbed. Radioactive decay of the long-lived parent results in the production of a short-lived daughter nuclide which is eluted or "milked" from the column by means of an appropriate eluant such as sterile, pyrogen-free saline. (1:478)

241. **B.** ^{99m}Tc is available commercially as a technetium-99m generator (various manufacturers) in which molybdenum 99 is the parent nuclide. The half-life of technetium (six hours) is long enough to allow completion of usual diagnostic procedures for which it is used, yet short enough to minimize the radiation dose to the patient. Lack of a beta component in its radiation further decreases the dose delivered to the patient. The 140 kev gamma energy is weak enough to achieve good collimation, yet strong enough to penetrate tissue sufficiently to permit deep-organ scanning. (1:478, 515)

242. **E.** The number of protons in the nucleus of an atom defines its atomic number. This is equal to the number of orbital electrons. The atomic weight or mass number of an element is equal to the number of protons and neutrons in the nucleus. Isotopes are species of nuclides which possess the same number of protons (i.e., atomic number) but a different number of neutrons (hence a different mass number). Isotopes represent the same chemical element and, therefore, have the same chemical properties. (1:474–75)

243. **B.** Decay rate is the rate at which atoms undergo radioactive disintegration. The rate of decay ($-dn/dt$) is proportional to the number of atoms (n) present at any time (t). Mathematically this may be expressed as

$$-dn/dt = \lambda N$$

where λ is a proportionality constant (the decay constant). The decay of radioactive atoms is, therefore, a first-order process. (1:481)

244. **A.** Alpha radiation is particulate radiation consisting of two protons and two neutrons. The range of alpha particles is about 5 cm in air and less than 100 micrometers in tissue. Beta radiation is also particulate radiation but exists as two types, the negative electron (negatron) and the positive electron (positron). They may have a range of over 10 feet in air and up to about 1 mm in tissue. Gamma radiation, x-rays, and ultraviolet radiation are forms of electromagnetic radiation and are radiated as photons or quanta of energy. These forms of radiation differ only in wave length and are the most penetrating types of radiation. Gamma rays are the most penetrating of all types of radiation and can easily penetrate more than a foot of tissue and several inches of lead. (1:474)

245. **B.** Technetium (^{99m}Tc) is eluted from the generator as sodium pertechnetate when sterile, pyrogen-free sodium chloride injection is used as the eluent fluid. Since it is possible for some of the alumina to be washed from the ion-exchange column, appropriate tests must be performed to indicate the amount of this substance and the amount of ^{99}Mo (as a radionuclidic impurity) before the product is used in patients. Maximum limits for both of these contaminants have been established. (15:645–46)

246. **D.** This relationship may be expressed mathematically by the following equation:

$$\frac{I_1}{I_2} = \frac{R_2^{\,2}}{R_1^{\,2}}$$

Where I_1 is the gamma intensity at distance R_1 from the source and I_2 is the gamma intensity at distance R_2. For example, the dose rate from a 1 millicurie point source of ^{24}Na is 18.4 r/hour at a distance of 1 centimeter. The dose rate at a distance of 10 centimeters can be calculated as:

$$\frac{18.4 \text{ r/hr}}{I_2} = \frac{(10)^2}{(1)^2}$$

$$I_2 = \frac{(18.4 \text{ r/hr}) \times (1)^2}{(10)^2}$$

$$= 0.184 \text{ r/hr} = 184 \text{ milliroentgens/h.}$$

It should be emphasized that this inverse square law is valid only for point sources of radiation with no shielding. (15:629)

247. **A.** Sodium iodide ^{131}I is one of the most widely used radiopharmaceuticals in the world. It is used in low doses (50 to 100 microcuries) to scan the thyroid gland. The thyroid scan is used to evaluate nodule localization and iodine uptake within a nodule. Nodules that do not take up iodine (cold nodules) are frequently cancerous and may be removed surgically. Nodules that take up radioiodine (hot nodules) to a greater extent than adjacent thyroid tissue are usually benign. In higher doses (i.e., millicurie doses), sodium iodide is also used therapeutically in the treatment of thyrotoxicosis and as an antineoplastic. (22:439, 440)
E. Because it gives off a much smaller radiation dose, sodium iodide ^{125}I is used primarily as a diagnostic agent in thyroid function tests and thyroid scanning. It is also used in the preparation of radioiodinated ^{125}I serum albumin. (22:439)

248. **D.** Scintillation counters are radiation detectors that measure the amount of fluorescence induced in a chemical (e.g., sodium iodide). The ion pairs produced by the radiation cause the orbital electrons of the interacting fluor to assume excited metastable energy states. When these higher energy (excited) electrons drop back to the ground energy state of the fluor, a photon is released in the visible region of the electromagnetic spectrum. This photon can be detected and amplified by a photomultiplier tube (PMT). The electrical signal from the PMT can be totalized with auxiliary electronics. (22:446)

249. **E.** Sodium Iodide ^{131}I capsules contain radioactive iodine that is essentially carrier-free. The capsules are formulated by evaporating a solution of radioactive sodium iodide ^{131}I on the interior wall of a gelatin capsule or by pipetting the solution onto a small absorbent pellet within the capsule. The capsule is sealed to prevent leakage and subsequent radioactive contamination of the product and the environment. The capsule may, therefore, contain a small amount of solid or may appear to be empty. (22:439)

250. **D.** The rad represents 100 ergs of energy absorbed per gram of tissue. (22:427)
A. The roentgen is a measure of radiation exposure. One roentgen in air represents the absorption of 87.7 ergs of energy per gram of air. (22:427)
C. The rem is used to equate the differences in biological responses produced by different radiations such as gamma, beta, neutron, and alpha. The rem dose is obtained by multiplying the rad dose by a quality factor (QF), such as a distribution factor or a specific toxicity factor. (22:427)
B. The curie refers to the rate of radioactive disintegration and is defined as 3.7×10^{10} disintegrations per second (dps). (22:427)
E. The electron volt describes the work done when one electron is accelerated by a potential difference of one volt. (22:426)

251. **D.** The United States Adopted Names Council establishes nonproprietary drug names. The Council is jointly sponsored by the AMA, United States Pharmacopoeial Convention, and the APhA. Since the USAN is not an official governmental agency, the chosen names are not formally recognized until they are published in the *Federal Register*. (1:447)

252. **B.** A "precaution" is intended to advise the physician of possible problems that may occur with the use of a drug. For example, the use of tetracycline may result in overgrowth of nonsusceptible microorganisms. A "warning" signifies a more serious problem with greater potential for harm to a patient. For example, renal impairment may require reduction in the drug dose. A "contraindication" is the most restrictive limitation since it refers to an absolute prohibition against the use of a drug under certain conditions. For example, the use of penicillin derivatives is prohibited in patients known to be sensitive to penicillin. (24:38)

253. **B.** (25:1–40)

254. **C.** (25:1–40)

255. **A.** (25:1–40)

256. **E.** (25:1–40)

257. **C.** (25:1–40)

258. **D.** (25:1–40)

259. **A.** (25:1–40)

260. **B.** (25:1–40)

261. **D.** (25:1–40)

262. **E.** (25:1–40)

263. **A.** (25:1–40)

264. **C.** (25:1–40)

265. **B.** (25:1–40)

266. **E.** (25:1–40)

267. **A.** (25:1–40)

268. **D.** (25:1–40)

269. **D.** (10)

270. **A.** (10)

271. **B.** (10)

272. **E.** (10)

273. **C.** (10)

274. **D.** (10)

275. **B.** (10)

276. **A.** (10)

277. **E.** (10)

278. **C.** (10)

279. **D.** (10)

280. **A.** (10)

281. **E.** (10)

282. **B.** (10)

283. **C.** (10)

284. **C.** (10)

285. **A.** (10)

286. **E.** (10)

287. **B.** (10)

288. **D.** (10)

289. **C.** (10)

290. **A.** (10)

291. **B.** (10)

292. **D.** (10)

293. **E.** (10)

294. **E.** (10)

295. **C.** (10)

296. **A.** (10)

297. **B.** (10)

298. **D.** (10)

299. **D.** (10)

300. **A.** (10)

301. **E.** (10)

302. **B.** (10)

303. **C.** (10)

304. **B.** (10)

305. **A.** (10)

306. **D.** (10)

307. **E.** (10)

308. **C.** (10)

309. **C.** (10)

310. **A.** (10)

311. **E.** (10)

312. **D.** (10)

313. **B.** (10)

314. **C.** Both Tylenol® No. 3 and Empracet® No. 3 contain 30 mg of codeine phosphate and 300 mg of acetaminophen. (3:702–25)

315. **A.** Ampicillin. (10)

316. **C.** Hydrochlorothiazide. (10)

317. **D.** Isosorbide dinitrate. (10)

318. **E.** Meprobamate plus tridihexethyl chloride. (10)

319. **B.** Phenformin hydrochloride. (10)

320. **D.** Erythromycin ethylsuccinate. (10)

321. **E.** Lithium carbonate. (10)

322. **A.** Erythromycin. (10)

323. **B.** Nystatin. (10)

324. **C.** (3:544)

325. **D.** (3:519)

326. **A.** (3:546)

327. **B.** (3:546)

328. **E.** (3:546)

329. **C.** (4:682)

330. **A.** Demecarium is a long-acting anticholinesterase. (4:682)

331. **E.** Physostigmine is a short acting anticholinesterase. (4:681)

332. **B.** Echothiophate iodide is a potent long-acting anticholinesterase marketed as a lyophilized powder for reconstitution. (4:681)

333. **D.** (6:389)

334. **B.** (6:390)

335. **E.** (6:390)

336. **A.** (6:390)

337. **C.** (6:388)

338. **A.** Despite its slow onset of action and low neutralizing capacity, aluminum hydroxide is a commonly used antacid because of its nonabsorbability, demulcent activity, and ability to adsorb pepsin. (2a:13; 4:1036)

339. **C.** Magnesium trisilicate appears to be longer acting than aluminum hydroxide. Also, magnesium trisilicate reacts with hydrochloric acid to form hydrated silicon dioxide which may coat ulcers, thereby providing symptomatic relief. (2a:13; 4:1040)

340. **B.** Magnesium hydroxide has been mixed with aluminum hydroxide in an attempt to reduce the incidence of constipation attributed to the aluminum ion. (2a:13; 4:1041)

341. **D.** Calcium carbonate is often considered the antacid of choice because of its rapid onset of action, high neutralizing capacity, and relatively prolonged action. Side effects include constipation, which may be prevented by combining calcium carbonate with either magnesium carbonate or magnesium oxide. Prolonged use of calcium carbonate may result in the formation of urinary calculi. Also, increased blood levels of calcium have been reported. (2a:9; 4:1036)

342. **E.** Dihydroxy-aluminum aminoacetate has been shown to possess antacid activity similar to that of aluminum hydroxide. (2a:13; 4:1036)

343. **C.** (13:309)

344. **E.** (13:309)

345. **D.** (13:309)

346. **A.** (13:309)

347. **B.** (13:309)

348. **E.** (13:309)

349. **A.** (13:309)

350. **C.** (1:954)

351. **D.** (1:953)

352. **B.** (1:952)

353. **A.** (1:955)

354. **D.** Alcohol USP, sometimes known as grain alcohol, contains 94.9% V/V of C_2H_5OH or 92.3% W/W. The remaining portion is water. (1:1252)

355. **A.** Diluted alcohol is prepared by mixing equal volumes of Alcohol USP and purified water. Because of some volume shrinkage, (about 3%), the final strength is somewhat higher than that calculated by simple alligation. (1:1254)

356. **B.** Rubbing alcohol is a form of denatured alcohol containing approximately 70% of absolute alcohol. This product is used as a germicide and an external rubefacient. (1:1088)

357. **B.** (18:6)

358. **E.** (18:6)

359. **C.** (18:6)

360. **D.** (18:6)

361. **A.** Two other solubility descriptors are "very slightly soluble," which indicates that 1000 to 10,000 parts of solvent are needed for one part of solute, and "practically insoluble" or "insoluble," which means that more than 10,000 parts of solvent are required. (18:6)

362. **C.** The needle hub can be made of plastic or metal. It is fitted onto the syringe body by either a locking system such as the luerlock or by a simple friction fit. (15:531–33)

363. **A.** The bevel is ground to sharpness except that the back portion (heel) of the bevel is left dull. A dull heel has been shown to decrease the incidence of coring of the rubber closure and the skin. (15:531–33)

364. **B.** Needle cannulae are made of various grades of steel. Both strength and flexibility are needed. (15:531–33)

365. **E.** (15:531–33)

366. **D.** This pleasantly flavored syrup is prepared from fresh ripe fruit. Its strength is based on its malic acid content which, along with other acids, gives the syrup an acidic pH. Benzoic acid is added during the manufacturing process to prevent fermentation. (19:788; 24:126)

367. **B.** Ipecac syrup contains several therapeutically active alkaloids including emetine, caphaeline, and psychotrine. During its manufacture, hydrochloric acid is added to form water soluble salts of the alkaloids. (1:800; 18:268)

368. **A.** Tolu balsam syrup is prepared by maceration of tolu balsam with magnesium carbonate which aids in dissolving the various resins present. Among the resinous ingredients are benzoic and cinnamic acids and their esters which are responsible for the pleasant odor of tolu balsam. (1:1236; 19:839; 24:127–28)

369. **E.** Wild cherry syrup (Syrupus Pruni Virginianae) is prepared from wild cherry bark. During its preparation, heat is avoided to prevent the decomposition of the enzyme emulsin. This enzyme is necessary for the hydrolytic conversion of prunasin into the active benzaldehyde and hydrocyanic acid. (1:1237; 24:128–29)

370. **E.** Coal tar is mixed with polysorbate 80 and then incorporated into zinc oxide paste. (1:1533)

371. **B.** This product contains 20% zinc undecylenate and 5% free undecylenic acid in PEG ointment. It is used in the treatment of fungal infections such as athlete's foot. (1:1261)

372. **C.** Simple ointment is officially known as white ointment. It contains 5% white wax in white petrolatum. It is used as an emollient vehicle for other ointments. A similar product is yellow ointment which differs only in color since yellow wax and yellow petrolatum are used. (1:1247)

373. **D.** Ichthammol is classified as an irritant and local antibacterial agent. (1:721)

374. **A.** (1:718)

375. **E.** (1:1180)

376. **C.** (1:721)

377. **B.** (1:1529)

378. **C.** (1:1529)

379. **B.** (1:1529)

380. **A.** (1:1529)

381. **C.** (1:1529)

382. **A.** (1:1529)

383. **E.** (1:1529)

384. **A.** (1:1529)

385. **B.** (1:1529)

386. **D.** (1:1529)

387. **D.** (1:1529)

388. **E.** White petrolatum is a bland base with a very low incidence of irritation to the eye. Also, due to the absence of water, it has low susceptibility to microbial growth. (24:328)

389. **E.** The decomposition of most antibiotics is enhanced by water. White petrolatum is anhydrous and contains few chemically reactive ingredients. (24:328)

390. **B.** Hydrophilic ointment is capable of absorbing serous fluid quite readily. Bases such as petrolatum and hydrophilic petrolatum which will form a hydrophobic film should be avoided, as they might prevent the desired seepage. (24:328)

391. **C.** Of all the bases listed, hydrophilic petrolatum will absorb the greatest quantity of water. (24:328)

392. **E.** The normal pH range for the blood is 7.36 to 7.40 for venous samples and 7.38 to 7.42 for arterial samples. It is essential that the blood pH remain within the range of 7.35 to 7.45. Normal acid-base balance is generally maintained by three homeostatic mechanisms utilizing chemical buffers (e.g., bicarbonate and carbonic acid), respiratory control, and renal function. An impairment in any of these mechanisms can result in either acidosis or alkalosis. (1:596; 13:163)

393. **E.** The pH of the lacrimal fluid is approximately 7.4 but varies with certain ailments. The eye can tolerate pH's from 6 to 8 with a minimum of discomfort. The buffering system of the lacrimal fluid is efficient enough to adjust the pH of most ophthalmic solutions. However some solutions, particularly those containing strongly acidic drugs, will cause discomfort. (1:1495)

394. **B.** The pH of the skin is usually based upon measurements taken in the lipid film that covers the epidermis. Although the value varies greatly between individuals and in various areas of the body, the average value reported is 5.5 with a range of 4.5 to 6.5. (1:1524)

395. **C.** (4:212)

396. **C.** (4:214)

397. **E.** (4:216)

398. **B.** (4:218)

399. **A.** (4:220)

400. **D.** (4:221)

CHAPTER 6

Biopharmaceutics and Pharmacokinetics

Biopharmaceutics is a scientific discipline concerned with the relationship between the physiochemical properties of a drug in a dosage form and the biological response observed after its administration. Much of the progress in the quantitative aspects of biopharmaceutics has been due to the development of pharmacokinetics, a discipline concerned with the characterization of the time course of drug absorption, distribution, metabolism, and excretion, as well as with the relationship of these processes to the intensity and time course of the therapeutic and toxicological effects of drugs (29). A knowledge of the principles of biopharmaceutics and pharmacokinetics is clearly fundamental to the rational selection of quality drug products and to the determination of appropriate dose and dosing schedules. This chapter questions and comments on aspects of these disciplines. Items to test this knowledge can be expected to appear on licensing examinations.

Directions: Each of the questions or incomplete statements below is followed by five suggested answers or completions. Select the BEST answer in each case.

1. The term *biological availability* or *bioavailability* refers to the relative amount of drug that reaches the
   - A. small intestine
   - B. stomach
   - C. systemic circulation
   - D. liver
   - E. kidneys (43:422)

2. The primary proof of a drug's availability is the
   - A. production of its pharmacological effect (clinical efficacy)
   - B. production of high blood levels
   - C. production of high urine levels
   - D. appearance of metabolites in the urine
   - E. appearance of metabolites in the blood (28:18)

3. To produce its characteristic pharmacological action(s), a drug must always
   - A. reach high blood levels
   - B. be absorbed from the gastrointestinal tract
   - C. achieve adequate concentration at its site(s) of action
   - D. be excreted unchanged in the urine
   - E. be formulated into a dosage form that produces the most rapid onset and duration of action (28:14)

4. Differences in bioavailability are most frequently observed with drugs administered by which of the following routes?
   - A. subcutaneous
   - B. intravenous
   - C. oral
   - D. sublingual
   - E. intramuscular (27:8–12)

5. The transfer of most drugs across biological membranes occurs by
   - A. active transport from a region of high concentration to one of low concentration
   - B. active transport from a region of low concentration to one of high concentration
   - C. passive diffusion from a region of high concentration to one of low concentration
   - D. passive diffusion from a region of low concentration to one of high concentration
   - E. facilitated diffusion regardless of concentration gradient (29:16)

6. When considering drug transport, a "passive transport process" implies that
   - A. all of the drug will pass from one compartment to another
   - B. the drug is highly lipid soluble
   - C. the net transfer of drug is from an area of

high concentration to an area of low concentration

D. the net transfer of drug is from an area of low concentration to an area of high concentration

E. the rate of drug transfer is constant (34:7)

7. Which one of the following statements concerning active transport is *not* correct? Active transport systems

A. consume energy

B. may be adversely affected by certain chemicals

C. are structure-specific

D. reach equilibrium faster than passive transport systems

E. can become saturated (34:34–35)

8. When the active transport system described in the previous question becomes saturated, the rate process will be

A. zero order

B. pseudo–zero order

C. first order

D. pseudo–first order

E. second order (34:35)

9. The rate of diffusion of drugs across biological membranes is most commonly

A. independent of the concentration gradient

B. directly proportional to the concentration gradient

C. dependent on the availability of carrier substrate

D. dependent on the route of administration

E. indirectly proportional to membrane thickness (31:177)

10. An absorption process is *not* involved when a drug is given by which one of the following routes of administration?

A. oral

B. intravenous

C. intramuscular

D. rectal

E. subcutaneous (29:4–5)

11. In general, the various oral dosage forms can be ranked in which of the following expected order of availability (fastest to slowest)?

A. aqueous solution, capsule, tablet, powder, coated tablet, suspension

B. capsule, tablet, coated tablet, powder, suspension, aqueous solution

C. aqueous solution, suspension, powder, capsule, tablet, coated tablet

D. suspension, aqueous solution, powder, capsule, coated tablet, tablet

E. aqueous solution, suspension, capsule, powder, coated tablet, tablet (29:43–50)

12. Whenever a drug is more rapidly and/or more completely absorbed from a solution than from a solid dosage form,

A. it is due to the fact that the solid dosage form did not disintegrate

B. a solution is the only practical oral formulation

C. it indicates that the solid dosage form is poorly formulated

D. it is likely that absorption is rate-limited by the dissolution process

E. none of the above (29:30)

13. When measuring the absolute (versus the relative) bioavailability of an oral dosage form compared with the same dose administered intravenously, it is essential that the reference IV preparation

A. be in a totally aqueous solvent system

B. contain the same diluents, fillers, etc. (in solution) that are present in the oral formulation

C. be administered when the subject is in a fasting state

D. be administered at approximately the same rate as the drug substance is absorbed from the oral formulation

E. have the same pH as the gastric contents (7:155)

14. The relative bioavailability of various drug products can be evaluated by comparing their serum concentration versus time curves (blood level curves). The three most important parameters of comparison that can be obtained *directly* from such curves are

A. peak concentration, biological $t_{1/2}$, elimination rate constant

B. biological $t_{1/2}$, time of peak concentration, absorption rate constant

C. peak concentration, time of peak concentration, total area under the curve

D. average serum concentration, area under curve, biological $t_{1/2}$

E. absorption rate constant, area under curve, elimination rate constant (27:17)

15. The peak of the serum concentration versus time curve approximates the

A. point in time when the maximum pharmacological effect occurs

B. point in time when absorption and elimination of the drug have equalized

C. maximum concentration of free drug in the urine
D. time required for essentially all of the drug to be absorbed from the GIT
E. point in time when the drug begins to be metabolized (43:422–23)

16. The rate of elimination of a drug that is excreted by first-order kinetics is greatest when the drug's
A. blood concentration is at its maximum
B. blood concentration is at its minimum
C. cumulative concentration in the urine is at its maximum
D. cumulative concentration in the urine is at its minimum
E. blood concentration is increasing (31:190)

17. Which of the following is the first process that must occur before a drug can become available for absorption from a tablet dosage form?
A. dissolution of the drug in the GI fluids
B. dissolution of the drug in the GI epithelium
C. ionization of the drug
D. dissolution of the drug in the blood
E. disintegration of the tablet (29:47)

18. The value of particle size reduction to enhance drug absorption is limited to those situations in which the
A. absorption process occurs by active transport
B. absorption process is rate limited by the dissolution of drug in GI fluids
C. drug is very soluble
D. drug is very potent
E. drug is irritating to the GI tract (29:36)

19. The rectal route of administration may be preferred over the oral route for some drugs because
A. the drug does not have to be absorbed
B. absorption is predictable and complete
C. a portion of the absorbed drug does not pass through the liver before entering the systemic circulation
D. inert binders, diluents, and excipients cannot interfere with absorption
E. the dissolution process is avoided (31:180)

20. According to pH partition theory, a weakly acidic drug will most likely be absorbed from the stomach because
A. the drug will exist primarily in the unionized, more lipid soluble form
B. the drug will exist primarily in the ionized, more water-soluble form
C. weak acids are more soluble in acid media
D. the ionic form of the drug facilitates dissolution
E. weak acids will further depress pH (29:27)

21. Gastric emptying is slowed by all of the following *except*
A. vigorous exercise
B. pain
C. hot meals
D. hunger
E. emotional stress (33b:36)

22. Drugs that are absorbed from the GI tract are generally
A. absorbed into the portal circulation and pass through the liver before entering the general circulation
B. filtered from the blood by the kidney, then reabsorbed into the general circulation
C. absorbed into the portal circulation and are distributed by an enterohepatic cycle
D. not affected by liver enzymes
E. stored in the liver (33b:33–37)

23. All of the following drugs are believed to undergo significant first-pass hepatic biotransformation *except*
A. acetylsalicylic acid
B. nortriptyline (Aventyl®)
C. reserpine (Serpasil®)
D. oxyphenbutazone (Oxalid®)
E. propanolol (Inderal®) (49:75, 83)

24. The volume of distribution of a drug is
A. a mathematical relationship between the total amount of drug in the body and the concentration of drug in the blood
B. a measure of an individual's blood volume
C. a measure of an individual's total fluid volume
D. an expression of total body volume
E. none of the above (29:2)

25. The volume of distribution (V_d) of a particular drug will be
A. greater for drugs that concentrate in tissues rather than in plasma
B. greater for drugs that concentrate in plasma rather than in tissues
C. independent of tissue concentration
D. independent of plasma concentration
E. approximately the same for all drugs in a given individual (7:6–7)

26. Which of the following is *not* a critical characteristic of an effective urinary tract antimicrobial drug?

A. high activity against gram-negative bacilli
B. high volume of distribution in the body
C. low level of protein binding
D. short biological half-life
E. all of the above are desirable characteristics (34:207–09)

27. At diffusion equilibrium, the concentrations of a drug in the various body compartments (body fluids, tissues, organs) are usually *not* equal because
A. all body compartments are not equal in size and weight
B. those compartments closest to the absorption site(s) will absorb most of the drug
C. the CNS is a body compartment that usually does not accumulate drugs
D. most drugs end up in the urine
E. the various body compartments are not equally accessible to the drug, nor do they have equal affinities for it (29:2)

28. Drugs that are poorly lipid soluble or extensively ionized at the pH of blood generally
A. penetrate the CNS very slowly and may essentially be eliminated from the body before a significant concentration in the CNS is reached
B. penetrate the CNS very slowly but are centrally active in much lower concentration
C. achieve adequate CNS concentrations only if given IV
D. must be metabolized to a more polar form before they can gain access to the CNS
E. can gain access to the CNS if other drugs are used to modify blood pH (29:84; 33:30)

29. The metabolism of drugs generally results in
A. less acidic compounds
B. more acidic compounds
C. compounds having a higher oil/water partition coefficient
D. more polar compounds
E. compounds with lower aqueous solubility (31:184)

30. The term "prodrug" refers to a
A. chemical substance that is part of the synthesis procedure in preparing a drug
B. compound that liberates an active drug in the body
C. compound which may be therapeutically active but is still under clinical trials
D. drug that has only prophylactic activity in the body
E. drug that is classified as being "probably effective" (34:216)

31. An example of a commercial product that is a prodrug is
A. Amoxil® (Beecham)
B. Cleocin® (Upjohn)
C. E-Mycin® (Upjohn)
D. Geocillin® (Roerig)
E. Prostaphlin® (Bristol) (10; 34:220)

32. The transfer of drugs from the blood to the urine and the biotransformation of drugs to inactive metabolites are usually both
A. related to creatinine clearance
B. irreversible processes
C. competitive processes
D. dependent on the rate constant for absorption
E. functions performed primarily by the kidneys (29:2)

33. The rate of metabolism or elimination for drugs that follow zero-order kinetics
A. is constant
B. changes with time but is *not* dependent on the concentration of drug in the blood
C. changes with time and is dependent on the concentration of drug in the blood
D. is independent of enzyme systems in the liver
E. none of the above (12:360; 34:36)

34. Most drugs are metabolized or eliminated from the body by first-order kinetics. This implies that the rate of metabolism or elimination
A. is constant
B. changes with time but is *not* dependent on the concentration of drug in the blood
C. changes with time and is dependent only on the concentration of drug in the blood
D. is independent of drug concentration in the blood
E. none of the above (31:190; 34:36)

35. The biological half-life of a drug
A. is a constant physical property of the drug
B. is a constant chemical property of the drug
C. may be increased in patients with impaired renal function
D. may be decreased by giving the drug by rapid IV injection
E. depends entirely on the route of administration (29:5; 31:195)

36. The biological half-life of many drugs is often prolonged in newborn infants because of
A. a higher degree of protein binding
B. microsomal enzyme induction

C. more complete absorption of drugs
D. incompletely developed enzyme systems
E. incompletely developed barriers to the distribution of drugs in the body (31:197)

37. The biological half-life of a drug that is eliminated by first-order kinetics is mathematically represented by ____, where k is the first-order rate constant for elimination.

A. $\frac{1}{k}$

B. log k

C. $\frac{0.693}{k}$

D. $\frac{2.303}{k}$

E. $\frac{\text{peak serum concentration}}{2}$

(31:192)

38. A reference source that has an extensive table listing biological half-lives of drugs is
A. *Perspectives in Clinical Pharmacy* (first edition)
B. *Parenteral Drug Information Guide* (first edition)
C. *Physical Pharmacy* (second edition)
D. *The United States Dispensatory* (twenty-seventh edition)
E. *United States Pharmacopoeia* (nineteenth edition) (30:292, 296–323)

39. If a drug appears in the feces after oral administration,
A. the drug cannot have been completely absorbed from the GI tract
B. the drug must not have completely dissolved in the GI fluids
C. the drug must have complexed with materials in the GI tract
D. parenteral administration of the drug may determine the contribution of the biliary system to the amount of drug in the feces
E. parenteral administration of the drug will be useful to determine the bioavailability of the oral formulation (33b:49)

40. When comparing a highly protein-bound drug to its less- or non-protein-bound analogue, the highly bound drug will probably have
A. a longer biological half-life
B. delayed elimination from the body
C. a more uniform distribution throughout body tissues
D. all of the above characteristics
E. none of the above characteristics (4:741–42; 49:101)

41. Which one of the following drugs does *not* bind to plasma protein to any significant extent?
A. allopurinol (Zyloprim®)
B. amitriptyline (Elavil®)
C. bishydroxycoumarin
D. furosemide (Lasix®)
E. sulfathiazole (49:101)

42. For many drugs, bioavailability can be evaluated using urinary excretion data. This is based on the assumption that
A. bioavailability studies can be done only on drugs that are completely excreted unchanged by the kidneys
B. drug levels can be measured more accurately in urine than in blood
C. a drug must first be absorbed into the systemic circulation before it can appear in the urine
D. all of the administered dose can be recovered from the urine
E. only drug metabolites are excreted in the urine (43:424)

43. In general, bioavailability estimations based on urinary excretion data are less satisfactory than estimations based on blood level data because accurate urinary excretion studies require
A. complete urine collection
B. normal or near normal renal function
C. that the drug being studied is completely excreted unchanged by the kidney
D. A and B
E. A and C (7:155, 594)

44. The excretion of a weakly acidic drug (i.e., pK_a 3.5) will be more rapid in alkaline urine than in acidic urine because
A. all drugs are excreted more rapidly in alkaline urine
B. the drug will exist primarily in the unionized form, which cannot easily be reabsorbed
C. the drug will exist primarily in the ionized form, which cannot be easily reabsorbed
D. weak acids cannot be reabsorbed from the kidney tubules
E. active transport mechanisms function better in alkaline urine (34:206)

45. The rate of change in the amount of drug in the body is a function of the
    A. rate of absorption
    B. rate of elimination
    C. size of the dose administered
    D. both A and B
    E. amount of unabsorbed drug in the GI tract (29:5)

46. The time of the peak serum concentration gives some indication of the relative rate of
    A. absorption
    B. distribution
    C. metabolism
    D. elimination
    E. complexation (43:422–23)

47. The area under the serum concentration–time curve represents the
    A. biological half-life of the drug
    B. amount of drug that is cleared by the kidneys
    C. amount of drug in the original dosage form
    D. amount of drug absorbed
    E. amount of drug excreted in the urine (43:422–23)

48. Two different oral formulations of the same drug having equal areas under their respective serum concentration–time curves
    A. deliver the same total amount of drug to the body and are, therefore, bioequivalent
    B. deliver the same total amount of drug to the body but are not necessarily bioequivalent
    C. are bioequivalent by definition
    D. are bioequivalent if they both meet USP disintegration standards
    E. are bioequivalent if they both meet USP dissolution standards (43:422–23)

49. If an oral capsule formulation of drug A produces a serum concentration time–curve having the same area under the curve as that produced by an equivalent dose of drug A given IV, it can generally be concluded that
    A. the IV route is preferred to the oral route
    B. the capsule formulation is essentially completely absorbed
    C. the drug is very rapidly absorbed
    D. all oral dosage forms of drug A will be bioequivalent
    E. there is no advantage to the IV route (31:194)

50. The properties of a drug may preclude its formulation into a sustained-release dosage form. Drugs with which of the following characteristics probably should not be so formulated?
    A. poor solubility
    B. very long half-life
    C. very high potency
    D. very short half-life
    E. all of the above (34:157)

51. Which of the following objectives is *not* desirable when developing a new antibiotic drug?
    A. increasing the minimum inhibitory concentration
    B. decreasing the tendency for protein binding
    C. increasing the biological half-life
    D. increasing drug distribution to tissues
    E. all are desirable objectives (34:185)

52. In vitro dissolution rate studies on drug products are useful in bioavailability evaluations only if they can be correlated with
    A. disintegration rates
    B. in vivo studies in humans
    C. in vivo studies in at least three species of animals
    D. the chemical stability of the drug
    E. USP disintegration limits (29:57)

53. Differences in bioavailability are especially significant when
    A. the drug is expensive
    B. the therapeutic index is high
    C. rather specific blood levels of the drug are required
    D. the drug is given IV
    E. the drug is rapidly absorbed from the gastrointestinal tract (35:23)

54. If bioavailability studies determine that brand #1 (a tablet formulation of drug A) is not equivalent to brand # 2 (another tablet formulation of drug A), what degree of inequivalence would make brand #1 a therapeutically unacceptable product?
    A. brand #1 has 95% of the availability of brand #2
    B. brand #1 has 90% of the availability of brand #2
    C. brand #1 has 75% of the availability of brand #2
    D. the degree of inequivalence that is therapeutically significant depends on other factors in addition to an absolute comparison of availability
    E. the USP limits (percent) for variations in drug content in the individual dosage form are also reasonable limits for therapeutically significant inequivalence (35:23)

55. Compartmental models are often used to illustrate the various principles of pharmacokinetics. A compartment is best defined as
    A. any anatomical entity that is capable of absorbing drug
    B. a kinetically distinguishable pool of drug
    C. specific body organs or tissues that can be assayed for drug
    D. any body fluid such as blood or urine that may contain drug
    E. any component of the blood, including blood proteins, that would have a tendency to absorb drug (34:44)

56. When describing a rate process, the two-compartment open model differs from the two-compartment closed model in that the open model
    A. describes elimination of drug from the system
    B. has more rate constants
    C. may not reach equilibrium between the two compartments
    D. all of the above are correct
    E. none of the above are correct (34:17)

57. If a fixed dose of a drug that is eliminated by first-order kinetics is administered at regular intervals, the time required to achieve a steady-state plasma level depends only on the
    A. dose of the drug
    B. volume of distribution of the drug
    C. half-life of the drug
    D. dosing interval
    E. fraction of dose absorbed (bioavailability) (6:22; 7:8)

58. A specific drug has a first-order biological half-life of four hours. This half-life value will
    A. be independent of the initial drug concentration
    B. increase when the concentration of the drug increases
    C. decrease when the concentration of the drug decreases
    D. decrease if the patient has renal impairment
    E. be the same whether the drug level is determined in the blood or by observing the pharmacological action (34:50)

59. If the rate of elimination of a drug is reduced because of impaired renal function, the
    A. half-life and the time required to reach steady state plasma levels will be increased
    B. half-life and the time required to reach steady state plasma levels will be decreased
    C. half-life will be increased and the time required to reach steady state plasma levels will be decreased
    D. half-life will be decreased and the time required to reach steady state plasma levels will be increased
    E. half-life and the time required to reach steady state plasma levels will remain the same (7:8–9)

60. Assuming complete absorption and an elimination half-life of four hours, how much of a drug will remain in the body twelve hours after administering a 400-mg dose?
    A. 200 mg
    B. 100 mg
    C. 50 mg
    D. 25 mg
    E. almost no drug will remain (34:50)

Questions 61 to 65
The following graph represents drug blood level curves. Answer the next five (5) questions based upon this graph.

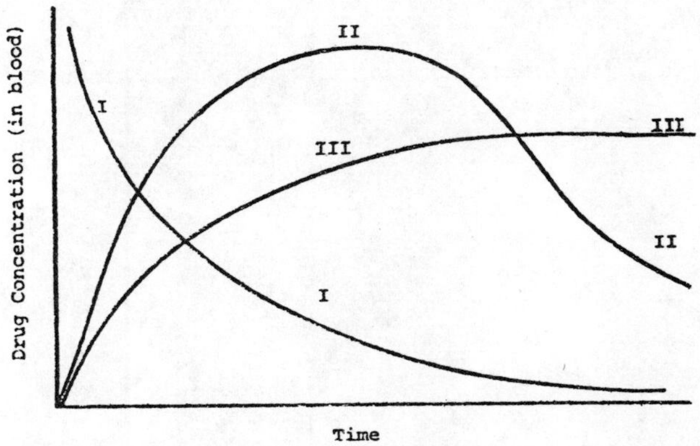

61. Curve I represents the blood level concentration of a drug administered by
    A. subcutaneous injection
    B. intramuscular injection
    C. intravenous injection
    D. either intramuscular or intravenous injection
    E. the oral route (34:79)

62. The upward slope of curve II could represent
    A. increased absorption of drug from a capsule dosage form
    B. absorption of drug from an intramuscular injection
    C. absorption of drug from a sustained-release tablet
    D. any of the above dosage forms
    E. none of the above dosage forms (34:80)

63. Which one of the following statements concerning the graph is completely true?
   A. once the peak in curve II has been reached, no further drug absorption is likely to occur
   B. doubling the administered dose will double the height of curve II
   C. the Y axis (concentration of drug in the blood) should be expressed as a log function
   D. the X axis (time) should be expressed as a log function
   E. none of the above are completely true (34:82)

64. Curve III would best illustrate a drug administered by
   A. intravenous push
   B. intravenous infusion
   C. intramuscular injection
   D. intrathecal injection
   E. either intravenous push or infusion (34:95)

65. The time needed to reach maximum drug blood levels (the plateau portion of curve III) during constant-rate intravenous infusion is
   A. directly proportional to the rate of infusion
   B. inversely proportional to the rate of infusion
   C. independent of the rate of infusion
   D. independent of the biological half-life
   E. not related to either the infusion rate or the biological half-life (34:95)

Answers and Commentary

1. **C.** For most drugs, a dose-response relationship can be correlated with the amount of drug that gains access to the general circulation. In many cases, the amount of drug that is present in the blood (blood level) is directly related to the intensity and duration of the pharmacological effect. The relative amount of drug that is biologically available compared to the total amount of drug in the dosage form administered is a measure of bioavailability. (43:422)

2. **A.** However, because of the great difficulty in quantitating pharmacological effects directly as a practical matter, the evaluation of the bioavailability of various drug products usually involves measurement of the concentration of a drug and/or its metabolites in a fluid compartment such as blood or urine where its presence can be correlated with a pharmacological response. (28:18)

3. **C.** Although the blood levels of various drugs are often utilized to compare different formulations of the same drug, it must be remembered that to exert a pharmacological effect, a drug must reach its site(s) of action in an adequate concentration. Some drugs (e.g., urinary tract anti-infectives) do not necessarily have to achieve high blood concentration to reach their site(s) of action. (28:14)

4. **C.** While differences in bioavailability of various drug products might be anticipated with any route of administration that requires the drug to be absorbed into the blood compartment, the oral route is most often involved because it is the most common route of administration and it presents the most difficult conditions in terms of chemical and biological obstacles. (27:8–12)

5. **C.** Although some drugs are absorbed from the gastrointestinal tract by active transport mechanisms against a concentration gradient or by facilitated diffusion with a concentration gradient, most drugs are passively absorbed from a region of high concentration to a region of low concentration (i.e., with a concentration gradient) (29:16)

6. **C.** Passive transport is the most common type of drug transport. It occurs when a drug is unevenly distributed between two compartments which are separated by a membrane or barrier that is permeable to the drug. Since the drug can pass freely through the membrane, it will do so until equilibrium is reached. (34:7)

7. **D.** As the name implies, active transport involves active participation of a membrane in transferring molecules from one side to the other. The "carrier," such as an enzyme in the membrane, aids in transporting the molecules of drug across the membrane. Since this transfer process is continuous, it can work against a concentration gradient and continue until all of the drug has been transported. Therefore, equilibrium does not occur.
B. Certain chemicals, known as poisons, may reduce active transport probably by destroying or inactivating the drug carriers.
C. Carriers are often very specific in respect to the drug they will transport. Only a certain chemical structure or similar chemical structures may be actively transported by a given carrier.
E. Because of the chemical specificity and limited capacity of carriers, active transport systems may become saturated. When this occurs, the active transport rate becomes a constant value until the drug concentration is reduced. (34:34–35)

8. **A.** A characteristic of a zero-order process or reaction is a constant rate of change. When the active transport system is saturated, there are not enough carriers to handle the large number of transferrable molecules. Therefore, the carriers work at maximum capacity, transferring molecules at a constant rate until the drug concentration is reduced to less than the capacity of the carrier system. At this time, the number of molecules transferred will be a fraction of those present for transfer (i.e., a first-order rate). (34:35)

9. **B.** The greater the difference between the concentration of a drug on one side of a biological membrane and that on the other, the greater will be the rate of transfer from the side having the higher concentration to the side having the lower concentration. (31:177)

10. **B.** When a drug is administered by the intravenous route, an absorption step is bypassed because the drug is injected directly into the bloodstream. All of the other routes of administration that are listed present the drug with various biological barriers through which the drug must pass to reach the blood. (29:4–5)

11. **C.** It is generally true that a drug must be in solution before it becomes available for absorption. An aqueous solution presents the absorption site(s) with the drug in the dissolved state. Even if the drug precipitates upon contact with fluid in the GI tract, it will do so in the form of very small particles that are eventually completely wetted and ready to be redissolved. Suspensions, while having larger particles of drug, are also wetted and ready for dissolution. A powder formulation must disperse in the GI fluids and become wetted

prior to dissolution. The gelatin shell of a capsule formulation must dissolve before the powder can disperse. Tablets must not only disintegrate from the tablet form but they must also disintegrate from the smaller granulation particles before the GI fluids have access to the drug. Coated tablets have the additional barrier of the coating material. (29:43–50)

12. **D.** When a drug is administered orally in a solid dosage form such as a tablet or capsule, it is frequently observed that the rate of absorption is controlled by the rate at which the drug dissolves in the fluids at the absorption site(s). When absorption is controlled by dissolution in this manner, absorptiòn is said to be dissolution rate–limited. If the dissolution step is eliminated by administering the drug in the form of a solution, it is quite likely that absorption will proceed more rapidly and/or more completely. (29:30)

13. **D.** When determining absolute (versus relative) bioavailability, it is important that the reference intravenous dose be administered at approximately the same rate as the drug substance is absorbed from the oral formulation. This procedure will minimize errors caused by different time–plasma concentrations. Large differences in time–plasma concentrations may be associated with differences in drug distribution, biotransformation, and renal excretion. (7:155)

14. **C.** (27:17)

15. **B.** Prior to the peak time, the rate of absorption is greater than the rate of elimination, and the curve ascends. After the peak, the rate of elimination is greater than the rate of absorption and the curve descends. If these rates are equal for some time interval, the curve will show a plateau rather than a distinct peak. (43:422–23)

16. **A.** The differential formula for a first-order process, $\frac{dc}{dt} = kc$, indicates that the rate of elimination is a direct function of drug concentration and, therefore, will be at maximum when the blood concentration of drug is at a maximum. 31:190)

17. **E.** The surface area of a drug is so limited in the intact tablet that dissolution of drug from the intact tablet is negligible except for very water-soluble drugs. Therefore, although a drug must dissolve before it can be absorbed, a tablet must generally disintegrate before the drug can dissolve. (29:47)

18. **B.** Making a drug dissolve faster (e.g., by particle size reduction) will not increase the rate of its absorption if the absorption process itself is the rate-limiting step in the overall transport of the drug from its intact dosage form to the blood. Furthermore, there are some circumstances in which particle size reduction may actually reduce the amount of drug absorbed. For example, for drugs such as penicillin G that are unstable in gastric fluids, more rapid dissolution would enhance degradation by increasing residence time of dissolved drug in the stomach and thereby result in reduced availability. (29:36)

19. **C.** Although it is desirable to bypass absorption into the portal circulation for certain drugs that are rapidly metabolized by the liver, the value of utilizing the rectal route for this purpose is limited. This is due to the fact that while the blood supply to the rectum is drained by three principal veins, only the middle and inferior hemorrhoidal veins actually bypass the liver. The superior hemorrhoidal vein enters the portal circulation via the inferior mesenteric vein. (31:180)

20. **A.** The ionic equilibrium that is established in the acid contents of the stomach will favor a relatively higher concentration of unionized drug in solution. The unionized molecule, because of the absence of a charge, is more lipid soluble than the ionic species and will be able to cross biological membranes more easily. If the drug reaches the more alkaline contents of the intestines before absorption is complete, the higher pH will then favor the ionic form of the drug, which has considerably less lipid solubility and is much less readily absorbed. It should be pointed out, however, that because of the extremely large surface area of the intestine, weakly acidic drugs can be absorbed from the intestine in spite of the unfavorable ion/molecule ratio. (29:27)

21. **D.** Gastric emptying appears to be an exponential process with a normal half-life of between 20 and 60 minutes. However, many factors can influence the rate of this process. It is slowed by the A, B, C, and E choices and is speeded by hunger, mild exercise, cold meals, dilute solutions, and lying on the right side. Since some drugs and some dosage forms (e.g., enteric coated tablets) are absorbed at rather specific sites along the gastrointestinal tract, alterations in the rate of gastric emptying may lead to erratic and unpredictable absorption. For example, if an acid labile drug that is preferentially absorbed from a portion of the small intestine is consumed as an enteric coated tablet, a greatly reduced gastric emptying rate may permit the tablet to dissolve in the stomach and be degraded by the acid fluids of the stomach. Similarly, if the gastric emptying rate is greatly increased, the tablet may not dissolve before it reaches its primary site of absorption. (33b:36)

22. **A.** Drugs are generally absorbed from the GI tract through capillaries that empty into the portal vein. This vessel carries the absorbed drugs to the liver, where they are subjected to varying degrees of metabolism before they are carried into the general circulation. This initial passage through the liver is therapeutically significant primarily for drugs that are metabolized to a less active or inactive form by the liver. (33b:33–37)

23. **A.** The term *first-pass* refers to the first passage of drug molecules through a designated organ such as the lungs or the liver. Biotransformation will often occur at this site, thereby altering the absolute bioavailability of a drug. Commercial preparations of such drugs are

formulated to contain sufficient quantities of drug to compensate for loss due to first-pass biotransformation. While acetylsalicylic acid does not appear to undergo a significant first-pass hepatic biotransformation, some drug loss does occur in the intestinal lumen or during absorption through the GI mucosa. (49:75, 83)

24. **A.** Volume of distribution (V_d) is an "apparent volume" measured in terms of a reference compartment that is usually the blood because of the accessibility of this compartment to sampling. This relationship, which is calculated by the expression:

$V_d = \frac{A_B}{C_b}$ where A_B = total amount of unchanged drug in the body and C_b = concentration of drug in the blood

is the total volume necessary to account for all of the absorbed drug, if the concentration of drug in this volume were equal to C_b. Knowledge of the volume of distribution for a particular drug permits calculation of the total amount of drug in the body (A_B) at any time by measuring the drug concentration in the blood since $A_B = V_d C_b$. (29:2)

25. **A.** Following a given dose of a drug, the greater its concentration in various tissue compartments, the smaller will be its concentration in plasma. Therefore, according to the relationship $V_d = \frac{A_B}{C_b}$ (see previous answer), the volume of distribution of a particular drug will be greater for those drugs that tend to concentrate in tissues compared with plasma. (7:6–7)

26. **B.** A high volume of distribution implies that the antimicrobial drug is being distributed in a large portion of the body. Since better antimicrobial activity would be anticipated if the drug were concentrated primarily in the urinary tract, a low volume of distribution would be preferred.
A. High activity against commonly infecting gram-negative microorganisms (*E. coli, Enterobacter aerogenes, Pseudomonas aeruginosa,* and *Proteus vulgaris*) is desirable.
C. Drugs that are bound to plasma protein are usually not available for therapeutic activity. It is generally the free form of the drug that is active.
D. For systemic antibiotics, a long biological half-life may be useful to maintain satisfactory blood or tissue levels. Urinary tract antibiotics, however, appear to be more effective if they reach the site of action (urinary tract) quickly and in a high concentration. A drug with a short half-life is more likely to have these properties. (34:207–09)

27. **E.** (29:2)

28. **A.** The "blood-brain barrier" appears to behave as a lipoid membrane toward foreign compounds. This barrier may be due to a sheath of glial cells surrounding the capillaries of the brain. The rate of entry of a drug can often be correlated with its oil/water partition coefficient and degree of ionization at plasma pH. (29:84; 33:30)

29. **D.** Drug metabolites are usually more polar and less lipid soluble than the parent compound. Because of these changes, metabolites are usually not as tightly nor as extensively protein-bound. They are ionized to a greater degree, and are less likely to cross biological membranes than the parent compound. Drug metabolism, therefore, is generally a process that inactivates a drug and changes it to a form that can be excreted more easily and rapidly. For some drugs, however, metabolism may result in activation of an inactive substance, or an active substance may be transformed into an active metabolite(s). In these cases, either further biotransformation takes place to inactive the metabolite(s) or it is excreted unchanged. (31:184)

30. **B.** In order to take advantage of certain desirable characteristics, some drugs are marketed as prodrugs. These are chemical modifications of biologically active drugs and may not be active themselves. However, the active form of the drug is liberated in the body by some biotransformation. Prodrugs may possess better water solubility, be more stable, have a less objectionable taste, or give higher blood levels than the parent compound. (34:216)

31. **D.** Geocillin® is the indanyl ester of disodium carbenicillin (Geopen®). Unlike Geopen®, Geocillin® is acid stable and will not be inactivated in the stomach. (10; 34:220)

32. **B.** Although a number of drugs can be reabsorbed into the systemic circulation from the kidney tubule, the elimination and biotransformation processes are irreversible for most drugs. (29:2)

33. **A.** The mathematical expression for a zero-order elimination process is

$$-\frac{dc}{dt} = k$$

$$-\frac{dc}{dt}$$

is the rate of change of drug concentration in the blood with respect to time, and k is the zero-order rate constant for elimination. Since the rate of such a process depends only on a rate constant, it remains constant. (12:360; 34:36)

34. **C.** A first-order process is one in which the rate is determined by a single factor. In this case, the single factor is the concentration of a drug in the blood. The general differential formula for a first-order process is

$$-\frac{dc}{dt} = kc$$

$$-\frac{dc}{dt}$$

is the rate of change of concentration with respect to time, k is the rate constant for the process, and c is the concentration of drug in the plasma. The rate of this process changes as the concentration of drug changes. (31:190; 34:36)

35. **C.** Generally, when a particular drug has a half-life of six hours, there is reasonable certainty that in spite of as much as a one- to two-fold intersubject variation, the mean biological half-life in any group of subjects will approximate six hours. Alterations in biological half-life can be expected when a particular drug is primarily excreted unchanged by the kidneys. The presence of renal impairment slows the process of excretion and thereby increases the biological half-life of the drug in the blood. (29:5; 31:195)

36. **D.** The metabolic pathways of newborn infants are incompletely developed at birth. Most notably deficient are the oxidative and conjugative mechanisms that are known to metabolize many drugs. The reduced capacity to metabolize certain drugs will, therefore, result in prolonged biological half-lives of these drugs in newborn infants. Because of inadequate metabolic inactivation, the plasma concentration of chloramphenicol is higher in infants under two weeks of age than in older infants. (31:197)

37. **C.** (31:192)

38. **A.** While some of the other references occasionally list biological half-lives, there is a chapter in *Perspectives in Clinical Pharmacy* devoted to this topic. The authors have included several pages listing values for commonly used drugs. Investigators are cautioned that variations in the biological half-life of a given drug may occur. Reasons for variation include patient's age, physical condition, and renal failure. (30:292, 296–323)

39. **D.** If an orally administered drug appears in the feces, it might be desirable to determine whether this is the result of incomplete absorption or the result of the drug's being secreted into the GI tract via biliary excretion. The clinical significance of biliary excretion or enterohepatic cycling of the drug depends on the fraction of the dose that is excreted in the bile. By administering the drug parenterally, this fraction can be determined. (33b:49)

40. **D.** Binding of drugs to blood components leads to a more even distribution throughout body tissues, thereby decreasing selective accumulation in specific body areas. Also, since only the unbound fraction of drug is available for biotransformation and excretion, protein-bound drugs have a tendency to remain in the body longer (i.e., delayed elimination and longer half-lives). For example, doxycycline is 93% protein bound and has a biological half-life of 15 to 17 hours. Its analogue, oxytetracycline, is approximately 34% protein bound and has a reported half-life of 9.5 hours. (4:741–42; 49:101)

41. **A.** When administered in therapeutic doses, allopurinol does not appear to bind to plasma proteins. The protein-bound fraction documented for the other drugs is 96%, 97%, 75%, and 70% respectively. The pharmacist should carefully monitor drug therapy when two or more drugs that exhibit significant protein-binding properties are prescribed. Relatively small changes in the degree of protein binding caused by competition for binding sites can result in significant changes in plasma concentration of free drug and in the intensity of the clinical response. (49:101)

42. **C.** After a drug gains access to the systemic circulation, it may be metabolized to varying degrees and/or be excreted unchanged. For most drugs and their metabolites, the kidneys are the primary organ of excretion. The presence of a drug and/or its metabolites in the urine must be preceded by the presence of drug in the blood. When an appreciable amount of drug is excreted in the urine, it is often possible to use urinary excretion data, such as cumulative amount of drug in the urine and maximum urinary excretion rate, to evaluate the systemic availability of various drug formulations. (43:424)

43. **D.** Urinary excretion studies require complete urine collection so that the total quantity of drug that is excreted in the urine can be determined. Normal or near normal renal function is also a prerequisite for accurate urinary excretion studies because sufficiently impaired renal function can alter the composition of various body fluids which, in turn, can alter the pharmacokinetic properties of many drugs. Although urinary excretion studies are usually performed on drugs that are primarily excreted unchanged by the kidney, it is not necessary that a drug be completely excreted unchanged by the kidney. (7:155, 594)

44. **C.** Just as shifting the ionic equilibrium in favor of the ionic species reduces the probability that a weakly acidic drug will be absorbed from the alkaline fluids of the intestines, it also reduces the probability that the drug will be reabsorbed from the renal tubules into the blood. Consequently, a greater fraction of drug in the tubules cannot be reabsorbed and will be excreted in the urine. (34:206)

45. **D.** Changes in the amount of drug in the body are directly influenced by the relationship between the rates of absorption and elimination. When the rate of absorption is greater than the rate of elimination, the amount of drug in the body increases with time. When the rate of absorption is less than the rate of elimination, the amount of drug in the body decreases with time. When these rates are equal, there is no change in the amount of drug in the body. Further, if the rate constant for absorption is significantly greater than the rate constant for elimination, the rate of absorption will reach zero much faster than the rate of elimination reaches zero. When this occurs, the rate of change in the amount of drug in the body is a function of the elimination rate only. (29:5)

46. **A.** For a given drug product the time interval between oral administration (zero time) and the time of the peak in the serum concentration versus time curve represents the time required for most of the drug to be absorbed into the blood. The shorter this interval is for a particular drug product, the faster is the rate of absorption for the drug. While the distribution, metabolism, and elimination processes all influence the shape of the curve, we cannot distinguish these processes directly from the curve because they are all postabsorptive phenomena. (43:422–23)

47. **D.** Since the serum concentration-time curve is a quantitative representation of the concentration of drug in the serum over a specific period of time, the area under the curve is a mathematical function of the amount of drug that has entered the blood. The total area under the curve, then, represents the amount of drug that has been absorbed. By comparing the areas under the curves of two formulations of the same drug, we can determine the relative amount of drug that is available from each formulation. (43:422–23)

48. **B.** Although equal areas indicate that the same total amount of drug was made available to the body, the areas alone give no information regarding the rate at which the drugs were made available. Two formulations of a drug can yield radically different serum concentrations versus time curves that have approximately equal areas. It should be emphasized that the concept of bioequivalence involves not only the amount of drug that is available but also the rate at which it becomes available. (43:422–23)

49. **B.** If the area under the respective curves are equal, it can be concluded that the total amount of drug delivered to the body by each dosage form was equal. Since the intravenous administration did not involve an absorption process, the fact that the same amount of drug administered in a capsule formulation delivered the same total amount of drug indicates that the absorption of the drug from the oral capsule was essentially complete. (31:194)

50. **E.** All of these drug characteristics are probably undesirable for a sustained- release dosage form.
A. For a successful sustained-release product, the rate-limiting step must be drug release from the dosage form. If the drug has poor solubility, the dissolution rate may become the rate-limiting step. Then the patient may not absorb the quantity of drug needed for desired blood levels and therapeutic activity.
B. Drugs with very long half-lives do not need to be formulated for sustained release since they inherently will be biologically present for a long period of time. Intelligent dosing, such as every 12 or 24 hours (depending on the actual half-life), will assure sufficient blood levels.
C. The release of drug from most sustained-release dosage forms is subject to individual biological variations. This patient-to-patient variability may result in the release of two or three times the normal dose in a particular patient. Therefore, a dangerous situation may develop if very large amounts of very potent drugs are formulated as sustained-release products.
D. A drug with a very short half-life is also a poor candidate for sustained release. A very large amount of drug would have to be included in the dosage form, and rapid release of the drug would be necessary. (34:157)

51. **A.** The minimum inhibitory concentration is that concentration of antibiotic that prevents the growth of microorganisms. The lower the value, the more effective the antibiotic is in respect to the concentration needed.
B. Binding of drug to plasma protein is generally undesirable since the bound fraction of drug is unavailable for therapeutic activity.
C. Increasing the biological half-life of an antibiotic increases the time that the drug remains in the body.
D. For therapeutic activity, the antibiotic must reach the site(s) of infection. Drug activity also may be required in the blood itself, and drug blood levels are convenient measurements of drug availability, but penetration of the antibiotic into infected tissue is an important characteristic. (34:185)

52. **B.** While in vitro dissolution rate studies may be useful in quality control procedures to evaluate batch to batch variability, they are of little value in bioavailability evaluations unless they can be correlated with in vivo studies in humans. More commonly, when several formulations of a particular drug are found to be biologically inequivalent through studies in humans, in vitro dissolution studies are performed to establish the basis for their inequivalence. (29:57)

53. **C.** If the therapeutic performance and/or toxicity of a particular drug is related to rather specific blood levels of the drug (e.g., digoxin), relatively minor differences in bioavailability may be extremely important. Under these circumstances, small differences observed in the area under the curves, the time of the peak concentration, and the height of the peak concentration may be significant enough to produce a therapeutic failure and/or toxic responses to the drug. (35:23)

54. **D.** Although methods to determine or even estimate the degree of bioinequivalence that is therapeutically significant have not been developed, it should be recognized that such determinations will depend on factors involving the patient, the condition being treated, and the drug itself. For example, the therapeutic response to a given drug can be altered by a patient's emotional attitude, his expectation of specific results, and the environmental conditions in which he is treated. The condition or disease being treated may alter the physical and chemical environment in which the drug must perform. Finally, the potency and/or toxicity of the drug itself make it impossible to establish rigid limits for acceptable difference in bioavailability. For drugs such as digoxin, where relatively small differences in bioavailability can be critical, the margin for acceptable inequivalence must be quite small. (35:23)

55. **B.** While various organs, tissues, and fluids in the body can be considered to be compartments for a specific drug, there is no requirement that a compartment must be an anatomical entity. Any body site or fluid that appears to contain drug may be described as a compartment or ''pool'' in the model. (34:44)

56. **D.** Describing a system as an open model implies that some of the drug is transferred or lost from one or more of the compartments. For example, a fraction of the drug in the blood compartment may be excreted while the drug is equilibrating between the blood and some other body compartment(s). The net result is that complete equilibrium does not occur. A closed, two-compartment model has two rate constants (drug transfer from blood to tissue and drug transfer from body tissue to blood). However, when the model is considered to be open, at least one additional rate constant is needed to describe the resulting drug elimination. (34:17)

57. **C.** For any drug that is eliminated by first-order kinetics, the time required to achieve steady-state plasma levels is dependent only on the biological half-life of that drug in a given individual. As a drug is repeatedly administered in constant dosage and at constant time intervals (that are short enough to preclude complete elimination of the drug), the elimination rate of the drug increases as the concentration of drug in plasma increases. The tendency of a drug to accumulate on repeated dosing is, therefore, balanced by increased amounts of drug being eliminated. Eventually, a steady state will be reached in which the amount of drug absorbed will equal the amount of drug being eliminated. The time to reach steady state corresponds to about four to five half-lives and is more completely described in the following table:

Time (half-lives)	Plasma Concentration (% of steady-state level)
1	50
2	75
3	88
4	94
5	97
6	98
7	99

(6:22; 7:8)

58. **A.** Most drugs have biological half-lives that follow first-order kinetics. A basic characteristic of first-order kinetics is that the rate constants for metabolism or excretion are independent of the intitial drug concentration. That is, a specific fraction of drug will be lost in a given time period. Doubling the drug concentration will not change the rate constant even though the amount of drug lost in a given time period would increase. (34:50)
D. Renal impairment may affect the biological half-life of drugs eliminated by the kidneys. However, the half-life would be expected to increase (not decrease) since the drug remains in the circulation for longer periods of time.
E. Two methods for determining half-life are to determine drug blood levels with respect to time and to quantify with respect to time actual biological responses to the drug. Ideally, the half-life values by each method should be identical. However, they will be identical only when there is a direct and measurable relationship between drug blood concentrations and the biological response. (34:50)

59. **A.** If the biological half-life of a drug is increased in patients with impaired renal function, the time required to reach steady state plasma levels will also be increased because the time required to reach steady state plasma levels is dependent only on the biological half-life of a given drug in a given individual. See answers to questions 35 and 58. (7:8–9)

60. **C.** One half (200 mg) of the administered dose will be eliminated in four hours. Of the remaining 200 mg, one half (100 mg) will be eliminated in the second four-hour period. In the next four-hour span, an additional 50 mg of drug will be lost. Therefore, after 12 hours (or three half-lives), only 50 mg of drug remains. (34:50)

61. **C.** Curve I shows an initial high concentration of drug in the blood with a steadily decreasing concentration. This curve is characteristic of drugs administered by rapid intravenous injection. (34:79)

62. **D.** Any of the above dosage forms could exhibit blood level curves similar to curve II. The first portion of the curve shows an increasing concentration of drug in the blood. This pattern would be expected whenever there is steady drug absorption (i.e., when absorption is greater than elimination) either from the GI tract or from a tissue injection site. (34:80)

63. **E.**
A. Two critical factors that affect the height and shape of a blood level curve are the rates of absorption and rates of elimination. Blood levels increase until a peak occurs where the rate of absorption equals the rate of elimination. Drug absorption will usually continue to occur even after the peak blood level has been reached. However, the blood level curve then begins to descend since the rate of elimination is greater than the rate of absorption.
B. Since most of the factors affecting pharmacokinetics are first order, doubling a drug dose will seldom double the height of a blood level curve. However, the total area under the drug curve can be expected to double since the area under the curve is directly proportional to the dose.
C. The pharmacokinetics of most drugs follow a first-order pattern. Therefore, if the concentration of drug in the blood is plotted as a log function on the Y axis, a straight line will be obtained rather than a curve, as shown.
D. The time factor is a constant variable which is plotted at regular intervals (hours, days, etc.). It is very seldom expressed as a log function. (34:82)

64. **B.** Administration of drugs by intravenous infusion, which implies slow administration into a vein, will result in a plateau effect in respect to drug blood levels.

The resulting steady state levels are directly proportional to the infusion rate.
A. An intravenous push (bolus dose) will give a curve similar to I.
D. The blood level curve for an intrathecal (spinal) injection will probably resemble curve II as the drug slowly diffuses into the blood. (34:95)

65. **C.** The time in which the maximum drug blood level is obtained is independent of the infusion rate. It is dependent only on the biological half-life of the particular drug. The time required to reach the plateau (steady state) is approximately four to five half-lives. (34:95)

CHAPTER 7

Clinical Pharmacy

Many have tried to define clinical pharmacy. A U.S. Supreme Court Justice, when challenged to define pornography, is said to have replied that maybe he could not define it, but that he sure recognized it when he saw it. With this example in mind, we have collected together in this chapter a series of test items which we believe can be called clinical pharmacy because they relate to patients, diseases, drugs, information, and pharmacists.

Directions: Each of the questions or incomplete statements below is followed by five suggested answers or completions. Select the BEST answer in each case.

1. Which of the following drugs is generally considered to be the drug of choice in status epilepticus?
   A. phenobarbital
   B. amobarbital (Amytal®)
   C. phenytoin (Dilantin®)
   D. paraldehyde
   E. diazepam (Valium®) (9:369–70)

2. A syndrome strongly resembling systemic lupus erythematosus (SLE) is an adverse reaction associated with
   A. hydralazine (Apresoline®)
   B. reserpine
   C. diazoxide (Hyperstat I.V.®)
   D. methyldopa (Aldomet®)
   E. guanethidine (Ismelin®) (6:706; 35:348)

3. The antihypertensive effect of guanethidine (Ismelin®) is inhibited by
   A. diazepam (Valium®)
   B. amitriptyline (Elavil®)
   C. hydrochlorothiazide (Hydrodiuril®)
   D. probenecid (Benemid®)
   E. nitrofurantoin (Furadantin®) (8:73; 17:110–12)

4. In terms of its major pharmacological effect metoprolol (Lopressor®) is most similar to
   A. isoproterenol (Isuprel®)
   B. metaproterenol (Alupent®)
   C. guanethidine (Ismelin®)
   D. hydrochlorothiazide (Hydrodiuril®)
   E. propanolol (Inderal®) (10)

5. When dispensing a new prescription for what drug should the pharmacist advise the patient that he may experience a large fall in blood pressure following the first dose?
   A. methyldopa (Aldomet®)
   B. prazosin (Minipress®)
   C. clonidine (Catapres®)
   D. reserpine (Serpasil®)
   E. propanolol (Inderal®) (17:113)

6. The ganglionic blocking agents are not extensively used as antihypertensive agents because
   A. they cannot be administered orally
   B. of their long duration of action
   C. they do not selectively block sympathetic ganglia
   D. their hypotensive effect is unpredictable and slow in onset
   E. both A and D are correct (9:130, 134; 17:100–02)

7. Diazoxide (Hyperstat®) is administered
   A. orally
   B. intramuscularly
   C. by rapid IV injection
   D. by IV infusion
   E. either C or D (17:113)

8. The antihypertensive drug of choice for patients with renal insufficiency is
   A. guanethidine (Ismelin®)
   B. methyldopa (Aldomet®)
   C. mecamylamine (Inversine®)

D. reserpine (Serpasil®)
E. hydralazine (Apresoline®) (17:112)

9. Which of the following antihypertensive agents would probably be the best choice to use in combination with hydrochlorothiazide in a hypertensive patient who is severely depressed?
   A. reserpine (Serpasil®)
   B. hydralazine (Apresoline®)
   C. guanethidine (Ismelin®)
   D. methyldopa (Aldomet®)
   E. clonidine (Catapres®) (7:491–93)

10. Benztropine (Cogentin®) is often given to patients taking the antipsychotic phenothiazines because benztropine
   A. reduces the dose of phenothiazine required
   B. is an anticholinergic drug that reduces the extrapyramidal side effects of the phenothiazine
   C. eliminates the unpleasant GI irritation caused by the phenothiazine
   D. is an antidepressant
   E. reduces gut motility to ensure that the phenothiazine is completely absorbed (17:260, 322)

11. Cholestyramine (Questran®, Cuemid®) will probably interfere with the gastrointestinal absorption of
   A. chlorothiazide
   B. phenylbutazone
   C. phenobarbital
   D. tetracycline
   E. all of the above (6:749)

12. A clinically noticeable drug interaction resulting from the displacement of drug A by drug B from common plasma protein-binding sites is most often seen when
   A. drug A has a high association constant (K) for binding the protein
   B. drug B has a high association constant (K) for binding the protein and is given in large doses
   C. drug B has a low association constant (K) for binding the protein and is given in large doses
   D. drug B is more toxic than drug A
   E. drug B is rapidly absorbed (33b:41)

13. The metabolism of which of the following compounds is altered in patients taking anticonvulsants?
   A. pyridoxine
   B. folic acid
   C. riboflavin
   D. renin
   E. tyrosine (33b:908)

14. When valproic acid (Depakene®) is prescribed for petit mal epilepsy in a patient who is already receiving phenobarbital
   A. the phenobarbital should be discontinued because phenobarbital will inactivate valproic acid
   B. the dose of phenobarbital may have to be decreased because valproic acid will increase phenobarbital blood levels
   C. ethosuximide (Zarontin®) should also be prescribed
   D. the valproic acid should be given in the morning and the phenobarbital should be given at bedtime
   E. the dose of both drugs may have to be higher than usual because each drug enhances the metabolism of the other (17:313)

15. Droperidol (Inapsine®) is a butyrophenone derivative that is used as an
   A. adjunct to anesthesia
   B. antipsychotic alternative to haloperidol
   C. antihypertensive
   D. analgesic
   E. emetic (4:307)

16. A microorganism that is particularly dangerous to the eye is
   A. *Aspergillus niger*
   B. *Bacillus subtilis*
   C. *Escherichia coli*
   D. *Pseudomonas aeruginosa*
   E. *Streptococcus thermophilus* (1:1498)

17. Purulent boils in the ear are usually caused by species of
   A. *Aspergillus*
   B. *Candida*
   C. *Pseudomonas*
   D. *Staphylococcus*
   E. *Streptococcus* (2:220)

18. The treatment of choice for herpes simplex infection of the eyelids and conjunctiva is
   A. thiabendazole (Mintezol®)
   B. idoxuridine (Stoxil®)
   C. amphotericin B (Fungizone®)
   D. bacitracin (Baciguent®)
   E. carbenicillin (Pyopen®) (7:1653)

19. Which of the following antifungal agents is ineffective against *Candida* organisms?
   A. nystatin (Mycostatin®)
   B. clotrimazole (Lotrimin®)
   C. tolnaftate (Tinactin®)
   D. amphotericin B (Fungizone®)
   E. miconazole (MicaTin®) (33b:939–40)

20. Methotrexate has been shown to be of clinical use in the management of
   A. psoriasis
   B. seborrhea
   C. acne
   D. fungal infections of the skin
   E. warts (7:1598)

21. Which of the following immunosuppressant drugs is a folic acid antagonist?
   A. azathioprine (Imuran®)
   B. methotrexate
   C. 6-mercaptopurine (Purinethol®)
   D. cyclophosphamide (Cytoxan®)
   E. nitrogen mustard (33b:684–85)

22. Which of the following agents is *not* administered intravenously?
   A. thiopental sodium
   B. halothane
   C. ketamine HCl
   D. methohexital sodium
   E. all of the above may be administered by the intravenous route (4:291)

23. An important potential complication of corticosteroid therapy is
   A. dissemination of local infection
   B. masking symptoms of an infection
   C. increased susceptibility to infection
   D. all of the above
   E. none of the above (7:1572)

24. A patient for whom you just dispensed a prescription for sulindac (Clinoril®) asks you if he should still take aspirin for his arthritis. You would point out that
   A. he should not take aspirin because aspirin will decrease the effectiveness of sulindac
   B. he should not take aspirin because aspirin will increase the likelihood of sulindac toxicity
   C. he should continue the aspirin because sulindac is intended for combined therapy with aspirin
   D. he should continue the aspirin because sulindac has anti-inflammatory but no analgesic activity
   E. it probably doesn't matter because there is no interaction (47:36–37; 10)

25. Which of the following arylalkanoic acid derivatives might be particularly useful in an arthritic patient who has difficulty remembering to take her medication during the day?
   A. tolmetin (Tolectin®)
   B. fenoprofen (Nalfon®)
   C. ibuprofen (Motrin®)
   D. naproxen (Naprosyn®)
   E. A and C (3:736–40)

26. When dispensing the fluorouracil solution, Fluoroplex®, the pharmacist should give the patient all of the following advice and warnings *except*
   A. apply with a nonmetallic applicator or fingertips
   B. avoid prolonged exposure to sunlight
   C. avoid exposure to ultraviolet light
   D. cover infected area with an occlusive dressing after application
   E. erythema will usually occur after application (4:910–11; 10)

27. Which of the following best describes the condition known as hypoprothrombinemia?
   A. a diminished blood supply to the brain
   B. blood clot formation in a peripheral blood vessel
   C. a reduced capability for blood to clot
   D. a low level of iron in the blood
   E. a decrease in the production of red blood cells by the bone marrow (7:1084)

28. The reversal of anticoagulant-induced hypoprothrombinemia is most rapidly accomplished by the administration of
   A. phytonadione (Aqua Mephyton®)
   B. menadione
   C. menadione sodium bisulfite (Hykinone®)
   D. menadiol sodium diphosphate (Synkayvite®)
   E. fresh blood or plasma

29. A patient complains of a reddish discoloration of his urine. Which of the following drugs would most likely produce such an effect?
   A. Gelusil®
   B. Pyridium®
   C. Gantrisin®
   D. Darvon®
   E. Mandelamine® (7:1650)

30. Clomiphene citrate (Clomid®) is used clinically in the treatment of

A. psoriasis
B. infertility
C. nausea
D. depression
E. dysmenorrhea

31. The in-home early pregnancy test (e.p.t.®) by Warner-Chilcott assays for the presence of
A. estradiol
B. human chorionic gonadotropin
C. progesterone
D. prolactin
E. none of these (10)

32. A positive e.p.t.® is indicated by
A. a blue color in the urine after consuming the tablets
B. a color change on the test paper that has been dipped into the urine
C. a dark donut-shaped brownish ring in the tube
D. the formation of a precipitate in the tube
E. a red color in the urine–test solution mixture (10)

33. The clinical investigation of a new drug consists of four phases. Phase I of the clinical testing involves administering the drug
A. to animals to determine side effects of the drug
B. to animals for toxicity studies
C. by select clinicians to healthy volunteers
D. by select clinicians to patients suffering from the disease
E. by general practitioners to patients suffering from the disease (24:15)

34. Which of the following best describes the common clinical manifestations of hypoparathyroidism?
A. hypocalcemia and hypophosphatemia
B. hypocalcemia and hyperphosphatemia
C. hypercalcemia and hypophosphatemia
D. hypercalcemia and hyperphosphatemia
E. none of the above (6:786–87)

35. Which of the following dyes has been found to be useful in the treatment and control of pinworm infestations in humans?
A. sulfobromophthalein
B. acriflavine
C. pyrvinium pamoate
D. fluorescein
E. methylene blue (6:1029–30)

36. Tubocurarine should *not* be used in patients taking
A. aspirin
B. morphine
C. indomethacin
D. levodopa
E. kanamycin (8:88–89)

37. Myxedema is what kind of state?
A. hypothyroid
B. hypoparathyroid
C. hyperthyroid
D. hyperparathyroid
E. normal parathyroid (17:344–45)

38. A person with normal thyroid function is called
A. myxedematous
B. basal
C. euthyroid
D. hypothyroid
E. none of the above (11:553)

39. Which of the following should *not* be used in patients who are allergic to aspirin?
A. Fiorinal®
B. Darvocet-N®
C. Butazolidin-Alka®
D. Liquiprin®
E. none of the above should be used (10)

40. Which of the following phrases best defines the clinical disorder known as hemosiderosis?
A. a lack of circulating antibodies
B. excessive storage of iron by the body
C. abnormally shaped red blood cells
D. diminished circulating blood volume
E. absence of pigmentation in circulating red blood cells (7:1058)

41. A reversible cholestatic hepatitis with fever and jaundice that may be a specific hypersensitivity to the drug has been observed as an adverse drug reaction in patients taking erythromycin
A. stearate (Erythrocin Filmtab®)
B. ethylsuccinate (Erythrocin Granules®)
C. free base (E-Mycin®)
D. estolate (Ilosone®)
E. gluceptate (Ilotycin®) (7:555; 33b:765)

42. Which of the following sulfonamides is primarily indicated for decreasing intestinal bacterial flora?
A. mafenide (Sulfamylon®)
B. sulfisoxazole (Gantrisin®)
C. succinylsulfathiazole (Sulfasuxidine®)
D. sulfamethizole (Thiosulfil®)
E. sulfamethoxazole (Gantanol®) (32:575)

43. The most important and, perhaps, the only indication for the use of vancomycin (Vancocin®) is in what type of serious infections that do not respond to other treatment?

A. pneumococcal
B. staphylococcal
C. streptococcal
D. gonococcal
E. pseudomonal (17:579–80)

44. Cimetidine (Tagamet®) inhibits gastric acid secretion as a result of what kind of activity?

A. anticholinergic
B. antiadrenergic
C. antihistaminic
D. antianxiety
E. anorectic (42:316)

45. Penicilloyl-polylysine is a substance used to

A. stabilize crystalline penicillin G preparations
B. counteract allergic reactions to penicillin
C. reduce the renal secretion of penicillin
D. skin test patients for penicillin allergy
E. manufacture the semisynthetic penicillins (37:910)

46. A tricyclic amine that is used as an antiviral agent is

A. desipramine (Norpramin®), Pertofrane®)
B. amantadine (Symmetrel®)
C. 5-flourouracil
D. cytosine arabinoside (cytarabine, Cytosar®)
E. idoxuridine (Dendrid®, Herplex®, Stoxil®) (17:592)

47. Assuming that the causative organism in a specific urinary tract infection is equally sensitive to the following antibiotics, which drug would probably be the *poorest* choice?

A. tetracycline HCI
B. oxytetracycline (Terramycin®)
C. methacycline (Rondomycin®)
D. doxycycline (Vibramycin®)
E. rolitetracycline (Syntetrin®) (4:742)

48. Spectinomycin (Trobicin®) is indicated primarily as

A. an alternative treatment for gonorrhea in patients who might be hypersensitive to penicillin or whose gonococci are resistant to penicillin
B. an antibacterial to treat urinary tract infections caused by organisms that are susceptible to gentamycin in patients with impaired renal function
C. a broad-spectrum antibiotic for topical application to protect the injection site in patients on parenteral hyperalimentation
D. an antitubercular drug to be used in combination with ethambutol or rifampin
E. a prophylactic antibiotic in patients with rheumatic heart fever (17:565)

49. The microbiological activity, clinical use, cautions, and dosage of hetacillin (Versapen®) are essentially identical to those of

A. penicillin V (Pen-Vee®)
B. ampicillin (Omnipen®, Penbriten®)
C. carbenicillin (Geopen®, Pyopen®)
D. methicillin (Staphcillin®)
E. oxacillin (Bactocill®, Prostaphlin®) (6:1145; 45:49)

50. The antibiotic tobramycin (Nebcin®) is most closely related both chemically and clinically to

A. chloramphenicol (Chloromycetin®)
B. doxycycline (Vibramycin®)
C. gentamicin (Garamycin®)
D. demeclocycline (Declomycin®)
E. erythromycin (Erythrocin®) (6:1175–76)

51. Isoniazid (isonicotinic acid hydrazide, INH, Rimicon®) is an antitubercular agent. Which of the following statements is correct for isoniazid?

A. cannot be used prophylactically in persons exposed to tubercular patients
B. one of the most potent antitubercular drugs
C. pyridoxine antagonizes the antitubercular action
D. not metabolized in the liver
E. must be used alone; other antitubercular drugs are inhibitory (1:1151; 6:1205; 33b:771; 39:708)

52. The purpose of combined drug treatment in tuberculosis is to

A. delay the emergence of drug resistance
B. reduce the number of organisms that leave the body via the feces
C. increase the tuberculostatic effects of the drugs
D. reduce the duration of active therapy
E. A and C (6:1214)

53. Patients taking the antitubercular drug rifampin (Rifadin®) should be told that the drug

A. may color their urine and sweat orange
B. may cause them to sunburn more easily
C. may produce nausea and vomiting if alcoholic beverages are consumed

D. may cause diarrhea
E. should be swallowed whole (i.e., not chewed) to prevent staining of the teeth (17:571)

54. Chloramphenicol (Chloromycetin®) is indicated primarily in
A. typhoid fever
B. rheumatic fever
C. tuberculosis
D. yellow fever
E. amebiasis (17:554–55; 37:913)

55. A penicillin derivative that is most closely related to ampicillin but has a much greater activity against *Pseudomonas* is
A. methicillin (Staphcillin®)
B. carbenicillin (Geocillin®)
C. nafcillin (Unipen®)
D. dicloxacillin (Dynapen®)
E. oxacillin (Prostaphlin®) (17:548)

56. Kanamycin produces additive toxic effects with
A. polymyxin B
B. streptomycin
C. ethacrynic acid
D. succinylcholine
E. all of the above (35:381)

57. When used to treat susceptible urinary tract infections, which one of the following anti-infective drugs will have its activity increased in an alkaline urine?
A. methenamine mandelate
B. nitrofurantoin
C. tetracycline
D. kanamycin
E. nalidixic acid (35:265)

58. A Fanconi-like syndrome has been associated with the use of outdated and degraded
A. ampicillin
B. doxycycline
C. tetracycline
D. cephaloglycin
E. clindamycin (6:1190)

59. The aminoglycoside antibiotics are
A. bactericidal for a wide range of gram-positive and gram-negative microorganisms
B. suitable for long-term treatment of chronic urinary tract infections
C. metabolized by the liver
D. more effective in urinary tract infections when the urine is alkaline
E. A and D (9:179)

60. The primary clinical advantage of cephamandol (Mandol®) over the older cephalosporins such as cephalothin (Keflin®) is the fact that cephamandol
A. has a wider antimicrobial spectrum
B. is resistant to beta-lactamase hydrolysis
C. is much less protein bound
D. can be given on a twice-a-day schedule
E. is relatively free of side effects (10; 47:44–45)

61. Which of the following cephalosporins is available in both oral and parenteral dosage forms?
A. cephalexin (Keflex®)
B. cephradine (Velosef®)
C. cefamandol (Mandol®)
D. cefazolin (Ancef®, Kefzol®)
E. cephapirin (Cefadyl®) (17:551–52; 47:42)

62. A disadvantage of using cromolyn sodium for asthma is
A. its brief duration of action
B. the development of rebound bronchoconstriction
C. the rapid development of tachyphylaxis
D. the possibility of an initial effect of bronchoconstriction
E. poor GI absorption after administration of the capsule dosage form (3:541–42; 10; 17:336)

63. An asthmatic patient who is currently taking Tedral® tablets (t.i.d.), prednisone 5 mg (q.i.d.), and Medihaler-Iso® (p.r.n.) gives you a prescription for Vanceril® Inhaler. The directions on the prescription are "one inhalation p.r.n. breathing difficulty." The most appropriate action for you to take is
A. fill the prescription
B. consult with the physician advising him that Vanceril® (beclomethasone) is a prophylactic drug that should be taken regularly
C. consult with the physician advising him that the prednisone should be discontinued before Vanceril® therapy is initiated
D. consult with the patient advising him to stop using the Medihaler-Iso®
E. carefully observe the patient for obvious signs of corticosteroid toxicity and consult with the physician if necessary (7:572)

64. A common name for the antidiuretic hormone elaborated by the posterior pituitary gland is

A. norepinephrine
B. renin
C. luteotropic hormone
D. vasopressin
E. secretin (6:855–56)

65. Which of the following is true of lithium carbonate (Eskalith®, Lithane®)?

A. indicated in the treatment of severe manic-depressive psychoses
B. may only be administered by the intramuscular route
C. onset of action occurs within two hours of the first administered dose
D. should be administered with a diuretic to minimize edema formation
E. usually given to adult patients in single daily doses (17:263–64)

66. Patients on lithium carbonate therapy should be advised

A. to drink plenty of water to avoid crystalluria
B. to stop taking the drug if they experience mild side effects
C. not to restrict their normal dietary salt intake
D. not to take the drug during the manic phase of their cycle
E. not to take the drug with food (33b: 867)

67. Hemolytic anemia due to erythrocyte deficiency of glucose-6-phosphate dehydrogenase (G-6-PD) would most likely be precipitated by

A. primaquine
B. ascorbic acid
C. isoniazid (INH®)
D. phenytoin (Dilantin®)
E. gentamicin (Garamycin®) (33a:541)

68. Phentolamine (Regitine®) is used as a diagnostic agent for

A. pheochromocytoma
B. gastric function
C. pituitary function
D. myasthenia gravis
E. glaucoma (17:97)

69. The range of values for clinical laboratory tests reported as normal may vary among different laboratories because of differences in

A. testing procedure
B. individuals examined
C. conditions under which the specimens are routinely collected
D. conditions under which the specimens are preserved
E. all of the above (31:111)

70. The anticoagulant action of heparin is monitored by

A. platelet counts
B. clotting times
C. prothrombin times
D. bleeding times
E. all of the above (17:177; 6:1362)

71. Two hours after receiving his last dose of heparin (9000 units IV), a patient begins bleeding from his gums after brushing his teeth. What is the most appropriate therapeutic action?

A. inject 10 mg of phytonadione (Aqua Mephyton®) intravenously
B. inject 60 mg of protamine sulfate intravenously
C. inject 30 mg of protamine sulfate intravenously
D. swab a small amount of epinephrine 1:100 onto the gum tissue to produce local vasoconstriction
E. wait for the anticoagulant effect to subside (6:1354–55)

72. The best choice of a drug with anticoagulant activity for an ulcer patient using antacids is

A. aspirin
B. dicumarol
C. warfarin
D. either dicumarol or warfarin
E. none of these should be used (26:11)

73. Which of the following would be considered to be a blood sugar concentration within normal limits for a fasting adult?

A. 100 mg/dl
B. 200 mg/dl
C. 300 mg/dl
D. 400 mg/dl
E. 500 mg/dl (1:588, 589)

74. Which of the following drugs can interfere with the diagnosis of pernicious anemia?

A. pyridoxine
B. menadione
C. thiamine
D. ascorbic acid
E. folic acid (4:105; 33b:632)

75. The direct van den Bergh test measures

A. conjugated bilirubin in the blood
B. unconjugated bilirubin in the blood

C. total bilirubin in the blood
D. unconjugated bilirubin in the urine
E. total bilirubin in the urine (16:220; 30:483)

76. A "White Cell Differential Count" is a laboratory procedure that
A. determines the relative proportions of the various white blood cells
B. determines the relative proportions of white cells to red cells
C. differentiates between iron-deficient and folic acid–deficient anemia
D. differentiates immature from mature white blood cells
E. differentiates normal from abnormal white blood cells (36:96)

77. A patient who has recently suffered a myocardial infarction will most likely have elevated serum levels of
A. creatine phosphokinase (CPK)
B. amylase
C. acid phosphatase
D. alkaline phosphatase
E. cholinesterase (31:135)

78. Even though a patient reaches a euthyroid state, his protein-bound iodine (PBI) value will be elevated if he has been treated with
A. desiccated thyroid
B. thyroglobulin
C. sodium levothyroxine (T_4)
D. sodium liothyronine (T_3)
E. all of the above (33a:311)

79. Urine determinations of catecholamines and their metabolites are useful in the diagnosis of
A. primary aldosteronism
B. pheochromocytoma
C. phenylketonuria
D. hyperthyroidism
E. Cushing's syndrome (33b:175)

80. The hematocrit (HCT) measures the
A. total number of blood cells per volume of blood
B. number of red blood cells per volume of blood
C. percentage of red blood cells per volume of blood
D. weight of hemoglobin per volume of blood
E. weight of red blood cells per volume of blood (1:578; 31:119)

81. Which of the following is *not* a white blood cell (or leukocyte)?
A. basophil
B. eosinophil
C. monocyte
D. reticulocyte
E. lymphocyte (36:85)

82. The bromsulphalein (BSP) excretion test is a measure of
A. liver function
B. thyroid function
C. pancreatic function
D. kidney function
E. circulation time (31:138)

83. Which of the following is an important and unique advantage of a decentralized unit dose drug distribution system over a centralized unit dose drug distribution system?
A. decentralized units are less costly to operate
B. messenger or delivery system is not required
C. the need for floor stock drugs is reduced
D. pharmacists are routinely in the patient care area
E. narcotics can be dispensed directly into the medication cart (30:79)

84. A unit dose package always contains
A. one discrete pharmaceutical dosage form (i.e., one tablet, one capsule, one ampule, etc.)
B. solid dosage forms only
C. the exact amount of drug that is to be administered to a patient during one complete nursing shift
D. a single dose of a drug intended to be self-administered by a hospitalized patient
E. the exact amount of drug ordered by a physician in a dosage form ready for administration (35:94)

85. The therapeutic value of electroconvulsive therapy (ECT) is due to the
A. convulsion itself
B. electric current itself
C. antipsychotic medication administered immediately after the convulsion
D. rapid succession of intense pain followed by intense relaxation
E. enhanced memory perception of the event that precipitated the psychosis (37:615)

86. Patients about to undergo electroconvulsive therapy (ECT) are usually given succinylcholine to
   - A. reduce the severity of the central nervous system (CNS) discharge
   - B. modify muscular contractions to prevent injury to the patient
   - C. lengthen the duration of the convulsion
   - D. prevent hyperventilation due to anxiety
   - E. make the patient unaware of the shock (32:139; 37:615)

87. The preferred route of administration of mercurial diuretics is
   - A. IV push
   - B. IM
   - C. SC
   - D. PO
   - E. IV infusion (17:165)

88. The intentional administration of intravenous fluids into subcutaneous tissue is called
   - A. infiltration
   - B. venoclysis
   - C. hypodermoclysis
   - D. hemodialysis
   - E. hemolysis (13:122)

89. Intermittent IV therapy is used to
   - A. avoid anticipated or potential stability or compatability problems
   - B. reduce the potential of thrombophlebitis
   - C. promote better diffusion of some drugs into tissues because of a greater concentration gradient
   - D. A and C only
   - E. all of the above (30:131, 147)

90. Parenterally administered electrolytes are usually ordered in
   - A. equivalents
   - B. milliequivalents (mEq)
   - C. milligrams percent (mg %, or mg/dl)
   - D. millimoles
   - E. micrograms (μg) (13:256)

91. A drug information source that consists of microfiche copies of papers published in medical and pharmaceutical journals is
   - A. *Current Contents/Clinical Practice*
   - B. de Haen Drug Information Systems
   - C. Index Medicus
   - D. International Pharmaceutical Abstracts
   - E. Iowa Drug Information Service (1:62–63)

92. Which of the following is the best example of an automated drug information retrieval system?
   - A. Medlars
   - B. Paul de Haen Drug Card Systems
   - C. Index Medicus
   - D. IPA
   - E. FDA Clinical Experience Abstracts (31:361)

93. Martindale's *Extra Pharmacopoeia* is most similar in content to
   - A. *Facts and Comparisons*
   - B. *Physicians' Desk Reference*
   - C. *National Formulary*
   - D. *United States Dispensatory*
   - E. *United States Pharmacopoeia* (27)

94. Generally, drug literature abstracts are most appropriately used to
   - A. provide the individual requesting the information with written documentation
   - B. provide detailed answers to specific questions
   - C. answer general questions
   - D. provide a rapid response to questions
   - E. identify those articles which are likely to contain the desired information (31:361)

95. Kernicterus is a drug-induced disorder that may occur in the neonate following therapy with which of the following drugs?
   - A. isoniazid (INH®)
   - B. sulfisoxazole (Gantrisin®)
   - C. phenytoin (Dilantin®)
   - D. gentamicin (Garamycin®)
   - E. promethazine (Phenergan®) (44:17)

96. Generally, the presence of impaired renal function or overt renal failure in a patient reduces his requirements for
   - A. all drugs
   - B. drugs that are reabsorbed from the kidney tubules
   - C. drugs that are directly excreted or whose active metabolites are excreted by the kidney
   - D. drugs that are metabolized by the liver but are excreted by the kidney
   - E. C and D (33a:64)

97. A common result of "slow metabolic acetylation" of isoniazid is
   - A. enhanced sensitivity to therapy and toxicity
   - B. peripheral neuropathy that is resistant to pyridoxine therapy
   - C. slow metabolism and reduced therapeutic response

D. slow metabolism and enhanced therapeutic response
E. slow acetylation but normal therapeutic response (33b:919–20)

98. The Limulus test is a rapid in vitro method for
A. testing for specific antibodies
B. pyrogen testing in parenteral solutions
C. determining the pH of blood
D. checking the tonicity of intravenous solutions
E. determining the sterility of intravenous solutions (13:36, 211)

99. Electrolytes should not be added to intravenous solutions of amphotericin B (Fungizone®) because
A. the solution is hypertonic by itself
B. they will precipitate (salt out) the drug
C. they will lower the pH and hasten the decomposition of the drug
D. all of the above
E. none of the above (4:824–26; 17:584)

100. Which of the following enzymes would be elevated in acute pancreatitis?
A. alkaline phosphatase
B. acid phosphatase
C. lactic dehydrogenase
D. creatinine phosphokinase
E. amylase (31:130)

101. The cation most prevalent in the extracellular fluid of the human body is
A. sodium
B. chloride
C. magnesium
D. phosphate
E. potassium (6:754–55)

102. The cation present in the highest concentration in intracellular water is
A. calcium
B. chloride
C. magnesium
D. potassium
E. sodium (13:250)

103. The blood level of which of the following cations would normally rise if a patient became hypophosphatemic?
A. sodium
B. magnesium
C. potassium
D. iron
E. calcium (31:141)

104. Pyrvinium pamoate (Povan®) tablets
A. may cause nausea, vomiting, diarrhea, or dizziness
B. should not be used in patients sensitive to aspirin
C. will usually stain the stools red for several days after treatment
D. should be swallowed whole, without chewing
E. all of the above (4:872; 17:675)

105. Patients who have a history of penicillin allergy should also be suspected of exhibiting a possible allergy to
A. sulfonamides
B. cephalosporins
C. tetracyclines
D. aminoglycosides
E. chloramphenicol (4:712–14; 17:550–52)

106. Which of the following agents is used only in the treatment of gram-positive and gram-negative infections of the urinary tract?
A. nitrofurazone
B. nalidixic acid
C. nitrofurantoin
D. phenazopyridine
E. furazolidone (6:1003, 1008, 1009, 1100)

107. Which of the following agents would be most dangerous to use in a patient already receiving high doses of gentamicin?
A. ethacrynic acid (Edecrin®)
B. tetracycline HCl
C. propantheline bromide (Pro-Banthine®)
D. Hydrodiuril®
E. pentobarbital sodium (8:88)

108. Which of the following would be *most* illogical to use concurrently in a patient?
A. penicillin G and tetracycline
B. penicillin VK and erythromycin
C. tetracycline and erythromycin
D. chloramphenicol and erythromycin
E. all of the above (6:1095, 1104)

109. A patient arriving in a hospital emergency room suffering from severe hypertensive crisis would most likely be treated initially with
A. guanethidine (Ismelin®)
B. methyldopa (Aldomet®)
C. reserpine (Serpasil®)
D. hydrochlorothiazide (Esidrix®)
E. diazoxide (Hyperstat®) (7:862)

110. Which of the following should be considered as part of the initial drug therapy of most hypertensive patients?
   A. reserpine (Serpasil®)
   B. methyldopa (Aldomet®)
   C. a thiazide diuretic
   D. hydralazine (Apresoline®)
   E. guanethidine (Ismelin®) (7:862)

111. Which of the following antihypertensive drugs should be administered by slow intravenous infusion?
   A. diazoxide (Hyperstat®)
   B. clonidine (Catapres®)
   C. hydralazine (Apresoline®)
   D. prazosin (Minipres®)
   E. nitroprusside (Nipride®) (6:715)

112. Food containing tyramine should not be part of the diet of patients taking which of the following antihypertensive agents?
   A. reserpine (Serpasil®)
   B. hydralazine (Apresoline®)
   C. pargyline (Eutonyl®)
   D. methyldopa (Aldomet®)
   E. rauwolfia (Raudixin®) (4:55)

113. Which of the following symptoms would be *least* likely to be exhibited by a patient suffering from diabetes mellitus?
   A. urinary retention
   B. excessive thirst
   C. glycosuria
   D. weight loss
   E. weakness (44:280)

114. Which of the following agents would most logically be given to a patient suffering from hypoparathyroidism?
   A. alpha tocopherol
   B. pantothenic acid
   C. ergocalciferol
   D. nicotinamide
   E. phytonadione (4:260)

115. Which of the following therapeutic agents is specifically contraindicated for use in patients who have bronchial asthma?
   A. propranolol (Inderal®)
   B. quinidine
   C. procainamide (Pronestyl®)
   D. digoxin
   E. chlorpromazine (Thorazine®) (6:552)

116. Which of the following phenothiazines is *least* likely to produce extrapyramidal side effects?
   A. chlorpromazine (Thorazine®)
   B. perphenazine (Trilafon®)
   C. prochlorperazine (Compazine®)
   D. thioridazine (Mellaril®)
   E. trifluoperazine (Stelazine®) (6:170;17:262)

117. Which of the following phenothiazine derivatives has been used in the treatment of Parkinson's disease because of its atropine-like (anticholinergic) effect?
   A. fluphenazine (Prolixin®)
   B. thioridazine (Mellaril®)
   C. ethopropazine (Parsidol®)
   D. perphenazine (Trilafon®)
   E. promethazine (Phenergan®) (6:237)

118. Which of the following potential adverse effects of the phenothiazines is thought to be irreversible?
   A. akathisia
   B. muscular rigidity
   C. tremor
   D. oculocutaneous pigmentation
   E. tardive dyskinesia (17:260–61)

119. Which of the following phenothiazine derivatives is used primarily for its analgesic effect?
   A. methotrimeprazine (Levoprome®)
   B. promethazine (Phenergan®)
   C. carphenazine (Proketazine®)
   D. triflupromazine (Vesprin®)
   E. propiomazine (Largon®) (17:260)

120. A middle-aged female patient is at the prescription counter to pick up her first refill on a chlorpromazine (Thorazine®) prescription. She is also about to purchase a bottle of aspirin which she says is for her fever. She also asks you what you would recommend for a "sore throat" she has had for several days. Having this information you would
   A. tell the patient that she is allergic to chlorpromazine and contact the patient's physician
   B. recommend a cough–cold preparation that does not contain a sympathomimetic
   C. contact the patient's physician and discuss the possibility of chlorpromazine-induced agranulocytosis
   D. tell the patient to see her doctor if her fever and sore throat do not improve in a day or two
   E. inquire about these symptoms the next time the patient comes in to refill the prescription (7:713, 812)

121. A pharmacist should suggest to the patient that suppositories made with what substance as the base be moistened with water before insertion?

A. Carbowax®
B. glycerinated gelatin
C. theobroma oil
D. hydrogenated vegetable oils
E. both A and B (15:268)

122. The expectorant dose of ipecac syrup for a four-year-old child would be approximately

A. 4 drops
B. 8 drops
C. 16 drops
D. 2 ml
E. 5 ml (1:800)

123. Which one of the following cough syrups should *not* be suggested to a diabetic patient?

A. Cerose DM®
B. Conar®
C. Coryban D®
D. Robitussin PE®
E. Trind® (2b:98–106)

124. A pharmacist is telling a young mother about clinical (fever) thermometers. He advises her to report both the degrees of temperature and whether the temperature was taken rectally or orally when she has to call the pediatrician. This is good advice because

A. oral temperature is about 1°F above rectal temperature
B. oral thermometers have degree calibrations which are different from rectal thermometers
C. rectal temperature is about 1°F above oral temperature
D. the normal temperature (marked with an arrow) is 99.6°F on the rectal thermometer and 98.6°F on the oral one
E. the bulb on the rectal thermometer is round and contains more mercury than is in the thin cylindrical bulb of the oral thermometer (1:1806; 15:480)

125. The best emergency advice that a pharmacist could give an individual who has just suffered a minor burn is to

A. apply butter to the burn
B. apply Vaseline® to the burn
C. contact a physician immediately
D. immerse the burn area in warm water followed by cold water
E. immerse the burn area in cold water (2b:335–36)

126. Narrow-angle glaucoma is present in approximately what percentage of the total glaucoma population?

A. 10%
B. 25%
C. 50%
D. 75%
E. 95% (37:88)

127. The miotic effect of pilocarpine after instillation into the eye is observed

A. immediately
B. within one minute
C. within five minutes
D. in 15 to 30 minutes
E. after one hour (4:923)

128. The number 20 in Ocusert Pilo-20® refers to the

A. duration of action of one Ocusert in days
B. strength of the preparation as a percentage
C. strength of the preparation in milligrams
D. rate of release of drug from the Ocusert
E. number of dosage units (Ocuserts) per original container (4:925–26)

129. Which of the following should *not* be administered to a patient being treated for narrow-angle glaucoma?

A. physostigmine
B. pilocarpine
C. phospholine iodide
D. homatropine
E. carbachol (6:529)

130. Advantage(s) of timolol maleate (Timoptic®) over pilocarpine for the reduction of elevated intraocular pressure include(s)

A. longer duration of activity
B. little or no effect on visual acuity or accommodation
C. little or no effect on pupil size
D. no systemic side effects
E. A, B, and C (47:39–40)

131. All of the following drugs are used to treat patients with open-angle glaucoma *except*

A. carbachol
B. cyclopentolate
C. demecarium
D. physostigmine
E. neostigmine (4:926–28, 945; 44:424–25)

132. Epinephrine is a useful drug for lowering intraocular pressure in open-angle glaucoma because it

A. increases outflow of aqueous humor and inhibits the formation of aqueous humor

B. causes miosis
C. causes mydriasis
D. inhibits carbonic anhydrase
E. dilates blood vessels in the eye (17:75–76)

133. Scabies is a contagious skin disease caused by a

A. flea
B. fungus
C. mite
D. protozoa
E. tick (1:1178)

134. Psoriasis is characterized by

A. granulomatous lesions
B. nodules
C. silvery gray scales
D. small red vesicles
E. small water-filled blisters (11:1281)

135. Which of the following is *not* a form of the malaria parasite?

A. gametocyte
B. granulocyte
C. merozoite
D. sporozoite
E. schizont (38:247–48)

136. The forms of prostaglandin currently available for clinical use are used to

A. induce abortion
B. relieve migraine headaches
C. lower blood pressure
D. decrease intestinal motility
E. increase gastric secretions (1:877–78, 6:644, 647, 872; 17:133–34)

137. Which one of the following statements concerning diethylstilbestrol is *not* true?

A. contraindicated in the treatment of senile vaginitis
B. contraindicated for the treatment of breast cancer in premenopausal women
C. contraindicated for the prevention of threatened or habitual abortion
D. useful in the management of cancer of the prostate
E. may be dispensed when a prescription requests stilbestrol (37:438; 5:420)

138. Tamoxifen citrate (Nolvadex®) is indicated primarily for

A. stimulation of ovulation
B. estrogen-dependent neoplasms
C. urinary tract infections
D. rheumatoid arthritis
E. bronchial asthma (46:57–58)

139. Most intravenous anesthetics are barbiturates. An *exception* is

A. ketamine
B. methohexital
C. thiamylal
D. thiopental
E. none of the above (4:298–99)

140. Ideally, an antacid should raise the pH of the stomach contents to a value of approximately

A. 3
B. 5
C. 6.5
D. 7 to 8
E. 9 or above (2b:5–9)

141. Which of the following drugs is used in conjunction with levodopa (Dopar®, Larodopa®) specifically to allow a reduction in the dose of levodopa?

A. pyridoxine
B. alpha-methyldopa hydrazine (carbidopa)
C. tyrosine
D. diphenhydramine (Benadryl®)
E. promethazine (Phenergan®) (10; 33b:895)

142. A patient with Parkinson's disease has been receiving levodopa (1 g four times daily) with fairly good response but excessive side effects. The patient's physician wishes to switch from levodopa to Sinemet®. An appropriate dose of Sinemet® would be

A. one 10/100 tablet daily
B. one 10/100 tablet four times daily
C. one 25/250 tablet daily
D. one 25/250 tablet four times daily
E. four 25/250 tablets four times daily (4:1007–08)

143. A patient is being effectively treated for Parkinson's disease with levodopa. Suddenly, all therapeutic benefits of the levodopa are lost and the adverse effects also disappear. Which of the following facts obtained from a medication history would most likely explain this phenomenon?

A. the patient has forgotten to take two doses of the medication
B. antacids were taken occasionally
C. trihexyphenidyl was added to the drug regimen for one week
D. over-the-counter multivitamins were taken to ward off a cold that winter
E. the patient occasionally drank a little whiskey (17:321)

144. If the patient in the preceding question was especially affected by early morning symptoms of stiffness and rigidity, which of the following anticholinergics might be of value?
A. benztropine mesylate (Cogentin®)
B. trihexyphenidyl HCl (Artane®)
C. ethopropazine HCl (Parsidol®)
D. cycrimine HCl (Pagitane®)
E. procyclidine HCl (Kemadrin®) (6:236)

145. Which of the following drugs is associated with the "gray syndrome" in infants?
A. phenytoin
B. chloramphenicol
C. demethychlortetracycline
D. amphotericin B
E. kanamycin (32:601)

146. Stomatitis refers to an inflammation of the
A. eyelid
B. nasal passages
C. oral mucosa
D. stomach wall
E. tongue (11:208, 633, 654, 1476)

147. An obese individual would most likely be suffering from
A. alopecia
B. hirsutism
C. polyphagia
D. urticaria
E. nystagmus
(11:61, 716, 1068, 1235, 1682)

148. Hypertrophy refers to
A. an abnormal increase in the number of cells in a tissue
B. an enlargement or overgrowth of an organ
C. excessive perspiration
D. increased motor activity
E. excessive sensitivity of the skin
(11:739, 740, 743, 744)

149. Dyspnea refers to
A. difficult or labored breathing
B. difficulty in swallowing
C. impairment of digestive function
D. painful or difficult urination
E. restlessness (11:485, 486, 488)

150. All of the following terms directly relate to body muscles *except*
A. myalgia
B. myocardia
C. myoclonus
D. myopia
E. myositis
(11:1004, 1009, 1010, 1012, 1013)

151. Ischemia refers to
A. a deficiency of blood in a part of the body
B. excessive collection of blood in an area
C. a jaundice condition
D. nodules usually located on the back
E. a red, inflamed patch of skin
(11:759, 799)

152. Stenosis refers to
A. hardening of tissues with a loss of elasticity
B. inflammation of the sternum
C. inflammation of the vertebrae
D. narrowing or stricture of a duct or canal
E. stoppage of blood flow in a part of the body (11:1389, 1457, 1468, 1470)

153. Phlebitis is most closely associated with which type of injections?
A. intradermal
B. intramuscular
C. intravenous
D. subcutaneous
E. both intramuscular and intravenous
(13:400)

154. The incidence of thrombophlebitis may be reduced by all of the following *except*
A. daily replacement of catheters
B. increasing the pH of acid solutions to neutrality
C. inclusion of heparin in the infusion fluid
D. use of plastic cannulas rather than metal cannulas
E. all are correct (i.e., no exceptions)
(13:401)

155. Which of the following diuretics would be least likely to produce a hypokalemic effect in a patient?
A. hydrochlorothiazide (Esidrix®)
B. triamterene (Dyrenium®)
C. chlorthalidone (Hygroton®)
D. furosemide (Lasix®)
E. ethacrynic acid (Edecrin®) (6:837–39)

156. Mannitol is used therapeutically primarily as a/an
A. cardiac stimulant
B. sucrose substitute
C. osmotic diuretic

D. anti-anginal agent
E. plasma expander (6:819–22)

157. The tricyclic antidepressant, imipramine (Tofranil®), has been approved by the FDA for use in

A. enuresis
B. Parkinson's disease
C. hypertension
D. peptic ulcer
E. mild anxiety states (10; 6:178–79)

158. Meperidine (Demerol®) is often administered with which of the following drugs as preoperative medication?

A. isoproterenol (Isuprel®)
B. pentazocine (Talwin®)
C. amobarbital (Amytal®)
D. promethazine (Phenergan®)
E. diazepam (Valium®) (17:260)

159. Analgesic nephropathy may result from chronic use of

A. pentazocine (Talwin®)
B. APC tablets
C. butorphanol (Stadol®)
D. propoxyphene (Darvon®)
E. codeine (33b:883)

160. A potentially serious complication of acetaminophen overdosage is

A. tinnitus
B. hepatotoxicity
C. gastrointestinal ulceration
D. hemorrhage
E. bronchoconstriction (33b:884)

161. Which of the following drugs has been used to treat acute acetaminophen toxicity?

A. cysteamine
B. naloxone (Narcan®)
C. penicillamine
D. thiamine (B_1)
E. Calcium Disodium Versenate (33b:884)

162. A potential problem of using butorphanol tartrate (Stadol®) in a patient who is dependent on codeine is the

A. additive respiratory depression
B. precipitation of narcotic withdrawal symptoms
C. increased tolerance to codeine
D. impaired renal excretion of codeine
E. excessive central nervous system stimulation (47:34–35)

163. The advantage naloxone (Narcan®) has over nalorphine (Nalline®) is

A. its more rapid onset of action
B. its lack of agonistic action
C. its availability as sublingual tablets
D. the fact that it does not have to be reconstituted immediately before use
E. it is not addictive (17:280)

164. Focal convulsions are usually associated with which of the following types of epilepsy?

A. grand mal
B. petit mal
C. Jacksonian
D. psychomotor
E. status epilepticus (37:573)

165. Polcythemia refers to an elevated number of

A. leukocytes
B. erythrocytes
C. thrombocytes
D. reticulocytes
E. granulocytes (36:91)

166. Phenylketonuria (PKU) is a

A. metabolic disorder
B. endocrine disorder
C. vitamin deficiency
D. amino acid deficiency
E. renal disorder (37:990)

167. In treating excessive heparin therapy with protamine sulfate, caution must be exercised to avoid using more protamine than is necessary because

A. protamine sulfate is toxic in small amounts
B. protamine sulfate is also an anticoagulant
C. the production of endogenous heparin will be stimulated
D. the strongly basic protamine will produce alkalosis
E. protamine sulfate is a local anesthetic (6:1355)

168. If a patient on oral anticoagulant therapy experiences mild to moderate bleeding, the desirability of administering vitamin K should be carefully weighed against the underlying need for anticoagulant therapy because

A. the use of vitamin K will make it much more difficult to retitrate the patient on the oral anticoagulant
B. vitamin K will displace the oral anticoagulant from protein-binding sites and

produce a transient increase in anticoagulant effect

C. it requires a minimum of 18 hours for vitamin K to become effective

D. rapid correction of vitamin K deficiency may precipitate thromboembolism

E. if anticoagulant therapy is to be resumed, an oral anticoagulant having a different mode of action will have to be used (6:1360)

169. Which of the following anticoagulants would be the best choice for use in a pregnant patient near the anticipated time of delivery?

A. bishydroxycoumarin (dicumarol)
B. warfarin (Coumadin®, Panwarfin®)
C. heparin
D. phenindione (Danilone®, Hedulin®)
E. diphenadione (Dipaxin®) (6:1352–53)

170. Sodium Heparin USP should always be ordered by the physician in units rather than milligrams because

A. heparin syringes are calibrated in units only
B. it is difficult to measure milligrams accurately
C. a conversion table is difficult to use
D. many different strengths are available
E. the use of a standard units/ml of preparation gives a more reproducible dose (33b:304; 18:229)

171. The prothrombin time of patients on anticoagulant therapy with coumarin or phenindione derivatives will be decreased by

A. clofibrate (Atromid-S®)
B. phenytoin (Dilantin®)
C. heparin
D. phenylbutazone (Butazolidin®)
E. vitamin K (17:171–76)

172. The Schilling Test is useful for the detection of pernicious anemia. This test utilizes orally administered

A. vitamin B_{12} labeled with ^{59}Fe
B. intrinsic factor labeled with ^{59}Fe
C. vitamin B_{12} labeled with ^{57}Co or ^{58}Co
D. red blood cells labeled with ^{59}Fe
E. intrinsic factor labeled with ^{57}Co (1:497)

173. Which of the following drugs is a dopamine agonist used to treat hyperprolactinemia?

A. chlorpromazine (Thorazine®)
B. bromocriptine (Parlodel®)
C. benztropine (Cogentin®)
D. diphenhydramine (Benadryl®)
E. ascorbic acid (10; 17:321)

174. The only insulin preparation that can be given intravenously is

A. globin zinc insulin
B. protamine zinc insulin
C. crystalline zinc (regular) insulin
D. isophane insulin
E. prompt insulin zinc (17:385)

175. Which of the following insulins would be expected to exert the longest duration of action?

A. semilente
B. NPH
C. protamine zinc
D. globin
E. regular (9:320)

176. The most common cause of diabetic ketoacidosis and coma in the diagnosed and treated diabetic is

A. insulin overdosage
B. failure of the patient to utilize insulin properly
C. electrolyte depletion
D. use of the wrong type of insulin
E. excessive physical activity (16:577)

177. Which of the following does *not* give a false positive test for glucose in the urine of patients taking cephalothin (Keflin®)?

A. Benedict's solution
B. Fehling's solution
C. Clinitest®
D. Tes-Tape®
E. none of the above (8:337; 3:1128)

178. A diabetic patient has been taking cephalexin (Keflex®) 500 mg q.i.d. for several days. In order to determine whether or not this drug is interfering with the patient's urine glucose test, a sample of urine is tested by *both* the Clinitest® and Tes-Tape® methods. The results are: 2 + (0.75%) with Clinitest®, 2 + (0.25%) with Tes-Tape®. The most appropriate conclusion from these data is that there is

A. no interference because a two-plus was obtained by both methods
B. a false-positive by the Clinitest® method
C. a false-negative by the Tes-Tape® method
D. an interference, but it cannot be determined which test has been affected
E. absolutely no conclusion can be made (48:284)

179. A mixture of regular insulin and PZI in a ratio of less than 1:1 would be expected to have about the same duration of action as
   A. the individual components of the mixture because there is no interaction
   B. NPH insulin because some free regular insulin will be present
   C. PZI alone because the excess protamine in PZI will bind essentially all of the regular insulin thereby converting it to PZI
   D. lente insulin because lente insulin is made from these components in this specific ratio
   E. PZI alone if neutral regular insulin is used (40:88)

180. What would be the most appropriate method of measuring a 25-unit dose of U100 insulin?
   A. use insulin-diluting fluid to make a stock solution (or suspension) of insulin having a concentration of 25 U/ml
   B. use a standard U100 syringe that is prefilled with 0.75 ml of insulin-diluting fluid
   C. use a special U100 syringe that has a maximum capacity of 50 units
   D. use a U40 insulin syringe
   E. use a standard U100 syringe, but make sure that there are no bubbles in the liquid after it has been drawn into the syringe (44:286)

181. Parenteral tolbutamide (Orinase®) is used to
   A. treat diabetes mellitus
   B. diagnose insulomas
   C. determine allergies to sulfonylureas
   D. differentiate ketosis-prone from ketosis-resistant diabetes
   E. treat diabetic ketoacidosis (17:388; 37:731)

182. Which of the following drugs is particularly useful for the treatment of acute hypoglycemic reactions when oral or intravenous administration of glucose is not possible?
   A. adrenocorticotropic hormone
   B. glucagon
   C. protamine
   D. pancreatin
   E. norepinephrine (17:391)

183. Compared with normal glucose tolerance, the blood glucose versus time curve of a diabetic has
   A. a higher peak that occurs later and decreases more rapidly
   B. a higher peak that occurs at about the same time but decreases more rapidly
   C. about the same height but occurs later and decreases more slowly
   D. a higher peak that occurs later and decreases more slowly
   E. about the same height but occurs earlier and does not level off (40:4)

184. Doses of 6-mercaptopurine (Purinethol®) should be reduced in patients taking allopurinol (Zyloprim®) because allopurinol
   A. enhances the absorption of 6-mercaptopurine
   B. inhibits the renal excretion of 6-mercaptopurine
   C. releases 6-mercaptopurine from protein binding sites
   D. inhibits the metabolism of 6-mercaptopurine
   E. inhibits tubular secretion of 6-mercaptopurine (33b:993; 17:491)

185. When administered concomitantly with allopurinol (Zyloprim®), the dose of 6-thioguanine (6-TG)
   A. should be reduced to 25 to 30% of the usual dose because 6-TG is detoxified by xanthine oxidase
   B. need not be reduced because 6-TG is primarily methylated, not oxidized, in the body
   C. should be reduced to 25 to 30% of the usual dose because 6-TG is metabolized to 6-mercaptopurine
   D. need not be reduced because 6-TG is not a purine analogue
   E. A and C (17:490–91)

186. Assuming that hospital policy permits generic substitution, what amount of ferrous sulfate would be dispensed if Feosol® (200-mg) tablets were prescribed?
   A. 60 mg
   B. 100 mg
   C. 200 mg
   D. 325 mg
   E. 400 mg (18:197; 25:1620)

187. The erythrocytes of an iron-deficient patient would be described as
   A. microcytic and hyperchromic
   B. macrocytic and hypochromic
   C. microcytic and hypochromic
   D. macrocytic and hyperchromic
   E. normocytic and hyperchromic (33b:631)

188. Which of the following agents has been used as an immunostimulant in cancer chemotherapy?

A. prednisone (Deltasone®)
B. 6-mercaptopurine (Purinethol®)
C. chlorambucil (Leukeran®)
D. BCG vaccine
E. Rho(D) immune globulin (RhoGAM®) (17:527)

189. Which of the following is considered to be the drug of choice for treating trigeminal neuralgia (tic douloureux)?

A. niacin (nicotinic acid)
B. pentazocine (Talwin®)
C. isoniazid (INH®)
D. carbamazepine (Tegretol®)
E. phenytoin (Dilantin®) (37:598)

190. Parkinsonism is a disease characterized by four clinical features. Which one of the following is *not* typical of parkinsonism?

A. tremor
B. mental deterioration
C. disturbances of posture
D. bradykinesia
E. rigidity (6:227)

191. Lomotil® should *not* be given to patients taking oral clindamycin because

A. toxic effects of clindamycin may be magnified
B. adsorption of clindamycin will occur
C. an insoluble complex will be formed
D. the rate of hydrolytic destruction of clindamycin in the GI tract will increase
E. none of the above (7:552)

192. An advantage of loperamide (Imodium®) over diphenoxylate (Lomotil®) as an antidiarrheal is the fact that loperamide

A. has a relatively short biological half-life and is, therefore, not likely to be abused
B. has a direct effect on the central nervous system and, therefore, works more rapidly than diphenoxylate
C. does not appear to have opiate-like effects
D. is not a controlled substance
E. can be given parenterally (3:1057–58)

193. Tricyclic antidepressants should be used with extreme caution in patients also taking

A. hydrochlorothiazide
B. methyldopa (Aldomet®)
C. hydralazine (Apresoline®)
D. guanethidine (Ismelin®)
E. furosemide (Lasix®) (6:553)

194. Side effects of cyclobenzaprine (Flexeril®) would be expected to be most similar to the side effects of

A. amitriptyline (Elavil®)
B. dantrolene (Dantrium®)
C. diazepam (Valium®)
D. meprobamate (Equanil®)
E. methocarbamol (Robaxin®) (3:957–58; 17:296)

195. A potential advantage of pemoline (Cylert®) over other stimulant drugs for use in hyperkinesis (minimal brain dysfunction, MBD) is that pemoline

A. can be given on a once-a-day schedule
B. has a more rapid onset of activity
C. has a strong sedative effect
D. stimulates (rather than inhibits) linear growth
E. is not a controlled substance (4:499–500; 33b:868–69)

196. Succinylcholine (Anectine®) should be administered with extreme caution to patients being treated with

A. phospholine iodide
B. pilocarpine nitrate
C. atropine sulfate
D. epinephrine bitartrate
E. phenylephrine HCl (8:206)

197. Drug-induced neonatal jaundice can be treated with

A. intravenous solutions to dilute the bilirubin
B. calcium gluconate
C. phenytoin (Dilantin®)
D. dexamethasone (Decadron®)
E. phenobarbital (6:119; 48:17–18)

198. The initiation of therapy with which of the following agents would be *least* likely to cause therapeutic problems in a patient already taking warfarin (Coumadin®)?

A. phenylbutazone (Butazolidin®)
B. chlorpheniramine maleate (Chlor-Trimeton®)
C. indomethacin (Indocin®)
D. aspirin
E. tolbutamide (Orinase®) (8:27, 43–44)

199. A patient taking pargyline (Eutonyl®) wishes to have you recommend an over-the-counter cold remedy. Which of the following cold remedy ingredients should this patient avoid?

A. chlorpheniramine maleate
B. aspirin
C. caffeine
D. acetaminophen
E. phenylephrine HCl (8:176)

200. A nutritional product is said to contain 18 g of protein, 14 g of carbohydrate, and 10 g of fat in each 100-ml serving. The caloric content of a serving would be

A. 218 kcal
B. 198 kcal
C. 238 kcal
D. 168 kcal
E. 378 kcal (33b:525)

201. Portagen® is a dietary product used to treat patients with

A. milk allergy
B. diabetes mellitus
C. steatorrhea
D. calcium deficiencies
E. kidney failure (2b:211, 216; 33b:462–63)

202. An electrolyte supplement used to replenish electrolytes lost as a consequence of a diarrheal condition is

A. Lytren®
B. K-Lyte®
C. Potassium Triplex®
D. Kaon®
E. Kayexalate® (4:234)

203. Parenteral administration of one liter of 5% dextrose in water provides the patient with approximately how many calories?

A. 100 to 125
B. 170 to 200
C. 400 to 450
D. 800 to 850
E. 1000 (33b:525)

204. Patients who are metabolically incapable of utilizing conventional dietary fats would most likely be given

A. Lipomul-Oral®
B. Lofenalac®
C. Lambase®
D. Nutramigen®
E. Portagen® (2b:211, 216; 33b:462–63)

205. Lofenalac® is a dietary product used in patients suffering from

A. celiac disease
B. pancreatic insufficiency
C. steatorrhea
D. phenylketonuria
E. hyperlipidemia (4:217; 37:990)

206. The therapeutic rationale for adding dicloxacillin (Dynapen®) to carbenicillin (Pyopen®) in the treatment of a mixed urinary tract infection is to

A. permit the reduction of the carbenicillin dose
B. compete with the carbenicillin for penicillinase secreted by resistant gram-negative organisms
C. kill resistant gram-positive organisms which secrete penicillinase
D. displace carbenicillin from plasma protein-binding sites
E. minimize the adverse drug reactions caused by carbenicillin (7:1698)

207. Which of the following would be a good alternative to penicillin V in a pregnant patient allergic to penicillins?

A. demeclocycline (Declomycin®)
B. erythromycin (Ilotycin®)
C. novobiocin(Cathomycin®)
D. tetracycline (Achromycin®)
E. any of the above (7:1732, 1741)

208. Which of the following sulfonamides is best suited for the topical prophylactic treatment of burns?

A. sulfacetamide (Sulamyd®)
B. sulfameter (Sulla®)
C. phthalylsulfathiazole (Sulfathaladine®)
D. sulfamethoxypyridazine (Kynex®)
E. mafenide (Sulfamylon®) (6:1120)

209. Because of the high cost and general unavailability of parathyroid hormone, it is not commonly used to treat postsurgical hypoparathyroid tetany.Which of the following drugs is more commonly used?

A. sodium dextrothyroxine (Choloxin®)
B. dihydrotachysterol (Hytakerol®)
C. methylprednisolone (Medrol®)
D. paramethasone (Haldrone®)
E. calcium gluconate (37:724)

210. Which of the following drugs used in the treatment of gout does *not* affect urate metabolism or excretion?

A. allopurinol (Zyloprim®)
B. probenecid (Benemid®)
C. colchicine

D. sulfinpyrazone (Anturane®)
E. none of the above (33b:691–92)

211. Metyrapone (Metopirone®) is useful as a/an

A. hypnotic
B. diagnostic agent for pituitary function
C. anti-inflammatory steroid
D. thyroid inhibitor
E. analgesic (17:367)

212. In addition to its use as an emetic, antimony potassium tartrate (tartar emetic) is a useful

A. thyroid inhibitor
B. anthelmintic
C. heavy metal chelator
D. topical keratolytic
E. antineoplastic (17:659; 48:50)

213. Nylidrin (Arlidin®) is useful as a/an

A. vasodilator
B. anticholinergic
C. skeletal muscle relaxant
D. anticonvulsant
E. antibiotic (17:91)

214. Which of the following drugs would most likely be best to use in treating grand mal seizures?

A. Paradione®
B. Mysoline®
C. Zarontin®
D. Tridione®
E. Milontin® (7:315)

215. Thiazides may produce

A. reduced glucose tolerance
B. hyperkalemia
C. decreased blood levels of uric acid
D. orthostatic hypotension
E. increased renal excretion of ammonia (17:163)

216. An important advantage of using dopamine (Intropin®) in cardiogenic shock is that dopamine

A. will not cross the blood-brain barrier and cause CNS effects
B. has no effects on alpha and beta receptors
C. produces dose-dependent increases in cardiac output and renal perfusion
D. will not increase blood pressure
E. can be given orally (33b:215, 218)

217. A patient suffering from acute alcohol withdrawal is given 100 mg of chlordiazepoxide (Librium®) intramuscularly. Because of an inadequate response, he is given another 100-mg IM dose in 30 minutes and a third 100-mg IM dose in another 30 minutes. Several hours later the patient becomes extremely ataxic and stuporous. These symptoms (ataxia and stupor) are most likely due to

A. the short duration of activity of the chlordiazepoxide
B. delayed absorption of relatively large amounts of drug
C. the combined effects of alcohol and chlordiazepoxide
D. the ineffectiveness of chlordiazepoxide in acute alcohol withdrawal
E. toxicity of the "special" diluent in which the drug is reconstituted (33b:846–47)

218. A congestive heart failure patient with normal kidney function and no other complicating disorders was discharged from the hospital on digoxin, furosemide, a salt-free diet, and Amphogel® (30 ml q. 2 h) for a recurrent ulcer. A potential problem of the prescribed therapy would be

A. diuretic therapy is unnecessary if the patient is placed on a salt-free diet
B. a low sodium intake will predispose the patient to digoxin toxicity
C. using Amphogel® in combination with a salt-free diet is therapeutically inconsistent
D. antacids interfere with the absorption of digitalis glycosides
E. none of the above (2b:13–16)

219. Dobutamine (Dobutrex®) is a

A. general anesthetic drug
B. hypoglycemic drug
C. beta-adrenergic agonist
D. antihypertensive drug
E. antirheumatic drug (25:1013; 33b; 216–17)

220. A patient for whom you dispensed a new prescription for amitriptyline (Elavil®) four days ago returns to your pharmacy and complains that the drug makes her very sleepy, makes her mouth very dry, and has not helped her depression at all. These symptoms

A. indicate that amitriptyline is not effective for this patient and you should so inform the prescribing physician
B. strongly suggest that an anticholinergic drug is indicated and you should point this out to the prescribing physician
C. are expected effects of early treatment of the drug and you would explain this to the patient

D. indicate early signs of toxicity and you would tell the patient to contact the prescribing physician
E. suggest that the patient is taking her entire daily dose (t.i.d.) at one time (q.d.) (17:295–96; 44:386–88)

221. A diabetic recovering from surgery has his insulin administered continuously by slow intravenous infusion in successive liter bottles of 5% dextrose in water. Urinary glucose tests indicate that blood glucose was markedly elevated after the first liter was administered. Similar testing after the second and third IVs were administered indicated noticeably improved control of blood glucose. Assuming that the insulin dose was initially adjusted for the stress of surgery, the hyperglycemia following the first IV was probably due to

A. inadequte insulin dosing
B. the initial loading of the circulatory system with glucose from the IV dextrose
C. error in quantity of insulin added to the first IV
D. adsorption of insulin on the bottle and tubing
E. rapid diuresis in response to the initial fluid load followed by an apparent hyperglycemia (40:90)

222. A diabetic patient tells you that she is planning a four-week trip to Europe and will not have continued access to a refrigerator in which to store her insulin. What information would you give her?

A. store the insulin in a small styrofoam box which can be kept cold with several ice cubes
B. be sure that insulin is available wherever you travel and purchase a fresh vial at least every third day
C. the insulin will remain stable at room temperature during the time period in which a single vial will be used
D. increase your insulin dose by 10% to account for any deterioration
E. see your doctor to prescribe a mixture of insulins that will be more stable (6:1516; 48:287)

223. The following "sliding scale" insulin coverage is ordered on a hospitalized diabetic

4+	10 units
3+	8 units
2+	6 units
1+	4 units

Four additional units of insulin are added for large amounts of ketones, two units for moderate amounts of ketones, and no additional insulin for small amounts of ketones. The patient's urine testing results are as follows:

	7 AM	11 AM	4 AM	11 PM
Glucose	3+	2+	4+	1+
Ketones	Mod	Sm	Mod	0

The patient's 4 PM insulin dose would be

A. 6 units of regular insulin
B. 12 units of regular insulin
C. 12 units of NPH insulin
D. 42 units of regular insulin
E. 42 units of NPH insulin (33b:529; 44:285)

224. Peripheral veins usually are *not* utilized for the administration of hyperalimentation fluids because

A. hyperalimentation fluids tend to infiltrate surrounding tissue
B. the blood flow in peripheral vessels is not great enough to protect the peripheral vessels from the hypertonic nutrient
C. large-bore needles must be used
D. the hypotonic solution causes local hemolysis
E. the vessels are easily occluded (30:147)

225. Which of the following complications associated with parenteral hyperalimentation (composed of amino acids or protein hydrolysates, glucose, electrolytes, and vitamins) is most likely to occur after the infusions have been discontinued?

A. alkalosis
B. hyperchloremic metabolic acidosis
C. hyperosmotic nonketotic hyperglycemia
D. hypoglycemia
E. pulmonary edema (45:405)

226. Which one of the following provides the greatest number of calories per gram?

A. ethanol
B. fats
C. anhydrous dextrose
D. hydrous dextrose
E. proteins (48:684)

227. Which one of the following TPN solutions does *not* contain a protein hydrolysate?

A. Amigen® (Baxter)
B. Aminosol® (Abbott)
C. CPH® (Cutter)
D. FreAmine II® (McGaw)
E. all contain protein hydrolysates (48:684)

228. Which one of the following ions will *always* present an incompatibility problem when added to TPN formulations?

A. bicarbonate
B. calcium
C. magnesium
D. phosphate
E. sulfate (48:684)

229. The term *essential amino acids* refers to amino acids that:

A. are available only in the form of conjugated proteins
B. are quickly lost during periods of stress
C. can be synthesized by the body only in limited quantities
D. are present in every protein molecule
E. must be supplied by the diet (1:428–29)

230. The level of potassium chloride usually included in each hyperalimentation solution bottle is

A. 2 mEq/l
B. 5 mEq/l
C. 10 mEq/l
D. 40 mEq/l
E. 80 mEq/l (30:148)

Directions: Each set of the following questions consists of several numbered items followed by a list of five lettered words or phrases. MATCH the lettered words or phrases most closely associated with the numbered item. Use each letter once only unless otherwise indicated.

Questions 231 to 235
MATCH the lettered meaning with the corresponding numbered prefix.

231. cata
232. dis
233. infra
234. meso
235. retro

A. apart
B. below
C. backward
D. middle
E. downward (11:271, 452, 781, 940, 1353)

Questions 236 to 240
MATCH the lettered area or organ most closely associated with the numbered root.

236. celi
237. cephal
238. col
239. cor
240. cost

A. abdomen
B. head
C. heart
D. large intestine
E. rib (11:279, 288, 341, 367, 1249)

Questions 241 to 243
MATCH the lettered body area or organ with the most closely related route of parenteral administration.

241. intra-articular
242. intrasynovial
243. intrathecal

A. artery
B. heart
C. joint
D. joint fluid
E. spinal fluid (13:9)

Questions 244 to 248
MATCH the lettered organ which is most closely related to the numbered disease.

244. goiter
245. Klinefelter's syndrome
246. acromegaly
247. Stein-Leventhal syndrome
248. Cushing's syndrome

A. testis
B. thyroid
C. pituitary
D. ovary
E. adrenal cortex (16:480, 507, 532, 600, 615)

Questions 249 to 253
MATCH the lettered portion of the body with the numbered disease which affects it.

249. Adams-Stokes disease
250. Addison's disease
251. Bright's disease
252. Hodgkin's disease
253. myasthenia gravis

A. adrenal glands
B. heart
C. kidney
D. lymph nodes
E. muscles (11:453, 454, 457, 1004)

Questions 254 to 257
MATCH each of the lettered diseases with the numbered description of symptoms.

254. pallor or cyanosis of the fingers or toes
255. enlarged thyroid gland, exophthalmos
256. watery blisters on skin and mucous membranes especially the lips
257. deafness, tinnitus, and dizziness

A. diabetes mellitus
B. Graves' disease
C. herpes simplex
D. Meniere's disease
E. Raynaud's disease

(11:457, 460, 707, 1180)

Questions 258 to 262
MATCH the lettered diagnostic agent with the numbered test most closely associated with it.

258. detection of achlorhydria
259. detection of amyloidosis
260. determination of kidney function
261. estimation of blood volume
262. test for liver function

A. azuresin
B. Congo red
C. Evans blue
D. phenolsulfonphthalein
E. sulfobromophthalein

(1:1214, 1216, 1217)

Questions 263 to 271
MATCH the lettered patient consultation most closely associated with the numbered drug brand name.

263. Pentids®
264. Indocin®
265. Colace®
266. Gantrisin®
267. Dulcolax®

A. take with a large volume of water
B. take with milk, antacids, or meals
C. take on an empty stomach
D. do not take with mineral oil
E. should be taken whole and not broken or chewed

(4:368, 385, 690, 773, 1074, 1080; 10)

268. Achromycin V®
269. Coumadin®
270. Pargyline®
271. Butazolidin®

A. do not ingest aged cheeses, beer, or chianti wine
B. do not use aspirin without the knowledge of your physician or pharmacist
C. do not take with milk or antacids
D. take with milk, antacids, or meals
E. this medication may alter urine color

(4:1035; 6:183, 341, 1338; 10)

Questions 272 to 278
MATCH the lettered drug with the most appropriate numbered statement. A letter may be used once, more than once, or not at all.

272. was occasionally used in brittle ketosis-prone diabetics to stabilize insulin requirements
273. reported to have significant uricosuric properties
274. more slowly absorbed than the other compounds
275. totally metabolized to an inactive form
276. metabolized to compounds having equal or greater hypoglycemic activity
277. has an antidiuretic effect which may be clinically useful in diabetes insipidus
278. may require several weeks to be completely eliminated from the body after the drug is discontinued

A. tolbutamide (Orinase®)
B. acetohexamide (Dymelor®)
C. tolazamide (Tolinase®)
D. chlorpropamide (Diabinese®)
E. phenformin (17:386–90; 33b:531)

Questions 279 to 288
A pharmacist must be fully acquainted with the contents of commonly used reference books so that drug information may be located quickly. MATCH the lettered reference source which should be consulted first for the answer to the numbered request for information. A letter may be used once, more than once, or not at all.

279. comparison of sodium content of a group of antacid liquids
280. discussion of the safe dose range and toxic doses of nitrofurazone
281. list of ingredients in Sominex® tablets
282. list of products manufactured by Paul B. Elder Co.
283. names of several vitamin tablets containing fluoride
284. pharmacological uses of a specific drug with literature references
285. possible identification of a capsule having a distinctive color combination
286. qualitative identification of a drug powder suspected to be imipramine hydrochloride
287. relative costs of several commercial antacid liquids
288. table listing the solubility of drugs in several solvents

A. *Facts and Comparisons*
B. *Handbook of Nonprescription Drugs*
C. *Physicians' Desk Reference*
D. *United States Dispensatory*
E. *United States Pharmacopoeia* and *National Formulary*
(1:61; 2b:3–17, 237; 3:62–64; 5:787; 18:248, 775; 19:1045; 25:1–36, 403–40; 3:988–99)

Questions 289 to 296
The following numbered laboratory tests are followed by a list of lettered organs. MATCH the lettered organ with the numbered laboratory test that provides information regarding the function or condition of the organ. A letter may be used once, more than once, or not at all.

289. creatinine clearance
290. bilirubin
291. protein-bound iodine (PBI)
292. amylase
293. alkaline phosphatase
294. blood urea nitrogen (BUN)
295. lactic dehydrogenase (LDH)
296. thymol turbidity

A. thyroid
B. heart
C. liver
D. kidney
E. pancreas (31:119–44)

Answers and Commentary

1. **E.** When administered intravenously, diazepam (Valium®) is a rapid-acting anticonvulsant that has less tendency to produce respiratory depression than do the barbiturates. Diazepam is effective in grand mal, focal motor, or petit mal status epilepticus. Because of its wide range of effectiveness, intravenous diazepam is probably the drug of choice for initial therapy of status epilepticus. Intravenous phenytoin is an important secondary drug but is likely to decrease heart rate and produce hypotension. Paraldehyde is also an effective drug but, as the barbiturates, is likely to cause respiratory depression. (9:369–70)

2. **A.** Chronic high-dose administration of hydralazine can produce an acute rheumatoid state in approximately 10% of patients taking the drug. A syndrome clinically indistinguishable from disseminated lupus erythematosus develops in a smaller percentage. This lupus-like syndrome (fever, arthralgia, splenomegaly, edema, and the presence of lupus erythematosus cells in the peripheral blood) has also been associated with procainamide. (6:706; 35:348)

3. **B.** Following slow uptake by the adrenergic nerve, guanethidine replaces norepinephrine in storage granules and accumulates in the nerve in place of norepinephrine. After several days of guanethidine administration, the sympathetic nerves no longer contain sufficient amounts of norepinephrine to maintain normal venomotor tone. Tricyclic antidepressants inhibit the uptake of guanethidine into the adrenergic neuron and, thereby, inhibit the antihypertensive effect of guanethidine. (8:73; 17:110–12)

4. **E.** Metoprolol (Lopressor®) blocks beta-adrenergic receptors. It differs from propranolol (Inderal®) primarily in that it has *some* preferential effect on $beta_1$ adrenoreceptors, which are chiefly located in cardiac muscle. This preferential effect is not absolute and, at higher doses, metoprolol also inhibits $beta_2$ adrenoreceptors, which are chiefly located in bronchial and vascular musculature. Although the mechanism of its antihypertensive effect is not known, the drug is indicated in the management of hypertension either alone or in combination with other antihypertensives. (10)

5. **B.** Prazosin is believed to be a direct vasodilator. Side effects of therapy may include a precipitous fall in blood pressure, possibly with tachycardia and loss of consciousness, following the first dose. The drug is equivalent to and a possible alternative to hydralazine (Apresoline®). The initial dose of prazosin is usually 1 mg three times a day and can be slowly increased to 10 mg twice daily. (17:113)

6. **C.** The ganglionic blocking agents are very potent antihypertensive drugs. They block the transmission of impulses in the autonomic nervous system by interfering with the action of acetylcholine at both sympathetic and parasympathetic ganglia. They are not widely used because of the many unpleasant effects that result from their parasympatholytic action (e.g., dryness of the mouth, constipation, impaired visual accommodation, urinary retention, etc.). (9:130, 134; 17:100–02)

7. **C.** Diazoxide has mild antihypertensive effects when given orally, but has a much greater effect when given by rapid IV injection. A slow injection or an infusion of the drug is essentially ineffective, possibly because diazoxide is readily bound to plasma protein. Diazoxide does not cause orthostatic hypotension and appears to lower blood pressure by a direct effect on arterioles. Cardiac output and renal blood flow are increased. (17:113)

8. **E.** Hydralazine does not adversely affect renal function and does not depend on renal function for its inactivation. It is believed that hydralazine initially increases renal blood flow. (17:112)

9. **B.** Hydralazine (Apresoline®) would be the best choice since depression is a principal side effect of reserpine, guanethidine, methyldopa, and clonidine. (7:491–93)

10. **B.** A significant and often dose-limiting side effect of the phenothiazines is the development of extrapyramidal symptoms that closely mimic parkinsonism (e.g., akinesia, muscular rigidity, and tremor). These bothersome side effects can often be controlled by the anticholinergic drugs used to treat Parkinson's disease (e.g., trihexyphenidyl, benztropine, etc.). (17:260, 322)

11. **E.** Cholestyramine is a basic anion exchange resin. This quaternary ammonium chloride compound exchanges the chloride ion for the cholate ion and, therefore, prevents the reabsorption of bile acids. Cholestyramine binds many organic acids, including all of the drugs listed in this question. (6:749)

12. **B.** If drug B has a greater affinity (i.e., higher association constant) for specific protein-binding sites than drug A, it will have a tendency to displace drug A

from these sites. Further, if drug B is given in large doses, the degree of this displacement will increase because there will be a greater amount of drug B competing with drug A for the binding sites. (33:41)

13. **B.** Each of the three major drugs used to treat convulsive disorders (phenobarbital, phenytoin, and primidone) can disturb folic acid metabolism. The hematological problems associated with folic acid deficiency are relatively easy to detect. However, the abnormal mental states that may develop are considerably more difficult to diagnose. These symptoms may range from mild confusion to psychoses resembling schizophrenia. (33b:908)

14. **B.** Valproic acid (Depakene®) is an effective anticonvulsant for petit mal and mixed types of epilepsy. This drug may be as effective as ethosuximide (Zarontin®), which has been considered to be the drug of choice for petit mal epilepsy. However, when valproic acid is added to a phenobarbital regimen, the serum levels of phenobarbital may increase by approximately 25%. Phenobarbital dosage may have to be reduced accordingly. It is not known whether this effect is due to modification of protein binding or metabolism of phenobarbital. (17:313)

15. **A.** Droperidol (Inapsine®) is used as an adjunct to anesthesia to produce sedation and to reduce the incidence of postoperative nausea and vomiting, especially in patients who have received strong analgesics. (4:307)

16. **D.** Penetration of the cornea by *Pseudomonas aeruginosa* will often lead to destruction of the cornea and interior portions of the eye. Blindness may result. *Pseudomonas aeruginosa* is a common contaminant in water. The need for sterility of ophthalmic products is well recognized. (1:1498)

17. **D.** Boils caused by staphylococcus organisms form in the anterior portion of the external auditory meatus. They are usually self-limiting, and treatment with antibiotic ointments will prevent spreading. (2:220)

18. **B.** Idoxuridine is an antimetabolite which inhibits the replication of viral DNA with greater selectivity than that of the host cell. It is used primarily in the treatment of simplex keratitis, a disease of viral origin which can cause blindness. (7:1653)

19. **C.** Although tolnaftate is effective against several types of fungi, it is ineffective against *Candida* organisms. Miconazole, clotrimazole, and nystatin appear to be broad-spectrum antifungal agents with activity against some species of *Candida*. Amphotericin B is also effective in the topical treatment of superficial candidiasis but is more commonly used in the treatment of systemic mycoses. (33b:939–40)

20. **A.** Methotrexate is useful in the treatment of psoriasis since it slows the proliferation of cells that are responsible for the psoriatic symptoms. (7:1598)

21. **B.** Methotrexate inhibits the enzyme dihydrofolate reductase and blocks the conversion of folic acid to tetrahydrofolic acid. Tetrahydrofolic acid acts as a coenzyme in one-carbon transfer reactions.
A., C. Azathioprine and 6-MP are purine antagonists.
D., E. Cyclophosphamide and nitrogen mustard are alkylating agents. (33b:684–85)

22. **B.** Halothane (Fluothane®) is a liquid, nonflammable, volatile anesthetic which is administered by inhalation. (4:291)

23. **D.** Complications of corticosteroid therapy are usually related to the length of time that they have been administered and the dosage used. Corticosteroids suppress normal tissue responses to infection, increasing susceptibility to infection and allowing further dissemination of existing infections. Since tissue responses to infection are suppressed, the subjective, objective, and laboratory manifestations of infection may be masked. (7:1572)

24. **A.** Sulindac (Clinoril®) is the result of several structural modifications of indomethacin (Indocin®). The intent was to retain the potent anti-inflammatory properties of indomethacin while reducing gastrointestinal irritation, CNS effects, and idiosyncratic reactions. One of the structural modifications involves the replacement of the para-chloro substituent of idomethacin with a para-methylsulfinyl (CH_3SO) moiety. Various clinical studies have indicated that this structural change produces an inactive drug (prodrug) which must be metabolized via reduction to the methylsulfide (CH_3S) to produce the active anti-inflammatory metabolite. Aspirin apparently interferes with the bioactivation of sulindac. Although the clinical significance of this interaction has not been determined, patients should be advised not to take aspirin with sulindac. (10; 47:36–37)

25. **D.** Perhaps the most significant difference among these drugs is the prolonged biological half-life of naproxen (13 hours). The other drugs have half-lives ranging from one to three hours. Because of this long biological half-life, naproxen can be administered on a twice-a-day regimen that may be of value to patients who have difficulty complying with more frequent dosing schedules. (3:736–40)

26. **D.** Fluorouracil is used topically for the treatment of multiple premalignant actinic keratoses. It prevents further development of existing lesions and results in cosmetic improvement. If an occlusive dressing is applied, there may be an increased incidence of inflammatory reaction in the adjacent normal skin. However, even without an occlusive dressing, such responses occasionally occur in skin that appeared clinically normal. This is due to the presence of subclinical actinic keratoses. (4:910–11; 10)
E. Normal progression of treatment includes erythema followed by scaling, tenderness, erosion, ulceration, necrosis, and reepithelization. Treatment

should be discontinued at the erosion stage. (4:910–11; 10)

27. **C.** In the condition known as hypoprothrombinemia, there is a reduction in the levels of prothrombin in the blood. This substance is essential in the blood-clotting mechanism. (7:1084)

28. **E.** Rapid reversal of drug-induced hypoprothrombinemia requires the use of a source of prothrombin such as fresh blood or plasma. The various vitamin K derivatives can be used if the situation is not urgent or as a supplement to one of the immediate sources of prothrombin (i.e., blood or plasma). Intravenously administered phytonadione acts more rapidly than the water-soluble menadione derivatives. (17:178–80)

29. **B.** Pyridium is a red dye which commonly causes discoloration of the urine. It is used primarily as a urinary tract analgesic. (7:1650)

30. **B.** Clomiphene citrate (Clomid®) is an agent which has moderate antiestrogenic activity. It has been successfully used to induce ovulation in many patients with amenorrhea and other conditions which cause anovulatory cycles. (6:1435)

31. **B.** Once conception has taken place, the body starts to produce chorionic gonadotropin. The e.p.t.® test assays for the presence of this hormone in the urine. (10)

32. **C.** The e.p.t.® kit consists of a test tube containing chemical reagents and a tube support. Three drops of urine from a morning specimen are placed into the test tube. Special purified water is added and the unit is set aside for two hours. Without touching the unit, the disc present in the tube is then observed. A positive test (pregnancy) occurs if a dark, donut-shaped, brownish ring is present. The test is negative if no ring or just a yellow-red deposit is observed. (10)

33. **C.** Animal work with a new drug has already been completed before the investigational new drug (IND) status is obtained for clinical work. The clinical work consists of phase I, the testing in healthy volunteers to determine drug tolerance, dosing schedules, side effects, and pharmacokinetics data. This is followed by phase II, which involves testing with the drug in actual patients suffering from the disease. Drug efficacy is observed, and side effects not evident in healthy volunteers may occur. Phase III involves administration of the drug to large numbers of patients by private practitioners. Phase IV is the continuous investigation or monitoring of the drug after marketing. (24:15)

34. **B.** Hypoparathyroidism usually presents itself as a disorder of calcium metabolism in which serum calcium levels of the patient decrease while levels of phosphate increase in an inversely proportional manner. Low serum calcium levels may precipitate a potentially serious condition known as tetany. To prevent the development of this disorder and in order to treat the hypoparathyroidism, calcium supplements such as calcium gluconate, calcium carbonate, calcium lactate, or calcium gluceptate are often prescribed. (6:786–87)

35. **C.** Pyrvinium pamoate (Povan®) is a cyanine dye which is administered in single oral doses in the treatment of pinworm infestations. It is not appreciably absorbed from the GI tract. Occupants of an entire household are often treated concurrently to minimize the risk of reinfestation by any single patient. (6:1029–30)

36. **E.** Kanamycin (Kantrex®) and other aminoglycoside antibiotics (gentamicin, neomycin, etc.) may produce neuromuscular blockage which may enhance the blockage of skeletal muscle relaxants such as tubocurarine. (8:88–89)

37. **A.** The hypothyroid state is characterized by marked retardation of mental and physical activity, hoarseness, dry sparse hair, thickening of the skin and subcutaneous tissues, constipation, cold intolerance, anemia, and dry, pale coarse skin. However, because of the nature of the general symptoms, hypothyroidism is usually recognized and treated before all the above symptoms develop. (17:344–45)

38. **C.** (11:553)

39. **A.** Fiorinal® is the only agent listed which contains aspirin. (10)

40. **B.** Hemosiderosis is defined as an increase in stored iron reserves of the body without accompanying tissue damage. Such a condition may be caused by a number of factors, one of which is the prolonged use of excessive doses of iron preparations. (7:1058)

41. **D.** The syndrome generally occurs when erythromycin estolate is given to susceptible individuals for more than 10 to 14 days. It is more common after multiple exposures to the drug, and full recovery usually follows discontinuation of the drug. The reaction is unpredictable, is apparently due to individual hypersensitivity, and has not been observed with erythromycin-free base or with other salts of erythromycin. Since there is no established clinical superiority of the estolate salt, there is little justification for using it in light of the possibility of this potential toxicity. (7:555; 33b:765)

42. **C.** Following oral administration, succinylsulfathiazole is hydrolyzed in the large intestine to yield free sulfathiazole, which is only slightly absorbed from this portion of the GI tract. Succinylsulfathiazole is administered in large doses prior to bowel surgery and for treatment of certain intestinal infections. (32:575)

43. **B.** Vancomycin is bactericidal for gram-positive bacteria in concentrations of 0.5 to 3 μg/ml. Most pathogenic staphylococci are killed by 10 μg/ml or less. However, since vancomycin is highly irritating to tissue, thrombophlebitis following IV injection is

common. Also the drug is ototoxic and nephrotoxic. Consequently, it is used only for serious staphylococcal or enterococcal infections in patients who fail to respond to other drugs. (17:579–80)

44. **C.** Conventional antihistamines, or H_1-receptor antagonists, inhibit histamine-mediated contraction of the bronchi and gut. They do not, however, block the stimulatory effect of histamine on gastric acid secretion. Cimetidine (Tagamet®), a selective H_2-receptor antagonist, blocks gastric acid and pepsin secretion in response to histamine, gastrin, food, distention, caffeine, vagal and other cholinergic agonists. (42:316)

45. **D.** In questionable cases of penicillin allergy, skin tests may be performed using penicilloylpolylysine and the minor determinants. Although a negative reaction to the test does not rule out the possibility of an allergic state, it does indicate that anaphylaxis is not likely to occur on administration of the drug. (37:910)

46. **B.** Amantadine (Symmetrel®) inhibits the replication of certain myxoviruses (e.g., influenza A, rubella, and some tumor viruses) in man. A daily oral dose of 200 mg for two to three days before and six to seven days after influenza A infection may effectively reduce the incidence, severity of symptoms, and the magnitude of the serologic response to the infection. (17:592)

47. **D.** Doxycycline and minocycline are two tetracycline derivatives that have much lower renal clearance rates than their congeners. Consequently, less drug is excreted in the urine. Tetracyclines having higher renal clearance rates would most likely be more effective in treating a urinary tract infection. (4:742)

48. **A.** A single 2-g dose injected intramuscularly is expected to result in a cure rate of 85 to 90%. (17:565)

49. **B.** Hetacillin is rapidly hydrolyzed to ampicillin (and acetone) in the body. Each milligram of hetacillin produces slightly less than one milligram of ampicillin. Since the activity of hetacillin results entirely from its conversion to ampicillin, there is no therapeutic advantage in using hetacillin in place of ampicillin. (6:1145; 45:49)

50. **C.** Tobramycin (Nebcin®) is an aminoglycoside antibiotic having the usual general indications and potential toxicities of this group. It remains to be seen if this drug has advantages over the other available aminoglycosides. (6:1175–76)

51. **B.** Some authorities state that isoniazid is the best tolerated, most effective, and most economical drug used in the management of active TB. However, it is commonly used with a second or even a third drug to reduce the development of resistant strains. Sodium PAS given orally, and streptomycin (IM injection) are used with it. (1:1151)

A. Isoniazid, without other drugs, is used prophylactically; it is given orally over a period of at least one year for this purpose. (33b:771)

C. Pyridoxine administered in doses of 50 mg daily will prevent development of peripheral neuritis, which is the most common adverse reaction caused by isoniazid. Pyridoxine does not interfere with the antitubercular action. (33b:771)

D. Isoniazid is converted to an acetylated form and to isonicotinic acid in the liver. These metabolic products and some unchanged drug are excreted through the kidneys. (6:1205; 39:708)

52. **E.** Combined drug treatment is usually required because of the rapid development of resistant organisms when a single agent is used. It has also been demonstrated that combined drug therapy enhances the tuberculostatic effects of the individual drugs. For example, a combination of streptomycin and isoniazid is significantly more tuberculostatic than either agent used alone. (6:1214)

53. **A.** The color change imparted to urine and sweat is a predictable and harmless side effect. Patients should be told to expect this effect so that they are not alarmed by it. (17:571)

54. **A.** Because of adverse reactions associated with chloramphenicol (e.g., bone marrow disturbances, aplastic anemia), it is currently indicated in only a few types of infections: (1) symptomatic salmonella infections (e.g., typhoid fever), (2) *Haemophilus influenzae* that does not respond to ampicillin, (3) gram-negative bacteremia caused by organisms resistant to other drugs, (4) severe rickettsial infection, (5) bacteroides and other anaerobic infections, (6) meningococcal infections in patients hypersensitive to penicillin, and (7) certain ophthalmic infections (topically). (17:554–55: 37:913)

55. **B.** (17:548)

56. **E.** Kanamycin produces additive neurotoxic and nephrotoxic effects with neomycin, polymyxin B and E, streptomycin, and viomycin. It may rapidly produce irreversible deafness, especially when given IV in combination with other ototoxic drugs such as ethacrynic acid. It may produce respiratory paralysis when used with curariform muscle relaxants such as decamethonium, succinylcholine, and gallamine. (35:381)

57. **D.** Methenamine mandelate, nitrofurantoin, and tetracycline are most active when the urine pH is 5.5 or less (i.e., acid). Drugs such as kanamycin, chloramphenicol, and streptomycin are most active in alkaline urine. On the other hand, some urinary tract anti-infectives, such as nalidixic acid, are not strongly affected by urinary pH. (35:265)

58. **C.** A clinical picture characterized by nausea, vomiting, polyuria, polydipsia, proteinuria, acidosis, glycosuria, and gross aminoaciduria (a Fanconi-like

syndrome) can be produced by anhydro-4-epitetracycline, one of the degradation products of tetracycline. The syndrome is reversible with symptoms disappearing in about one month after termination of consumption of degraded drug. (6:1190)

59. **E.** (9:179)
B. Because of the well-established nephrotoxicity and ototoxicity of the aminoglycosides, they are not suitable for long-term treatment of chronic urinary tract infections. (9:179)
C. After parenteral administration, the aminoglycosides are excreted unchanged in the urine at varying rates. (9:179)

60. **A.** Although cephamandol is somewhat more resistant to beta-lactamase inactivation than the earlier cephalosporins, its primary clinical advantage is a wider spectrum of antimicrobial activity. (10; 47:44–45)

61. **B.** Cefamandol, cefazolin, and cephapirin are not adequately absorbed from the gastrointestinal tract and, therefore, must be administered parenterally for systemic therapy. Although both cephalexin and cephradine are adequately absorbed from the gastrointestinal tract, only cephradine is commercially available in both oral and parenteral dosage forms. Cephalexin is available only in an oral dosage form. (17:551–52; 47:42)

62. **D.** Cromolyn sodium is available as 20-mg capsules (Intal®). The drug is administered by inhalation of the powder through a mechanical inhaler (Spinhaler®). The particle size of the powder is small enough (2 to 6 μm in diameter) to reach the alveoli and may cause an initial bronchoconstriction severe enough to require that isoproterenol be administered concomitantly. It should be emphasized to the patient that the drug is not effective by the oral route and the capsules should not be swallowed. (3:541–42; 10; 17:336)

63. **B.** A major advance in steroid therapy for asthma has been the development of corticosteroid aerosols such as beclomethasone (Vanceril®). Like cromolyn (Intal®), beclomethasone is a prophylactic agent that must be used regularly. It is not suitable for an acute asthmatic attack. The primary value of steroid therapy by inhalation is to avoid systemic side effects in patients who require steroids for the first time or to permit significant dosage reductions of oral steroids in patients on maintenance therapy. (7:572)

64. **D.** Vasopressin, which is a purified preparation of antidiuretic hormone, is used therapeutically in the treatment of diabetes insipidus, a disease of pituitary origin. When administered in any one of a number of available dosage forms (IM, IV, SC, and nasal insufflation or spray), vasopressin will usually reverse the symptom of excessive urination (polyuria) which is the primary symptom of patients suffering from this disease. The initially observed action of the hormone was vasoconstriction, which led to the name vasopressin, which is still the official USP designation. (6:855–56)

65. **A.** Lithium carbonate (Lithane®, Eskalith®) is primarily indicated for treating manic episodes in patients with manic-depressive psychoses. It is administered orally in daily doses of 600 mg to 1.8 g and generally should *not* be administered with diuretics, since retention of lithium may occur. (17:263–64)

66. **C.** The rate of excretion of lithium carbonate is generally independent of urine flow and dietary sodium. However, in the presence of sodium deficiency, the excretion of lithium is markedly decreased and toxic levels can accumulate rapidly. (33b:867)

67. **A.** Glucose-6 phosphate dehydrogenase controls the initial step in the pentose phosphate pathway, bringing about the oxidation of glucose-6-phosphate to 6-phosphogluconate, a reaction coupled to the reduction of NADP to NADPH. Many oxidant drugs, (e.g., primaquine, sulfisoxazole, probenecid) increase the rate of oxidation of glutathione. This increases the intracellular demand for NADPH to maintain glutathione in the reduced form. In patients with a deficiency in erythrocyte G-6-PD, oxidized glutathione accumulates, and, by some unknown mechanism, disrupts erythrocyte membrane integrity with subsequent hemolysis. (33a:541)

68. **A.** Pheochromocytomas are tumors composed of chromaffin tissue that usually originate in the adrenal medulla. These tumors secrete large quantities of epinephrine and norepinephrine into the systemic circulation and cause paroxysmal or even sustained hypertension. They are important to diagnose since they represent a form of hypertension that is surgically curable. Phentolamine is an alpha-adrenergic blocking agent that, when administered IV in a dose of 5 mg, usually causes only a minor fall in blood pressure in patients with essential hypertension. A fall of 35/25 mmHg within two minutes of administration is presumptive evidence of pheochromocytoma. Since false positive tests are fairly frequent, this test must be followed by assays of urinary catecholamines or their metabolites. (17:97)

69. **E.** Not only do individual testing procedures vary from one laboratory to another, but individual population variations in normal ranges may occur because of age, sex, or race. The time of day the specimens are routinely obtained in relation to meals and the time elapsed before the tests are performed on the specimens may influence the results. The conditions under which the specimens are stored (refrigeration, room temperature, etc.) before the tests are performed may also influence the results. (31:111)

70. **B.** The effect of heparin is quantitated by clotting time. The Lee-White method measures the rate at which whole venous blood clots in a glass tube without additives. In the usual therapeutic range, the clotting time is two to three times greater than the normal

(control) value. It is an insensitive and often inaccurate test. With distinction to the bleeding time test (a measurement of the duration of bleeding from an incision in the earlobe or forearm), clotting time does not provide an indication of the ability of small vessels to constrict. (6:132; 17:177)

71. **E.** Because of heparin's brief duration of action, mild hemorrhaging is usually treated simply by withdrawal of the drug. In the presence of severe hemorrhage, the use of a specific heparin antagonist (e.g., protamine sulfate) is imperative. Usually 1 mg to 1.5 mg of protamine sulfate will neutralize 100 units of heparin. However, after the intravenous administration of heparin, the quantity of protamine required decreases rapidly with time. Only 0.5 mg of protamine is required to neutralize 100 units of heparin 30 minutes after IV administration of heparin. (6:1354–55)

72. **C.** The absorption and therapeutic effect of warfarin does not appear to be affected by antacids. However, the ulcer patient should still be monitored for signs of GI tract bleeding.
A. Aspirin's propensity for causing stomach irritation should preclude its use in peptic ulcer patients.
B. Dicumarol's absorption is adversely affected by magnesium and aluminum hydroxides. (2b:11)

73. **A.** Normal fasting blood sugar values for adults are 80 to 120 mg/100 ml (or 80 to 120 mg%). When the fasting blood sugar levels exceed 120 mg/100 ml, diabetes mellitus should be suspected. Levels below 60 mg/100 ml may suggest insulin overdosage, glucagon deficiencies, and (or) hypoactivity of various endocrine glands. (1:588, 589)

74. **E.** The administration of pharmacologic doses (0.4 mg/day or more) of folic acid can stimulate reticulocytosis and improve the anemia associated with vitamin B_{12} deficiency. However, folic acid administration does not prevent the development or progression of the neurological manifestations of pernicious anemia. Consequently, the FDA has restricted the content of folic acid in over-the-counter products to a maximum of 0.1 mg. (4:105; 33b:632)

75. **A.** The van den Bergh test is a serum test that can be used to differentiate between conjugated and unconjugated bilirubin. The direct test is performed in an aqueous medium and is a measure of the more soluble conjugated bilirubin. If alcohol is added, both the conjugated and the less soluble unconjugated bilirubin will react, giving a measure of total bilirubin.The total minus the direct reading will give the indirect level, a measure of unconjugated bilirubin. When the ability of the liver to excrete bilirubin is impaired by obstruction, it is believed that the excess bilirubin in the blood is relatively free of attached protein (i.e., is unbound). When increased levels of bilirubin are due to increased red cell destruction (i.e., hemolysis), it is believed that the bilirubin is attached to plasma protein (i.e., bound). Since the direct van den Bergh test measures the amount of conjugated bilirubin (which is free of attached protein) and the indirect van den Bergh test measures the amount of unconjugated bilirubin (which is tightly bound to protein) a comparison of these values gives some indication as to whether a patient's illness is due to obstruction or hemolysis. (16:220; 30:483)

76. **A.** By revealing the relative proportions of the various white blood cells, the "White Cell Differential Count" may direct the physician's attention toward a particular disease or group of diseases. For example, eosinophils are increased in parasitic infections and allergic conditions; neutrophils are increased in most bacterial infections, basophils may be increased in certain blood dyscrasias, and monocytes are often greatly increased in chronic infections such as tuberculosis. (36:96)

77. **A.** CPK is an enzyme that is found primarily in muscle tissue. It is released into the blood in response to muscle injury. Serum concentrations of CPK are elevated in disorders involving muscle damage such as myocardial infarction, muscular dystrophy, muscle trauma, and muscular inflammation. The normal values may vary with the assay method used. (31:135)

78. **D.** The normal thyroid produces both levothyroxine (T_4) and liothyronine (T_3). Both T_3 and T_4 have biological activity, but only T_4 is measured by the PBI determination. The PBI will be elevated in patients treated with T_4 because relatively more T_4 must be used to achieve a euthyroid state than if a combination of T_3 and T_4 are used. Desiccated thyroid and thyroglobulin contain both T_3 and T_4 and generally maintain PBI within normal limits. (33a:311)

79. **B.** Pheochromocytoma is a rare tumor of the adrenal medulla or of other cells of neural crest origin. The definitive diagnosis of pheochromocytoma is made by measuring the urinary excretion of catecholamines and their metabolites. Urinary excretion of these substances is abnormal in more than 95% of patients having this disorder. (33b:175)

80. **C.** Whole blood treated with anticoagulant is centrifuged in a calibrated hematocrit tube. The volume ratio of the packed red blood cells to total blood volume is determined. The hematocrit is normally 40 to 54 for men and 36 to 47 for women. It gives some indication of both the number and size of the red blood cells present in an individual. (1:578; 31:119)

81. **D.** A reticulocyte is an immature erythrocyte. (36:85)

82. **A.** BSP is a synthetic dye which, when injected (usually 5 mg/kg IV), measures the excretory function of the liver. The dye is removed from the blood by the liver and is excreted in the bile. The normally functioning liver will remove 95% of the dye in 45 minutes. (31:138)

83. **D.** The routine presence of a pharmacist in the patient care area will promote closer communications between the pharmacist and both nurses and physicians. A decentralized system allows the pharmacist to perform clinical activities requiring his presence in the patient care area while maintaining close contact with the drug distribution system. (30:79)

84. **E.** Choice A, known as a single unit package, can be considered a unit dose package only when the physician happens to order that particular amount of drug. (35:94)

85. **A.** Although it is not known precisely why ECT works, it is known that the therapeutic value lies in the convulsion itself rather than the electric current. (37:615)

86. **B.** ECT consists of producing a convulsive seizure by means of a controlled electric current through electrodes placed on the patient's temples. It is useful for many types of depression and certain types of schizophrenia. The electric shock can produce violent muscular contractions that are capable of collapsing a vertebral body or even fracturing a long bone. To minimize this possibility, muscle relaxants such as IV succinylcholine are administered prior to the shock treatment. (32:139; 37:615)

87. **B.** The major limitation of the mercurial diuretics is their poor absorption following oral administration and the gastrointestinal irritation they usually cause. (17:165)

88. **C.** Hypodermoclysis is used on rare occasions in infants or obese patients in whom veins are inaccessible.
B. Venoclysis refers to the administration of solutions by rapid IV injection or infusion. (13:122)

89. **E.** The administration of a drug by intermittent (rather than continuous) intravenous injection is accomplished over a period of minutes (rather than hours). Stability and/or compatibility problems are less likely to occur because the drug does not remain in contact with a large-volume IV fluid for long periods of time. The potential for thrombophlebitis is reduced because the drug is not in constant contact with the blood vessel tissue at the site of the injection. Finally, the greater concentration gradient produced by a more rapid injection may promote better diffusion of some drugs into tissues. (30:131, 147)

90. **B.** The use of the milliequivalent unit takes into consideration the chemical combining capacity of various ionic species. (13:256)

91. **E.** Important papers from leading medical and pharmaceutical journals are microfilmed and sent to subscribers on a monthly basis. The microfiche cards are subdivided into drugs and disease conditions categories. Each paper is cross-indexed and descriptor terms are included to further define the paper's contents. (1:62–63)
A. This weekly publication reproduces the tables of contents from journals devoted to clinical aspects of health care. By perusing this journal, the pharmacist will see the titles of all papers published in specific journals. Then, either the actual journal can be obtained for reading or a reprint request can be sent to the listed author. (1:62)
B. The de Haen Drug Information Systems consists of several specialized services which present data from biomedical journals on file cards. Cards are available on drugs in prospect, drugs in research, drugs in use, new drug releases, etc. (1:63)

92. **A.** The *Med*ical *L*iterature *A*nalysis and *R*etrieval *S*ystem (MEDLARS) is available through the National Library of Medicine. This computer-based information system is usually tied in with medical school libraries and is an excellent source of comprehensive literature searches. (31:361)
D. International Pharmaceutical Abstracts (IPA) is a manual information retrieval system. (31:361)

93. **D.** The *Extra Pharmacopoeia*, better known as Martindale, is probably the most comprehensive, international, one-book reference on drugs and drug products. Its scope of coverage is even more extensive than the *United States Dispensatory*. The Martindale is divided into three parts. The first part consists of monographs on drugs and ancillary substances. Although drugs that are manufactured in the United Kingdom are stressed, generic and proprietary products from many other countries are included. The discussion includes physiochemical data, storage, incompatibilities, uses, doses, and toxic effects. The second part contains a supplementary discussion of new drugs, obsolete drugs, and miscellaneous substances. The third part lists formulas of OTC products sold in the United Kingdom. There is also a directory of worldwide pharmaceutical manufacturers. (27)

94. **E.** Although literature abstracts often appear to provide sufficient detail to answer certain questions, it must be recognized that an abstract may contain statements taken out of context and that supporting detail and/or qualifications for such statements have been excluded. It is the obligation of the individual providing the information to retrieve the entire article to ascertain whether the information he provides is accurate and complete. (31:361)

95. **B.** Kernicterus is a neurological syndrome in which bile pigments are deposited in and damage the basal ganglia in the central nervous system. It may develop in the neonate following therapy with the sulfonamides. Bilirubin is a normal breakdown product of hemoglobin and is generally conjugated in the liver to a water-soluble glucuronide that is excreted in the bile. Because of a deficiency in the enzyme glucuronyl transferase, neonates have a limited capac-

ity to metabolize bilirubin. Sulfonamides are implicated in this disorder because of their ability to displace unconjugated bilirubin from protein-binding sites. Sulfonamides should be avoided in pregnancy near term because these drugs cross the placenta, and by nursing mothers because they are excreted in breast milk. (44:17)

96. **C.** Although the presence of impaired renal function or renal failure does not contraindicate the use of drugs that are directly excreted or whose active metabolites are excreted by the kidney, it does modify the dose required to produce a given therapeutic effect. Renal impairment or renal failure will allow these drugs or their metabolites to accumulate in the blood. Drug accumulation in these situations can be avoided by reducing the dose and/or the dosage schedule of the drug. Careful monitoring of drug concentrations in the blood and of remaining renal function should also be done. (33a:64)

97. **E.** No significant difference in clinical response can be identified between patients who acetylate isoniazid slowly and those who do so rapidly. (33b:920)
B. Although slow acetylators of isoniazid are more likely to develop peripheral neuropathy from the drug, they respond equally well to pyridoxine therapy as rapid acetylators. (33b:919)

98. **B.** The amebocytes or circulating blood cells of the horseshoe crab (Limulus polyphemus) contain a protein that clots in the presence of bacterial endotoxin (pyrogens). When present in solution with pyrogens, the lysate will produce a visible gelatin of the solution within 30 minutes. The Limulus method appears to be more sensitive than the official USP method for pyrogen detection. (13:36, 211)

99. **B.** For systemic use, amphotericin B is available as a colloidal dry powder combined with sodium deoxycholate. The colloidal solution is sensitive to heat, light, low pH, and substances (i.e., additives) that will precipitate the drug. (4:824–26; 17:584)

100. **E.** Amylase is an enzyme secreted by the pancreas that is involved in the breakdown of starches. In certain diseases of the pancreas such as acute pancreatitis, digestive enzymes of the pancreas escape into surrounding tissue, producing pain and inflammation, and into the blood, producing elevated serum levels. (31:130)

101. **A.** The relative concentration of different anions and cations varies considerably between intracellular and extracellular fluids of the body. Intracellular body fluids contain high concentrations of potassium (a cation) and phosphate (an anion), whereas extracellular fluid contains high concentrations of sodium (a cation) and chloride (an anion). (6:754–55)

102. **D.** The usual concentrations of cations in intracellular water in mEq/l are sodium 15, potassium 150, calcium 2, and magnesium 27. Anions include chloride 1, bicarbonate 10, phosphate 100, sulfate 20, and proteinate 63. (13:250)

103. **E.** There is a reciprocal relationship between the concentration of calcium and phosphorus in the blood. For example, hypoparathyroidism is characterized by low serum calcium and high serum phosphorus, whereas hyperparathyroidism is characterized by low serum phosphorus and high serum calcium. (31:141)

104. **E.** Pyrvinium pamoate is usually well tolerated but may cause nausea, vomiting, diarrhea, or dizziness in some individuals. The red vomitus will stain clothing. (4:872)
B. The tablets should not be prescribed for patients who are sensitive to aspirin because of the cross-sensitivity between the chemical, tartrazine, contained in the Povan® tablet coating, and aspirin. Povan® suspension should be used for these patients. (17:675)
C. Patients should be told that their stools may be stained a bright red. (17:675)
D. If the tablets are chewed, the red dye will stain the teeth, mouth, and tongue. The stain cannot be removed; it gradually wears off. (4:872)

105. **B.** Because of the structural similarity between the penicillins and the cephalosporins, cross-sensitivity may be a problem in these patients. Although the possibility exists, relatively few such cross-sensitivity reactions have been reported in the literature. Patients allergic to penicillin should, however, be watched carefully upon initiating cephalosporin therapy. (4:712–14; 17:550–52)

106. **C.** Nitrofurantoin (Furadantin®, Macrodantin®) is used in the treatment of severe urinary tract infections of both gram-negative and gram-positive origin that have proven to be refractory to other agents. (6:1008–09)
A. and E. Nitrofurazone (Furacin®) and furzolidone (Furoxone®) are similar to nitrofurantoin but are used for their topical and local actions respectively. (6:1003, 1100)

107. **A.** Ethacrynic acid (Edecrin®) is capable of producing ototoxicity which would enhance the similar toxicity produced by gentamicin. (8:88)

108. **B.** While combinations of bactericidal and bacteriostatic antibiotics (choices A and B) are to be avoided, they may be used to treat a mixed infection if their spectrum of antimicrobial activity differs. The combination of penicillin VK and erythromycin, however, is irrational since these agents have virtually identical spectrums of activity. Choices C and D may be rational since both are combinations of bacteriostatic drugs which have different mechanisms of action. Such combinations may be used in situations where the offending organism is sensitive to both agents and

where the use of the combination is more effective than using each agent alone. (6:1095, 1104)

109. **E.** Diazoxide (Hyperstat®) is a drug which is administered parenterally only in the emergency treatment of acute hypertensive crisis. It causes a rapid fall in blood pressure which may last from three hours to seven or eight days. (7:862)

110. **C.** A thiazide diuretic should form the basis of antihypertensive therapy since it will potentiate the action of other antihypertensive agents and will in itself often be sufficient to control many cases of mild to moderate hypertension. (7:862)

111. **E.** Sodium nitroprusside is a powerful vasodilator that acts directly on the smooth muscle of blood vessels. Because of its rapid conversion to thiocyanate in the body, the effects of nitroprusside are quite transient. Following termination of the drug infusion, blood pressure begins to rise immediately and reaches the pretreatment level in one to ten minutes. It is extremely important that the blood pressure and the flow rate of the solution be carefully monitored. Although the dose range is quite large, the average adult dose is 3 μg/kg/minute. Nitroprusside is used when short-term, rapid reduction in blood pressure is necessary. (6:715)

112. **C.** Pargyline (Eutonyl®), the only agent listed which is a monamine oxidase (MAO) inhibitor, may interact with pressor amines such as tyramine in some cheeses, wines, beers, etc., to produce a hypertensive crisis which may be life-threatening. (4:55)

113. **A.** Frequent urination (polyuria) is a common symptom of diabetes mellitus. (44:280)

114. **C.** Ergocalciferol or vitamin D_2 is one of a number of active compounds collectively called vitamin D. Administration of vitamin D to a patient suffering from hypoparathyroidism is indicated since it will tend to elevate serum calcium levels and lower serum phosphate levels of the patient to acceptable levels. (4:260)

115. **A.** Propranolol (Inderal®) is used primarily for its ability to block beta-adrenergic activity and is, therefore, useful in treating patients suffering from cardiac arrhythmias and angina pectoris. However, since beta-adrenergic blockage also tends to increase airway resistance, the drug is usually contraindicated for use in patients suffering from asthma or severe allergies. (6:552)

116. **D.** The phenothiazine group of drugs can be subdivided into three groups according to chemical structure: dimethylaminopropyl derivatives (e.g., chlorpromazine), piperazine derivatives (e.g., perphenazine, prochlorperazine, and trifluoperazine), and the piperidyl derivatives (e.g., thioridazine). Generally, the piperidyl group is the least likely to produce extrapyramidal symptoms and the piperazine group is the most likely to do so. (6:170, 17:262)

117. **C.** Although extrapyramidal effects are associated with the phenothiazine derivatives in general, the anticholinergic effect of ethopropazine is great enough to make this drug useful to treat the tremor and rigidity of parkinsonism. (6:237)

118. **E.** Tardive (late-occurring) dyskinesia (involuntary muscular movements) is a drug-induced neurological disorder that appears to be irreversible and unresponsive to drug treatment. It is characterized by involuntary movement of the lips, tongue, or jaw and is commonly observed as a smacking of the lips, rhythmical movement of the tongue, or facial grimaces. This disorder may be due to hypersensitivity of dopaminergic receptors to endogenous dopamine after long-term blockade by antipsychotic drugs.
A. Akathisia is a feeling of restlessness or of compelling need for movement. (17:260–61)

119. **A.** The analgesic properties that are present to a negligible degree in phenothiazines such as chlorpromazine (Thorazine®) are greatly increased in methotrimeprazine (Levoprome®). When administered parenterally, it is nearly as potent as morphine. (17:260)

120. **C.** Monitoring for phenothiazine side effects is best done by close observation rather than routine use of laboratory tests. Although it is a rare side effect, agranulocytosis characteristically occurs within the first eight weeks of phenothiazine therapy. Sore throat with mucosal ulcerations, chills, and fever are among the early symptoms. Phenothiazine-induced agranulocytosis seems to be due to a direct toxic effect on bone marrow cells. It is particularly likely to occur in women over the age of 40. In the case outlined, the physician should be made aware of the patient's symptoms and the possible relationship to agranulocytosis. With early diagnosis and withdrawal of the drug, granulocyte recovery usually takes place in a week or more. (7:713, 812)

121. **E.** Because of their hygroscopic nature, glycerinated gelatin and Carbowax® suppositories may cause a stinging sensation when first inserted. This can be avoided by dipping the suppository into water just prior to insertion. (15:268)

122. **B.** A useful formula for estimating a child's expectorant dose of ipecac syrup is five drops for the first year of age plus one drop for each additional year. The average adult dose is only 1 to 2 ml. The emetic dose is 10 to 30 ml. (1:800)

123. **E.** All of the other listed syrups are known to be sugar-free. Trind® may contain sugar and does contain 15% alcohol, which would contribute calories. While a stabilized diabetic could tolerate the additional calories, the brittle diabetic might not. (2b:98–106)

124. **C.** A satisfactory approximation of the temperature of the internal organs can be made by inserting a

clinical thermometer into either the mouth or rectum. These are both closed cavities with good blood supply. The accepted average oral temperature is 98.6°F with recognition that both individual and diurnal variations regularly occur. The rectum is about 1°F warmer. Rectal and oral thermometers have the same temperature scales and markings, differing only in the shape of the bulb. To avoid the potential confusion and errors in subtracting or adding degrees from readings, physicians prefer that the actual temperature and the method be reported, i.e., 102.5°F, taken rectally. (1:1806; 15:480)

125. **E.** Immediate counteraction to the burn is recommended. Application of cold water will often reduce the severity of the burn. The burn area should be kept in cold water until no further pain is experienced whether in or out of the water. If necessary, a physician may then be contacted. (2b:335–36)

126. **A.** (37:88)

127. **D.** Pilocarpine appears to be well absorbed through the cornea. Miosis occurs in 15 to 30 minutes with maximum reduction in ocular pressure in two to four hours. The duration of miotic action is usually four to eight hours. (4:923)

128. **D.** The Ocusert pilocarpine unit is a relatively new drug delivery system that has a centrally located reservoir of pilocarpine. The Ocusert is placed in the upper or lower cul-de-sac of the eye. Pilocarpine then diffuses across two outer polymeric layers that serve as rate-controlling membranes. The Ocusert is a clear, oval device with a visible white margin to aid in placement and removal. The unit is available in two strengths, Pilo-20 and Pilo-40, for use in chronic open-angle glaucoma. The numbers designate the rate of release of drug, 20 μg/h and 40 μg/h respectively. Each Ocusert unit contains sufficient drug for one week. (4:925–26)

129. **D.** While each of the other choices will produce a constriction of the iris (miosis) and will most likely aid in reducing the patient's intraocular pressure, homatropine will produce mydriasis which will further aggravate the patient's condition and possibly lead to blindness. (6:529)

130. **E.** The usual categories of drugs used to treat glaucoma include cholinomimetics (e.g., pilocarpine), sympathomimetics (e.g., epinephrine), and carbonic anhydrase inhibitors (e.g., acetazolamide). The most widely used cholinomimetic, pilocarpine, is relatively short acting, causes accommodative spasm and miosis. Timolol maleate (Timoptic®), a beta-receptor antagonist, represents a major advance in the treatment of chronic open-angle glaucoma. It is believed to reduce elevated intraocular pressure via its beta-blocking activity. It apparently antagonizes the action of endogenous catecholamines at ocular beta adrenoreceptors. Timolol exerts it maximal effect within one to two hours and maintains significant effects for as long as 24 hours following a single topical dose. There seems to be little or no effect on pupil size, visual acuity, or accommodation. (47:39–40)

131. **B.** Cyclopentolate (Cyclogyl®) is a mydriatic and cycloplegic used for refraction work and ophthalmoscopy. (4:945)
A. Carbachol is used as a replacement when resistance or intolerance to pilocarpine occurs. (4:926)
C. Demecarium is a long-acting anticholinesterase used to treat primary open-angle glaucoma, glaucoma in aphakia, and accommodative esotropia. (4:928)
D. Physostigmine is a short-acting anticholinesterase used in treatment of primary open-angle glaucoma and for emergency treatment of angle-closure glaucoma. (4:927)
E. Neostigmine is similar in action to physostigmine. (44:424–25)

132. **A.** Epinephrine effectively reduces intraocular pressure in open-angle (chronic) glaucoma by both increasing the outflow of aqueous humor from the anterior chamber of the eye and inhibiting the formation of aqueous humor. Because of its mydriatic action (pupillary dilation), epinephrine is contraindicated in narrow-angle glaucoma. Dilation of the pupils may precipitate acute-angle closure. (17:75–76)

133. **C.** (1:1178)

134. **C.** The distinctive lesion is a vivid red macule, papule, or plaque covered by silvery, lamellated scales. Usually the scalp, elbows, knees, and shins are affected first. (11:1281)

135. **B.** A granulocyte (polymorphonuclear leukocyte) is a form of white blood cell.
A., C., D., E. Four species of plasmodium (protozoan parasites) can cause malaria in man. Each has a multistage life cycle requiring two hosts, man, and a mosquito of the genus *Anopheles*. Sporogony, the sexual phase in the mosquito, consists of union of male and female gametocytes and finally the production of sporozoites, which are the form injected into bitten humans. In schizogony, the asexual phase in humans, sporozoites develop into schizonts in tissue cells. Schizonts segment to form merozoites, which invade the red blood cells (erythrocytes), where they become trophozoites, then erythrocytic schizonts, which form new merozoites that are liberated (when the erythrocyte bursts) to invade other erythrocytes. At times, some trophozoites develop into male and female gametocytes which circulate in the blood, available for ingestion by mosquitoes. Antimalarials are sometimes classified in terms of the plasmodial stage which they kill. Quinine, for example, is an erythrocytic schizontocide. (38:247–48)

136. **A.** Dinoprost tromethamine, a solution containing the equivalent of 5 mg of prostaglandin F_2 per milliliter, is available for intra-amniotic administration to induce abortion. (1:877–78; 6:872)

C. PGEs and PGAs are vasodilators, but this property does not seem to be of practical use in reducing hypertension. Analogues may yield valuable antihypertensive drugs, however. (6:647; 17:133)
D. PGs increase intestinal motility. Diarrhea, cramps, nausea, and vomiting are common side effects in patients given prostaglandins for abortion. (6:644)
E. PGE inhibits gastric secretion stimulated by histamine or food and has antiulcer activity. Derivatives may prove therapeutically useful. (6:647; 17:134)

137. **A.** A dose of 0.5 mg of diethylstilbestrol is used in treatment of senile vaginitis in adults. Both vaginal suppository and ointment dosage forms are used.
C. There have been several reports of vaginal adenocarcinoma in young women whose mothers had been treated with diethylstilbestrol to prevent threatened abortion. Diethylstilbestrol is presently contraindicated in all pregnancies. (5:420)

138. **B.** Tamoxifen citrate (Nolvadex®) is a nonsteroidal estrogen antagonist (antiestrogen). It is believed to antagonize endogenous estrogen binding to cytoplasmic receptors. This, in turn, inhibits cellular synthesis of RNA and protein, ultimately resulting in an inhibition or reversal of the growth of estrogen-dependent cells. (46:57–58)

139. **A.** Ketamine hydrochloride is a nonbarbiturate anesthetic that is administered by either intravenous or intramuscular routes. It is used for both diagnostic and minor surgical anesthesia. Commercial products are Ketalar® and Ketaject®. (4:298–99)

140. **B.** Buffering the pH of stomach contents to a pH value of 4 to 5 will result in sufficient neutralization of hydrochloric acid. Higher pHs (above 5) may stimulate the production of more hydrochloric acid, commonly known as "acid rebound." The pH range of 4 to 5 is also high enough to inhibit pepsin production which has been cited as a possible factor in the development of peptic ulcers. (2b:5–9)

141. **B.** Alpha-methyldopa hydrazine inhibits dopa decarboxylase peripherally but does not cross the blood-brain barrier. Inhibiting the peripheral metabolism of levodopa leaves a greater fraction of intact levodopa available to cross the blood-brain barrier where metabolism to dopamine is desired. If a larger fraction of a given dose of levodopa reaches the brain, then a smaller original dose can be used with a reduction in side effects of therapy. This combination of alpha-methyldopa hydrazine (carbidopa) and levodopa is commercially available as Sinemet® tablets. (10; 33b:895)

142. **D.** Sinemet® is a combination product containing carbidopa and levodopa in a ratio of 1:10. Because carbidopa inhibits the peripheral decarboxylation of levodopa, much smaller doses of levodopa can be used. This, in turn, generally reduces the peripheral side effects associated with high doses of levodopa. Dosage levels of levodopa can be decreased by approximately 75%. (4:1007–08)

143. **D.** The administration of pyridoxine even in the small doses (5 mg or more) contained in ordinary vitamin preparations is equivalent to a reduction in dosage of levodopa. Pyridoxine is believed to be a cofactor for the enzyme dopa decarboxylase, which is responsible for the peripheral metabolism of levodopa. The decarboxylated metabolic product cannot enter the brain, which is the desired site of action. (17:321)

144. **A.** While the anticholinergic agents are qualitatively similar in their actions and side effects, a desirable feature of benztropine mesylate is its long duration of action. This property makes the drug very useful as bedtime medication to reduce the early morning symptoms. (6:236)

145. **B.** The gray syndrome occurs in premature and term newborn infants when chloramphenicol is administered during the first few days of life. The syndrome results from the inability of the infant to metabolize the drug because of a deficient enzyme, glucuronyl transferase, which is required to detoxify the drug by changing it to the glucuronide. Symptoms consist of cyanosis, vascular collapse, and elevated chloramphenicol levels in the blood. (32:601)

146. **C.** (11:1476)
A. Inflammation of the eyelid is blepharitis. (11:208)
D. Gastritis is an inflammation of the stomach wall. (11:633)
E. Inflammation of the tongue would be known as glossitis. (11:654)

147. **C.** Polyphagia is defined as an excessive craving for food. (11:1235)
A. Alopecia is baldness. (11:61)
B. Hirsutism is abnormal hairiness. (11:716)
D. Uriticaria is commonly called hives. (11:1682)
E. Nystagmus is an involuntary rapid movement of the eyeball which may be horizontal, vertical, rotatory, or mixed. (11:1068)

148. **B.** (11:744)
A. Abnormal increase in cell number of a tissue is hyperplasia. (11:743)
C. Excessive sweating is hyperhidrosis. (11:740)
D. Increased motor activity (excessive movement) is called hyperkinesia. (11:740)
E. Excessive sensitivity to stimulation is hyperesthesia. (11:739)

149. **A.** (11:486)
B. Difficulty in swallowing is dysphagia. (11:485)
C. Impairment of digestive functioning is dyspepsia. (11:485)
D. Painful or difficult urination is dysuria. (11:488)
E. Restlessness is dysphoria. (11:485)

150. **D.** Myopia is the condition of nearsightedness. (11:1012)
A. Myalagia is pain in a muscle. (11:1004)
B. Myocardia pertains to the heart muscle. (11:1009)
C. Myoclonus is muscular twitching or contraction. (11:1010)
E. Myositis is inflammation of a voluntary muscle. (11:1013)

151. **A.** The deficiency is usually due to a constriction or actual obstruction of a blood vessel. For example, myocardial ischemia is a deficiency of the blood supply to the heart muscle. (11:799)
C. Icterus is a synonym for jaundice. (11:759)

152. **D.** For example, aortic stenosis is the narrowing of the aortic orifice of the heart. Pyloric stenosis is obstruction of the pyloric orifice of the stomach caused by hypertrophy of the pyloric muscle. (11:1470)
A. Sclerosis is generally caused by overgrowth of fibrous tissue. (11:1389)
C. Refers to spondylitis. (11:1457)
E. Refers to stasis. (11:1468)

153. **C.** Phlebitis indicates vein inflammation. It is due to injury to the endothelial cells of a blood vessel, usually the vein at an intravenous injection site. The earliest sign is tenderness at the site. The area around the vein then becomes red, warm, and painful, often with edema and stiffness. In some instances thrombophlebitis occurs. This term implies that a clot (thrombus) has formed in the blood vessel at the site of the inflammation. Breakage of the thrombus from the site of formation may lead to an embolism (i.e., obstruction or occlusion of a blood vessel at some site removed from the site of clot formation). (13:400)

154. **D.** Several papers have indicated that the incidence of infusion phlebitis is greater when plastic cannulas are used instead of metal units. Both the chemical composition and larger size of the plastic cannulas have been suggested as reasons for the increased incidence. (13:401)

155. **B.** Under normal circumstances, diuresis induced by triamterene is accompanied either by no or only slight increase in potassium excretion. However, a sharp reduction in potassium output is observed when triamterene is given with other natriuretic drugs. This potassium sparing action is the rationale for concomitant drug therapy with triamterene. Because of the possibility of inducing serious hyperkalemia, potassium supplements should not be given to patients being treated with triamterene. Spironolactone (Aldactone®) is an aldosterone antagonist which also is used to decrease the potassium loss that occurs secondary to the use of other diuretics. (6:837–39)

156. **C.** Mannitol is usually administered intravenously as a hypertonic 10 to 25% solution (an isotonic solution is about 5.5%). The introduction of a hypertonic solution provokes urine flow. Mannitol solutions have found application in prophylaxis of acute renal failure, in the evaluation of acute oliguria, and for the reduction of the pressure and volume of the intraocular and cerebrospinal fluids. (6:819–22)

157. **A.** Since many patients taking imipramine for depression reported difficulty in urination, it was reasoned that the drug might be of value in treating enuresis. After imipramine was used for enuresis for some years, the FDA approved the use for this purpose in children. It is not recommended for children under six. It is interesting to note that imipramine now is widely used to treat hyperkinetic children without explicit FDA approval. (6:178–79; 10)

158. **D.** Narcotic analgesics and phenothiazines both produce sedation. However, the effect of injecting a mixture of the two (e.g., meperidine and promethazine)is more than additive. It is believed that the analgesic effects of these drugs are also potentiated. (17:260)

158. **D.** Narcotic analgesics and phenothiazines both produce sedation. However, the effect of injecting a mixture of the two (e.g. meperidine and promethazine) is more than additive. It is believed that the analgesic effects of these drugs are also potentiated. (17:260)

159. **B.** Although the occurrence of analgesic-induced nephropathy is controversial, there is some evidence that it may be associated with several analgesics such as aspirin, antipyrine, aminopyrine, and phenacetin. Aspirin alone, however, is rarely associated with nephropathy, even when it is taken in high doses for long periods of time. Phenacetin seems to be the necessary ingredient for nephropathy, regardless of whether it is the sole toxic agent or whether it acts synergistically with aspirin. Since phenacetin does not enhance the analgesic efficacy of APC preparations, it would seem appropriate not to recommend its use. Early in 1980 phenacetin was removed from the Empirin Compound® formulation; the new product is Empirin®. (33b:883)

160. **B.** Acetaminophen hepatotoxicity is being reported more frequently with the increased availability and use of this OTC drug. The hepatic lesion associated with acetaminophen is caused by microsomal enzyme–induced metabolism of the drug to a highly active intermediate metabolite that covalently binds to liver cell macromolecules. This is not a problem when the drug is used in thereapeutic doses because this intermediate metabolite is rapidly inactivated by preferential conjugation with glutathione and is excreted in the urine. When large amounts of acetaminophen are consumed, there is not enough glutathione to inactivate this hepatotoxic metabolite. (33b:884)

161. **A.** See commentary on question 160.
Since it is believed that acetaminophen hepatotoxicity occurs because there is not enough endogenous glutathione to inactivate the toxic intermediate

metabolite, it was reasoned that administering precursors of glutathione, such as cysteamine, might be effective in dealing with this problem. Cysteamine rapidly enters the cells and supplies enough glutathione to inactivate large amounts of the toxic acetaminophen metabolite. The drug has been used successfully when given intravenously in an initial dose of 2 g followed by three subsequent doses of 400 mg at intervals of four, eight, and eight hours. (33b:884)

162. **B.** Butorphanol tartrate is a partial opiate antagonist that is capable of relieving moderate to severe pain. Although it lacks euphoriant effects, the drug has sedative effects and produces mild, non-dose-related respiratory depression. The narcotic antagonist activity of butorphanol can precipitate withdrawal symptoms in narcotic-dependent patients (e.g., cancer patients). (47:34–35)

163. **B.** If nalorphine is administered to patients who have not received narcotics (i.e., after an overdose of barbiturates), its actions are similar to those of morphine and it may intensify respiratory depression. In addition to being more potent than nalorphine, naloxone lacks the agonistic actions common to other narcotic antagonists and will not intensify the respiratory depression induced by non-narcotic drugs. If the ingested drug is not known to be a narcotic, it is safer to administer naloxone. (17:280)

164. **C.** Jacksonian epilepsy consists of a focal convulsion during which consciousness is often maintained. The seizure itself may be motor, sensory, or autonomic in nature. It usually begins in part of a limb or the face as a localized clonic spasm, then spreads in a somewhat orderly fashion. (37:573)

165. **B.** Mild polycythemia is normal in persons who exercise excessively and in persons who live at high altitudes. Polycythemia vera is a disease state in which the rate of red cell production is far greater than normal, even though there is no apparent physiological need for the increased production. It is believed that this disease may result from some sort of tumor of the bone marrow. Phlebotomy whenever the hematocrit rises above 55% may suffice as the only treatment for patients who do not have severe thrombocytosis. Drugs used include busulfan (Myleran®) and radioactive phosphorus, ^{32}P. (36:91)

166. **A.** Phenylketonuria is an inherited metabolic disorder due to the absence of the enzyme phenylalanine hydroxylase, which converts phenylalanine to tyrosine. Phenylalanine accumulates in the blood and, if untreated, leads to mental retardation and schizoid changes, usually in the presence of normal physical growth. Routine testing of newborn infants for PKU is common in the United States. (37:990)

167. **B.** Protamine is a strongly basic substance that combines with the strongly acidic heparin to produce a stable salt and a loss of anticoagulant activity. Because protamine itself possesses anticoagulant properties, it is unwise to administer more than 100 mg of protamine over a short period of time unless it is known that there is a definite need for a larger amount. (6:1355)

168. **A.** Administration of vitamin K_1 (phytonadione) will correct oral anticoagulant-induced bleeding within a few hours. This form of treatment, however, should only be used in severe cases of hemorrhage since the patient may become temporarily refractory to renewed oral anticoagulant therapy. (6:1360)

169. **C.** Although the risk of hemorrhage in the fetus can be minimized by closely monitoring the prothrombin time of the mother, it is probably best to use heparin if anticoagulant therapy is necessary under these circumstances. Since heparin is a high-molecular-weight mucopolysaccharide, it does not cross the placenta. (6:1352–53)

170. **E.** Heparin is not a uniform molecular species and, therefore, should be prescribed in units rather than milligrams. The old equivalence of 100 mg = 10,000 units is a poor approximation because the U.S.P. specifies the potency to be not less than 120 U/mg when derived from lung tissues and not less than 140 U/mg when derived from other tissues. Potency must be within 90 to 110% of what is stated on the label. If a physician orders 100 mg of heparin, it is not clear whether he means 10,000 units, 12,000 units, or some other quantity. (18:229; 33b:304)

171. **E.** Prothrombin time (PT) is a measure of the time it takes for fibrin to gel in plasma after addition of calcium and thromboplastin. The PT of patients on coumarin drugs is prolonged because of the reduced activity of several blood factors. Vitamin K antagonizes the action of these anticoagulants and therefore shortens PT. The other drugs all will increase PT. (17:171–76)

172. **C.** In normal individuals, over 50% of an oral dose of vitamin B_{12} is absorbed from the gastrointestinal tract. This absorption only occurs in the presence of the intrinsic factor of Castle, with which the vitamin must presumably combine in order to pass through the intestinal walls. By means of radioactive cobalt–labeled cyanocobalamin, it has been shown that over half of an oral dose soon appears in the blood. Normally, only a small amount of radioactivity appears in the urine. However, if a large "flushing" dose (1000 μg) of vitamin B_{12} is given parenterally within an hour of the tagged oral dose, the renal threshold for B_{12} is exceeded and radioactivity is observed in the urine. In patients with pernicious anemia, there is a deficiency in intrinsic factor which results in poor absorption of the radioactive B_{12}. Most of the radioactivity in these patients will be detected in the feces. (1:497)

173. **B.** Bromocriptine is an ergot alkaloid derivative that acts on the anterior pituitary gland to suppress prolac-

tin secretion. The drug may be indicated in the treatment of amenorrhea and galactorrhea associated with hyperprolactinemia. It is available as 2.5-mg tablets, and the usual therapeutic dose is one tablet two or three times daily.

A. Chlorpromazine is a dopamine antagonist.

C. Benztropine is an anticholinergic drug.

D. Diphenhydramine is an antihistaminic drug. (10; 17:321)

174. **C.** Insulin injection (regular or crystalline zinc) is used in situations where rapid onset and brief duration of action are desired. It is the only preparation that can be given intravenously, and it is so used in the treatment of diabetic ketoacidosis. In this emergency situation, it is often used in conjunction with subcutaneously administered, longer acting insulin preparations. (17:385)

175. **C.** Protamine zinc insulin exerts an action for as long as 24 to 36 hours. The shortest duration is exhibited by regular insulin, which may act only for six to eight hours. (9:320)

176. **B.** Diabetic ketoacidosis is a direct result of the lack of insulin. The omission of insulin doses or errors in adjusting the insulin dosage in response to changes in food intake or physical activity is probably the most common cause of diabetic ketoacidosis. Other common causes include infections and myocardial infarctions. (16:577)

177. **D.** The glucose oxidase test for the presence of glucose in the urine is apparently not affected by cephalothin. (3:1128; 8:337)

178. **B.** Copper reduction tests are more quantitative measures of glucosuria than are the glucose oxidase tests. It is documented in the literature that the cephalosporin antibiotics *may* cause false positives with copper reduction tests. If the more quantitative copper reduction test is desired for a patient who is taking a cephalosporin (as in the case described), it is useful to determine whether or not the drug is interfering with the test. This can be done by testing a urine sample by both methods. If the resulting percentages of glucose are the same (e.g., Clinitest® 1+ or 0.5% and Tes-Tape® 3+ or 0.5%) then it is reasonable to conclude that there is no interference. If the percentage is higher by the Clinitest® method, it is likely that the cephalexin is causing a false-positive test. (48:284)

179. **C.** (40:88)

180. **C.** There is a commercially available U100 syringe which measures a maximum of 50 units. This syringe is approximately the same length as the standard 1-ml U100 syringe but has a smaller inside diameter and, consequently, has a capacity of 0.5 ml. It is calibrated in one-unit increments to a maximum of 50 units. This syringe makes it possible for the patient to measure small amounts of insulin with greater accuracy. (44:286)

181. **B.** Sodium tolbutamide (Orinase®) is available for intravenous use in the diagnosis of islet-cell adenomas and borderline abnormalities of glucose tolerance. One gram of sodium tolbutamide, diluted with 20 ml of diluent, is administered intravenously over a two-minute period. Most patients with insulin-producing tumors of the pancreas will respond with profound and prolonged hypoglycemia. (17:388; 37:731)

182. **B.** The usual method of treating an acute hypoglycemic reaction is to give glucose orally, or, in unconscious patients, intravenously in concentrated solutions. If, however, these routes cannot be used, 0.5 to 1 mg of glucagon may be given subcutaneously or intramuscularly as well as intravenously. Glucagon is an endogenous hormone produced by the alpha cells of the pancreatic islets of Langerhans. Glucagon increases blood glucose by stimulating hepatic gluconeogenesis and glycogenolysis. (17:391)

183. **D.** Three parameters of significance in a glucose tolerance curve are: the peak concentration of glucose in the blood, the time required for this peak to occur, and the rate at which the blood glucose level declines with time. In an individual who definitely has diabetes mellitus, the blood glucose peak is higher, occurs later, and declines more slowly than a corresponding blood glucose curve for a normal individual. This is illustrated in Fig. 1. (40:4)

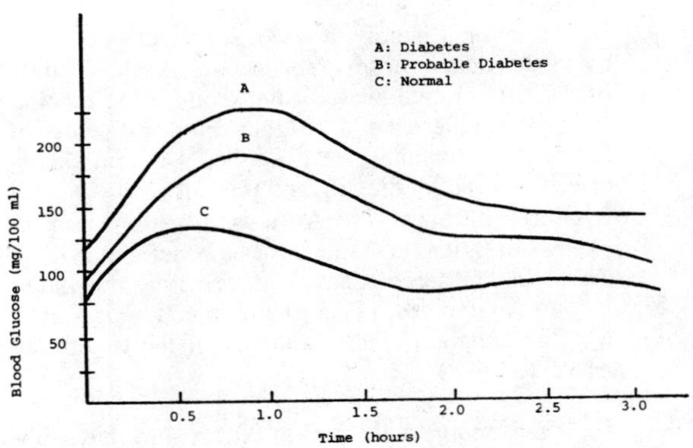

Figure 1. Typical Glucose Tolerance Curves

184. **D.** Since 6-mercaptopurine is metabolized by the enzyme xanthine oxidase, concomitant administration of allopurinol, which is a xanthine oxidase inhibitor, will decrease the rate of metabolism of 6-mercaptopurine. This will potentiate the effects and toxicity of 6-MP unless the dose of 6-MP is reduced to 25 to 30% of its usual therapeutic level. (17:491; 33b:993)

185. **B.** Although 6-TG is a purine analogue (as is 6-mercaptopurine), it is not primarily detoxified by xanthine oxidase as is 6-TG. Because so much of 6-TG is excreted as the methylated metabolite, the dose of 6-TG need not be reduced when given con-

comitantly with xanthine oxidase inhibitors (e.g., allopurinol). (17:490–91)

186. **D.** Feosol® tablets are available as dried ferrous sulfate ($FeSO_4 \cdot 2\ H_2O$) in a 200-mg strength. This quantity of dried ferrous sulfate contains 65 mg of elemental iron. This is considered to be equivalent to 325 mg ferrous sulfate ($FeSO_4 \cdot 7\ H_2O$), which also contains 65 mg of elemental iron. (18:197; 25:1620)

187. **C.** In the iron deficient state, the iron storage compartment becomes depleted. This is followed by a reduction in plasma transferrin saturation. Subsequently the number and size of the red cells as well as their hemoglobin content will be decreased. (33b:631)

188. **D.** Bacillus Calmette-Guerin (BCG) vaccine is a viable strain of *Mycobacterium bovis* which has been used for immunization against tuberculosis. More recently, it has been used as a nonspecific adjuvant or immunostimulant in cancer chemotherapy. A possible mode of action is the activation of macrophages to make them more effective killer cells in conjunction with lymphoid cells. Macrophage activation with BCG also appears to increase the rate of clearance of immune complexes (e.g., antibody-soluble tumor antigen) from the blood. (17:527)
A., B., C., E. These drugs are useful immunosuppressants in cancer chemotherapy.

189. **D.** Trigeminal neuralgia is a disorder characterized by sudden attacks of severe pain along the distribution of the fifth cranial nerve. Attacks are often precipitated by stimulation of a "trigger zone" in the area of the pain. Carbamazepine (Tegretol®) is remarkably effective in both relieving and preventing the pain of trigeminal neuralgia. Anticonvulsants such as phenytoin (Dilantin®) may also be beneficial in some cases. Other drugs that have been effective are vitamin B_{12} in massive doses (1 mg) and injection of alcohol into the ganglion or the branches of the trigerminal nerve. (37:598)

190. **B.** Aged people with parkinsonism may have impairment of memory and judgment or have mental disturbances due to other disease states or social isolation, but not caused by the disease per se.
A. Tremor is a rhythmical alternating contraction of a given muscle group and its antagonist.
C. Positive disturbances include difficulty in maintaining an upright position of the trunk while standing or walking. Also retropulsion (tendency to walk backward) or festination (an involuntary increase or hastening in gait, generally in a stooped position) may be present.
D. Bradykinesia is slow or retarded movement. In parkinsonism, there is diminished spontaneous movement, loss of normal associative movement, and slowness in initiation of all voluntary movements.
E. Rigidity is an increased muscle tone that is resistant to passive movement of an extremity. (6:227)

191. **A.** The development of inflammatory conditions of the colon (e.g., nonspecific colitis or a more severe pseudomembranous colitis) has been associated with antibiotic therapy. Although many antibiotics have been implicated, there have been a disproportionate number of reports specifically involving clindamycin and lincomycin. Colitis has been associated with both oral and parenteral administration of these drugs and no clear predisposing conditions have been identified. Antimotility drugs (e.g., diphenoxylate) used to treat the resulting diarrhea seem to prolong the disease, so they should not be used. (7:552)

192. **C.** Loperamide (Imodium®) is a schedule V controlled substance. It inhibits peristaltic activity by a direct effect on the musculature of the intestinal wall. Loperamide appears to be devoid of opium-like effects. Even after chronic administration of loperamide, the injection of the narcotic antagonist naloxone does not produce pupillary dilation. Furthermore, because of its long biological half-life (approximately 40 hours) it may be possible to use single daily doses to control chronic diarrhea. (3:1057–58)

193. **D.** Tricyclic antidepressants such as imipramine (Tofranil®) and amitriptyline (Elavil®) may block the uptake of guanethidine by adrenergic nerves, thereby inhibiting its antihypertensive action. (6:553)

194. **A.** Cyclobenzaprine (Flexeril®), an analogue of amitriptyline, is available for the treatment of acute voluntary muscle spasm. Because they are so alike in chemical structure, cyclobenzaprine and amitriptyline have essentially the same side effects and toxicity. (3:957–58; 17:296)

195. **A.** Although dextroamphetamine was the preferred drug for MBD for many years, methylphenidate (Ritalin®) has become the drug of choice, largely because of unjustified fears that the use of dextroamphetamine may predispose one to subsequent abuse. Pemoline (Cylert®), a schedule IV controlled substance, has been recently introduced for the treatment of MBD. While it is no more effective than either dextroamphetamine or methylphenidate, it certainly approaches these drugs in terms of efficacy and has the advantage of a longer biological half-life, permitting once-a-day dosing. This is desirable because multiple daily dosing often creates problems associated with drug administration while the child is in school (e.g., who administers the drug?).
B. Pemoline has a slower onset of clinical activity than either dextroamphetamine or methylphenidate. Improvement may not be observed for three to four weeks. Consequently the drug should not be discontinued before it has been given a reasonable therapeutic trial. (4:499–500; 33b:868–69)

196. **A.** Phospholine iodide is used in the treatment of glaucoma. Prolonged use of this agent results in reduced activity of pseudocholinesterase, the enzyme responsible for the metabolism of succinylcholine.

The action of succinylcholine as a muscle relaxant is enhanced in patients getting this combination, thereby possibly causing apnea and death. (8:206)

197. **E.** Although exchange transfusions have traditionally been used to manage hyperbilirubinemia, this treatment rarely decreases the bilirubin level to even half its pretransfusion level and exposes the neonate to the hazards of blood transfusion. More recently, phenobarbital has been found to be effective in lowering serum bilirubin levels. Apparently, phenobarbital enhances glucuronidation by stimulating synthesis of hepatic microsomal enzyme and by inducing production of bilirubin-binding Y protein. The dosage of phenobarbital is 5 mg every eight hours beginning six to eight hours after delivery for three to five days until serum bilirubin levels fall to below 10 mg/dl. Complete failure of this treatment can probably be attributed to discontinuing the drug prematurely. (6:119; 48:17–18)

198. **B.** Chlorpheniramine maleate will not displace warfarin from its protein-binding sites and has, therefore, less of a tendency to cause a therapeutic problem in this patient. All of the other choices have a high affinity for plasma proteins. (8:27, 43–44)

199. **E.** Phenylephrine is an adrenergic stimulant which is normally metabolized in the liver by the enzyme, monamine oxidase (MAO). In the presence of an MAO inhibitor such as pargyline, much higher and more toxic blood levels of phenylephrine will result, thereby causing an elevation in the patient's blood pressure. (8:176)

200. **A.** Each gram of protein supplies about 4 kcal; each gram of carbohydrate supplies about 4 kcal; and each gram of fat supplies about 9 kcal. It is obvious, therefore, that strictly on a weight basis, fats are better caloric sources than other nutrients. (33b:525)

201. **C.** Portagen® is a product used when conventional dietary fats may not be well absorbed, digested, or utilized. Its fat content consists of more than 95% medium-chain triglycerides which are more rapidly absorbed than the triglycerides of long-chain fatty acids present in conventional food fats. Patients suffering from steatorrhea (excessive loss of fats in the feces) are ideal candidates for dietary supplementation with Portagen®. (2b:211, 216; 33b:462–63)

202. **A.** Lytren® is an orally administered electrolyte solution containing dextrose, potassium chloride, and sodium, calcium, and magnesium salts. It is used to supply water and electrolytes in a balanced proportion in order to prevent serious deficits from occurring in patients suffering from mild to moderate fluid loss. (4:234)

203. **B.** Each gram of carbohydrate supplies 4 cal of energy to a patient. Since a liter of dextrose 5% solution contains 50 g of dextrose, the administration of the liter will supply the patient with approximately 200 cal. (33b:525)

204. **E.** Portagen® is a dietary product which contains protein, carbohydrate, and fat. More than 95% of the fat content consists of medium-chain triglycerides which are more rapidly absorbed than the long-chain fatty acids found in most conventional dietary fat sources. (2b:211, 216; 33b:462–63)

205. **D.** PKU or phenylketonuria is a condition characterized by the accumulation of high levels of phenylalanine in the blood due to a congenital metabolic defect. If left unmanaged, mental retardation or death may ensue. Treatment consists of following a carefully regulated low-phenylalanine diet that should be started in the first few weeks of life. Lofenalac® is a dietary product which contains a low concentration of phenylalanine. (4:217; 37:990)

206. **C.** Dicloxacillin is useful in the treatment of infections caused by penicillinase-producing gram-positive organisms. Since carbenicillin is not penicillinase-resistant, such a combination would be a rational one. (7:1698)

207. **B.** Of the drugs listed, erythromycin has the lowest degree of toxicity and the spectrum of action most similar to penicillin. Demeclocycline and tetracycline may inhibit skeletal growth in fetuses. Deposition of tetracyclines in the teeth of fetuses has been associated with enamel defects and staining of the teeth. Novobiocin may disturb liver function of the fetus and newborn infant. (7:1732, 1741)

208. **E.** Sulfamylon® cream applied topically to burns has been found to be quite effective in inhibiting the invasion of the affected site by both gram-positive and gram-negative bacteria. The cream is usually applied to a thickness of about 1/16 inch twice daily over the entire burned surface. Silver sulfadiazine is also used topically for the same purposes. (6:1120)

209. **B.** Parathyroid hormone exerts a major effect on bone metabolism because of its effect on calcium and phosphorus in the body. Parathyroid hormone produces an increase in renal excretion of phosphorus and a direct decalcification of bone. It is indicated only as replacement therapy after accidental removal of the parathyroid glands following thryroidectomy. Dihydrotachysterol and vitamin D are more commonly used to treat hypoparathyroidism. Both of these sterols are effective by mouth. Dihydrotachysterol is somewhat more effective and has a more rapid onset of action than vitamin D, which has a longer duration of action and is less expensive. (37:724)

210. **C.** Colchicine is one of the most valuable drugs available for the treatment of an acute attack of gout. The mechanism of action is not known but is believed to be interference with the inflammatory response of gout. Colchicine may alter other inflammatory states,

but the effects are less dramatic. The uricosuric drugs used in gout act by either increasing the rate of uric acid excretion by the kidney (i.e., probenecid and sulfinpyrazone) or by decreasing the rate of synthesis of uric acid (i.e., allopurinol). (33b:691–92)

211. **B.** Metyrapone is an inhibitor of 11-hydroxylation in the adrenal cortex. Through this inhibition, metyrapone interferes with the adrenal synthesis of cortisol and corticosterone. This, in turn, leads to the secretion of the precursor 11-deoxycortisol. In the presence of normal pituitary function, there is a compensatory increase in ACTH production. This stimulates the adrenal cortex, but because of the inhibition of 11-hydroxylation, cortisol production remains low and 11-deoxycortisol is produced in greater quantities. This response is a measure of the capacity of the anterior pituitary to produce ACTH. (17:367)

212. **B.** Tartar emetic is an intravenously administered anthelmintic agent. It is employed against *Schistosoma japonicum, S. mansoni,* and *S. haematobium.* It was once considered an outstanding emetic. However, it is no longer widely used for this purpose because of its slow action and toxicity. Doses of 200 mg (usual emetic dose is 30 mg) have been fatal. (17:659; 48:50)

213. **A.** Nylidrin is an indirect-acting cardiac stimulant and vasodilator. It acts by enhancing the cardiac stimulant and vasodilating properties of endogenous epinephrine. (17:91)

214. **B.** All of the other agents listed are useful in the treatment of petit mal but not in grand mal seizures. (7:315)

215. **A.** Glucose tolerance is impaired by the thiazides even though certain other sulfonamide derivatives are hypoglycemic agents. The degree of hyperglycemia induced by the thiazides is unimportant in patients with normal carbohydrate tolerance but may intensify the hyperglycemia of diabetes or precipitate glycosuria in persons predisposed to diabetes. (17:163)

216. **C.** Dopamine (Intropin®) is a sympathomimetic drug that acts directly on alpha and beta receptors and produces indirect effects due to release of norepinephrine. Dopamine also dilates renal and mesenteric vessels through a dopamine receptor. The hemodynamic effects of dopamine are dose related. At low infusion rates (1–5 μg/kg/min) dopamine increases renal blood flow without much change in cardiac output or total peripheral resistance. In higher doses (5–20 μg/kg/min), cardiac output and heart rate increase, the increase in renal perfusion persists, and total peripheral resistance is variable. At higher infusion rates, renal vasoconstriction occurs, total peripheral resistance rises, and blood pressure increases. Consequently, the infusion rate must be adjusted and carefully monitored to achieve the desired response. (33b:215, 218)

217. **B.** Because of the relatively poor aqueous solubility of chlordiazepoxide, the drug is reconstituted in a "special" diluent that consists primarily of propylene glycol. When injected intramuscularly, the drug is believed to precipitate at the injection site, forming a depot from which it slowly redissolves and becomes available for absorption. Compared to equal oral doses, intramuscular chlordiazepoxide is absorbed more slowly and produces lower blood levels. If large intramuscular doses of the drug are given repeatedly over a short period of time, it is quite likely that the patient will demonstrate symptoms of overdose several hours later when large amounts of the drug are absorbed from the multiple injections. (33b:846–47)

218. **C.** Amphogel® has a fairly high sodium content (7.0 mg/5 ml) and would be a poor choice for patients on salt-free diets. The use of a low sodium antacid, such as Riopan® (0.7 mg/5 ml), would be a more rational selection. (2b:13–16)

219. **C.** Dobutamine (Dobutrex®) is a beta-adrenergic agonist that is available for intravenous use as an inotropic drug. Although dobutamine is similar to isoproterenol (Isuprel®) in terms of its inotropic effect, dobutamine is relatively less potent than isoproterenol as a stimulator of peripheral beta receptors that mediate vasodilation. Consequently dobutamine produces an inotropic effect with comparatively little effect on preload, afterload, or heart rate. (25:1013; 33b:216–17)

220. **C.** The full therapeutic effect of the tricyclic antidepressants often takes several weeks to develop. During this period, many patients subjectively feel that their depression has worsened. On the other hand, the side effects of these drugs, sedation and anticholinergic effects, usually begin shortly after therapy is initiated. The pharmacist should discuss these anticipated effects with the patient. He should also consult the prescribing physician if it is apparent that an intensified depression may be serious enough to lead to suicide. (17:295–96; 44:386–88)

221. **D.** The theoretical advantage of administering insulin in IV glucose is that both insulin and glucose are delivered in constant proportions. Administration of insulin in this manner, however, can result in undesirable fluctuations in blood glucose levels. As much as 20% of the insulin added to an IV is bound to the flask and tubing. Proportionally greater binding occurs with lower doses of insulin. If the same administration set is used for subsequent infusions, the binding sites on the set may be saturated with insulin. This would be observed clinically as some improvement in control of blood glucose since subsequent binding would be to the IV bottle alone. Furthermore, even if the insulin dose is adjusted for binding by the flask, hyperglycemia may still occur after the administration set is changed. This, of course, does not mean that insulin should not be administered by IV infusion, but that the absorption of insulin by IV bottles and tubing

should be considered in accounting for unusual changes in blood glucose levels and in determining insulin doses, especially when low doses are contemplated. (40:90)

222. **C.** In general, all insulins are reasonably stable at room temperature (75°F). Regular insulin may lose 10% of its activity at room temperature after 18 months. Modified insulins will coagulate within a few days if they are stored at temperatures above 75°F. Although this does not result in a total loss in potency, it is markedly more difficult to withdraw a uniform dose and to predict the onset of action and duration of response. Traveling diabetics should be advised to avoid prolonged exposure of their insulin to very high temperatures, and that it is not necessary to refrigerate the vial in use. Insulin vials stored in pharmacies are required to be refrigerated because it is possible that they may be kept in stock for a long time. (6:1516; 48:287)

223. **B.** The sliding scale (or rainbow scale) is a method of determining insulin dosing based on periodic determinations of glucose and ketones in the urine. The physician prescribes the regular insulin dosage as a function of the number of pluses determined by the copper reduction (Clinitest®) glucose determination and the presence of urinary ketones. He may prescribe a fixed number of units for each plus (e.g., 4 units for each plus) or a more variable schedule (as in the problem above). At 4 PM the patient had a 4+ for glucose, for which 10 units of regular insulin are ordered. The patient also had moderate (Mod) amounts of ketones present, for which 2 units of regular insulin are ordered.

Total 4 PM dose: 10 units
2 units
12 units of regular insulin

C., E. Since the "sliding scale" is generally used to determine the 24-hour insulin requirements of a ketotic diabetic, the modified insulins (e.g., NPH) are not used. (33b:529; 44:285)

224. **B.** Hyperalimentation fluids are generally very hypertonic and hyperosmotic. Until the technique of subclavian vein catheterization was perfected, it was too irritating and inflammatory to use the usual sites of intravenous administration. Peripheral veins are not used in the administration of hypertonic nutrient solutions because of blood flow insufficient to provide the necessary dilution of the fluid to protect the intima of the vessel. (30:147)

225. **D.** Sudden discontinuation of dextrose solution may cause a rebound hypoglycemia in response to the sudden elimination of the sustained glucose load of the hyperalimentation solution. It is best to maintain the patient on a nominal amount of dextrose such as D5W.

B. Hyperchloremic metabolic acidosis may occur during hyperalimentation therapy when the total chloride ion content is high. The amino acids in the protein salts are usually chloride or hydrochloride salts. Additional amounts of chloride are obtained when sodium or potassium chlorides are added to the hyperalimentation solutions. It may be useful to supply either sodium or potassium as acetate salts.

C. Hyperosmotic nonketotic hyperglycemia is a result of infusing an overload of glucose. Causes include a too rapid infusion rate, dextrose solutions that are too concentrated, and malfunction of pancreatic secretion of insulin. (48:405)

226. **B.** Fats provide approximately 9 calories per gram. Because of their isotonicity, fat emulsions can be safely administered through peripheral veins. A commercial example of a fat emulsion is Intralipid®, a 10% soybean emulsion.

A. Ethanol provides 7 calories per gram. Disadvantages associated with ethanol are the fact that too-rapid infusion can cause heartburn and/or intoxication, and the fact that it cannot be used in patients with GI disease such as pancreatitis.

D. Hydrous dextrose provides 3.4 calories per gram. It is the usual source of calories in TPN formulations because of its safety, economy, and availability to the body.

E. Proteins provide 3 to 4 calories per gram. (48:684)

227. **D.** FreAmine II® differs from the other listed products in that it is a mixture of crystalline amino acids. While the product is more expensive than the other products, there is better control over the choice and amounts of specific essential amino acids present. Also the content of electrolytes is lower. (48:684)

228. **A.** The pH of a TPN formula is usually in the range of 5 to 6. The addition of akaline sodium bicarbonate will cause a loss of bicarbonate through the formation of carbon dioxide. (48:684)

229. **E.** Amino acids are the building blocks for body protein. For adequate nutrition, a diet must include a variety of amino acids, usually in the form of proteins. While many amino acids can be synthesized by the body, some amino acids cannot be synthesized. Their designation as "essential amino acids" implies that they are essential constituents in a protein diet.

A. Conjugated proteins are those found in nature combined with a nonprotein substance. Examples include the lipoproteins such as lecithin and the sterols, which consist of proteins combined with lipids. (1:428–29)

230. **D.** A dose of 40 mEq/l of potassium chloride will assist in maintaining normal serum levels and provide the 3.5:1 ratio of potassium to nitrogen necessary for protein synthesis. (30:148)

231. **E.** Downward—*cata*bolism indicates any destructive process by which complex substances are converted by living cells into more simple compounds. (11:271)

232. **A.** Apart—*dis*articulation is amputation or separation at a joint. (11:452)

233. **B.** Below—*infra*orbital refers to lying under or on the floor of the orbit. (11:781)

234. **D.** Middle—*meso*bronchitis indicates inflammation of the middle coat of the bronchi. (11:940)

235. **C.** Backward—*retro*grade means to retrace a former course. (11:1353)

236. **A.** For example, *celi*otomy is an incision into the abdominal cavity. (11:279)

237. **B.** *Cephal*algia is a headache. (11:288)

238. **D.** A coloproctitis is an inflammation of the colon and rectum. (11:341)

239. **C.** The pre*cor*dium is the region over the heart. (11:1249)

240. **E.** The term inter*cost*al means located between two ribs. (11:367)

241. **C.** (13:9)

242. **D.** (13:9)

243. **E.** (13:9)

244. **B.** Goiter is a condition characterized by the enlargement of the thyroid.

245. **A.** Klinefelter's syndrome is a series of symptoms related to diminished development of the seminiferous tubules of the testes.

246. **C.** Acromegaly is a disease caused by the presence of a pituitary tumor which results in the production of excess growth hormone.

247. **D.** Stein-Leventhal syndrome is a collection of symptoms related to the hypersecretion of androgens by the ovarian stroma.

248. **E.** Cushing's syndrome is a series of clinical symptoms related to the excessive secretion of cortisol by the adrenal cortex. (16:480, 507, 532, 600, 615)

249. **B.** Adams-Stokes disease or syndrome is caused by heart block. It is characterized by sudden attacks of unconsciousness, sometimes with convulsions. (11:453)

250. **A.** Addison's disease is due to hypofunction of the adrenal glands. It is characterized by a bronze pigmentation of the skin, progressive anemia, low blood pressure, diarrhea, and severe prostration. (11:453)

251. **C.** Bright's disease is a term used to describe kidney disease characterized by proteinuria and glomerulonephritis. (11:454)

252. **D.** Hodgkin's disease affects lymphoidal tissue. There is progressive enlargement of lymph nodes, spleen, and other lymphoid tissue. (11:457)

253. **E.** Myasthenia gravis is characterized by fatigue and exhaustion of muscles. Although progressive paralysis of muscles occurs, there are no sensory changes or atrophy. (11:1004)

254. **E.** (11:1180)

255. **B.** Graves' disease is a thyroid disorder of unknown etiology. Other symptoms include acceleration of pulse rate, sweating, nervousness, psychic disturbances, emaciation, and increased metabolic rate. (11:457)

256. **C.** (11:707)

257. **D.** This is a nonsuppurative disease of the labyrinth. (11:460)

258. **A.** A gastric secretion stimulant (caffeine) is given one hour before the administration of azuresin. If gastric secretion is normal, hydrochloric acid displaces the dye from the resin portion of azuresin. The dye is then absorbed and excreted in the urine within two hours. The concentration of excreted dye can be estimated by comparison to a color chart. (1:1217)

259. **B.** Congo red is injected into the blood. Disappearance of the dye from the blood indicates retention by abnormal amyloid deposits. (1:1217)

260. **D.** Phenolsulfonphthalein (phenol red) is injected by either the IM or IV route. Approximately 80% of the dye is excreted within two hours when kidney function causes either delayed or more incomplete elimination of the dye. (1:1216)

261. **C.** After IV injection, Evans blue combines with plasma protein. A blood sample is withdrawn and assayed to estimate total blood volume. (1:1217)

262. **E.** The dye solution is injected intravenously and a blood sample is withdrawn after 30 minutes for comparison with a standard. A normally functioning liver will excrete most of the dye within that 30-minute period. (1:1214)

263. **C.** In order to limit destruction by acid hydrolysis, penicillin G tablets should be taken on an empty stomach when gastric acid is at its lowest level. Pentids® should be taken one hour before or two hours after meals. (4:690; 10)

264. **B.** Indocin® should be taken with food, immediately after meals, or with antacids to reduce gastric irritation. (4:368, 385; 10)

265. **D.** Colace® is a surfactant and may increase the absorption of mineral oil if given concurrently. (4:1080; 10)

266. **A.** Sulfonamides are taken with a large volume of water to insure a volume of urine adequate to keep the excretory products in solution. Crystalluria has occurred with some sulfonamides. (4:773; 10)

267. **E.** Dulcolax® tablets are enteric coated to prevent gastric irritation. (4:1074; 10)

268. **C.** Milk and antacids reduce the absorption of tetracyclines by forming insoluble complexes. (4:1035; 10)

269. **B.** Large doses of salicylates have often been associated with bleeding problems, especially in patients taking oral anticoagulants. The bleeding may be due to direct gastric irritation, suppression of platelet functions, or a true hypoprothrombinemic effect. (6:1338; 10)

270. **A.** Foods or beverages containing significant amounts of tyramine must be avoided by individuals taking MAO inhibitors such as Pargyline®. Because of hepatic MAO inhibition, ingested tyramine escapes the normal deamination and releases an excessive amount of norepinephrine from storage granules at nerve endings. The hypertensive crisis which results leads to headaches, fever, and sometimes death due to intracranial bleeding. (6:183; 10)

271. **D.** The presence of food or antacids in the stomach lessens the gastric irritation caused by Butazolidin®. (6:341; 10)

272. **E.** (17:390)

273. **B.** (33b:531)

274. **C.** (17:386)

275. **A.** (17:386)

276. **B.** (17:386)

277. **D.** (17:388)

278. **D.** (17:386)

279. **B.** The chapter that discusses antacids lists commercial products with the sodium content of each where the data were available. (2b:3–17)

280. **D.** *The United States Dispensatory* usually presents a more detailed discussion of drug doses, ranges, and toxicity than that found in the USP or NF. For example, the toxicity section for nitrofurazone lists data obtained in both animals and human beings. (5:787)

281. **B.** Each of the chapters in the *Handbook* covers a specific group of OTC products. Usually the anatomy and physiology of the body area affected is discussed. Also the pharmacological action of ingredients commonly included in the OTC products is considered. Tables are present that list commercial products, manufacturers, ingredients, and levels of ingredients when known. For example, the ingredients in Sominex® are listed in the section discussing sleep aids. (2b:237)

282. **C.** *The Physicians' Desk Reference* is divided into several sections, one of which lists pharmaceutical companies with the products manufactured by each. (1:61; 25:1–36)

283. **A.** *Facts and Comparisons* lists prescription and some nonprescription drug products by pharmacological classifications. Those prescription-only vitamins that contain fluoride are listed together so that the pharmacist can compare formulas and levels of ingredients. (3:62–64)

284. **D.** The USD usually presents detailed discussions of the pharmacology of a drug, often with literature citations. For example, the section on the action and therapeutic uses of nitrofurazone contains several references for further information. Although the book emphasizes USP and NF drugs, important nonofficial drugs are also discussed. (5:787)

285. **C.** The PDR has a colored-plate reference section that pictures products for easy identification. The section is subdivided by individual manufacturers. (25:403–40)

286. **E.** Most drug monographs list identification tests which will aid in the qualitative identification of a drug. For example, the USP monograph for imipramine HCl describes three identification tests. (18:248)

287. **A.** *Facts and Comparisons* features a cost index which indicates the relative cost of similar products based upon cost per ml, per tablet, or other common dosage base. (3:988–89)

288. **E.** The approximate solubilities of USP articles are listed in table form. Among the solvents listed are water, boiling water, alcohol, chloroform, and ether. A similar table is presented in the NF for articles official in that book. (18:775; 19:1045)

289. **D.** (31:119–44)

290. **C.** (31:119–44)

291. **A.** (31:119–44)

292. **E.** (31:119–44)

293. **C.** (31:119–44)

294. **D.** (31:119–44)

295. **B.** (31:119–44)

296. **C.** (31:119–44)

CHAPTER 8

Post-Test

You have come a long way through over 1350 test items. This post-test should confirm what you may already feel, i.e., confidence that your time and effort have been well spent. You should be able to answer 40 or more questions without guessing.

Of course, the post-test is also a learning and self-assessment experience. As with the pretest, each answer has a notation directing your attention to a related question in one of the chapters. For missed questions look back at the similar ones in the chapter and study the commentaries and the reference sources.

Directions: Each of the questions or incomplete statements below is followed by five suggested answers or completions. Select the BEST answer in each case.

1. A pharmacist adds 1 g of calcium chloride ($CaCl_2 \cdot 2H_2O$) to a 500-ml bottle of D5W. How many mEq of calcium chloride are present in each ml of dilution? (atomic wt. Ca = 40; MW $CaCl_2$ = 11; H_2O = 18)
   A. 0.014
   B. 0.027
   C. 0.036
   D. 0.041
   E. 13.6

2. The administration of which of the following agents may antagonize the action of methenamine mandelate (Mandelamine®)?
   A. tetracycline HCl
   B. sulfisoxazole
   C. morphine sulfate
   D. ascorbic acid
   E. aspirin

3. The presence of ascorbic acid in the urine will give a false-positive result with
   A. Tes-Tape®
   B. Ketostix®
   C. Clinistix®
   D. Benedict's solution
   E. Acetest® Tablets

4. Which of the following is true?
   A. digitoxin cannot be administered intravenously
   B. digoxin has a longer serum half-life than digitoxin
   C. digitoxin is more lipid soluble than digoxin
   D. digitoxin has a more rapid onset of action than digoxin
   E. none of the above are true

5. How many grains of pilocarpine nitrate are needed to prepare two fluid ounces of a 7.5% solution?
   A. 4.5 gr
   B. 6.8 gr
   C. 7.2 gr
   D. 68 gr
   E. 72 gr

6. Phenobarbital is a metabolite of
   A. succinimide
   B. phenytoin
   C. glutethimide
   D. primidone
   E. ethchlorvynol

7. Glucagon increases blood glucose levels by
   A. inhibiting insulin release
   B. inhibiting glucose uptake by insulin-dependent tissues
   C. stimulating lipolysis in fat tissue
   D. stimulating hepatic gluconeogenesis and glycogenolysis
   E. increasing gastrointestinal absorption of glucose

8. A pharmacist has a stock bottle containing 1% W/V sodium fluoride in purified water. How

much of this solution should be used to prepare the following prescription?

Rx
Sodium Flouride q.s.
Purified Water q.s. 30 ml
Sig: gtt xx dil to one quart contains 6 ppm NaF

A. 3 ml
B. 9 ml
C. 17 ml
D. 18 ml
E. none of these

9. Bentonite magma exhibits which two rheological properties?

A. plastic and thixotropic
B. pseudoplastic and thixotropic
C. pseudoplastic and Newtonian
D. Newtonian and thixotropic
E. thixotropic and dilatant

10. Equal doses of two brands of drug A are administered by the following routes: oral, intravenous, intramuscular, sublingual, and subcutaneous. We would expect that

A. if inequivalence is demonstrated in the oral formulations, it will also be demonstrated in all of the other dosage forms
B. actual differences in bioavailability could be demonstrated in only the oral and the sublingual dosage forms
C. actual differences in bioavailability would be present only in the oral formulation
D. no difference in bioavailability would be demonstrated by intravenous administration
E. meaningful differences could be demonstrated only if the formulations for each of the above dosage forms were identical

11. In comparison with boric acid, salicylic acid has

A. a higher pK_a
B. the same pK_a
C. a lower pK_a
D. a lower K_a
E. a lower pK_b

12. In patients with excessive serum levels of copper, which of the following agents would be indicated?

A. penicillamine
B. cholestyramine resin
C. Kayexalate®
D. barium sulfate
E. magnesium sulfate

13. A physician needs 60 ml of an isotonic solution of 2% tetracaine hydrochloride. How many mg of sodium chloride should be included in the formula? (The E value for tetracaine hydrochloride is 0.18.)

A. 160
B. 270
C. 320
D. 540
E. none of these

14. Terbutaline sulfate (Brethine®) would be expected to exert which of the following effects?

A. bronchodilation
B. increased heart rate
C. increased blood pressure
D. beta-adrenergic stimulation
E. all of the above

15. The antihypertensive agent most likely to produce severe depression is

A. methylodopa (Aldomet®)
B. hydralazine (Apresoline®)
C. reserpine (Serpasil®)
D. mecamylamine (Inversine®)
E. veratrum alkaloids

16. A hospital pharmacy has a 1-pint bottle of Hydrochloric Acid USP labeled 36.5% W/W, specific gravity 1.18. How many ml of Diluted Hydrochloric Acid USP (10% W/V; specific gravity 1.04) can be prepared?

A. 1300
B. 1463
C. 1726
D. 2040
E. 5580

17. Equal doses of a drug are given by oral and intravenous routes. The area under the serum concentration–time curves is determined to be equal for both routes of administration. We can conclude that

A. oral administration will produce the same blood levels as will intravenous administration
B. the total amount of drug available is the same by both routes
C. the oral route will produce as rapid a response as will intravenous administration
D. different oral formulations of this drug will be bioequivalent
E. the oral route will be as effective as the intravenous route

18. Which type of isomerism is illustrated by the structures I and II shown below?

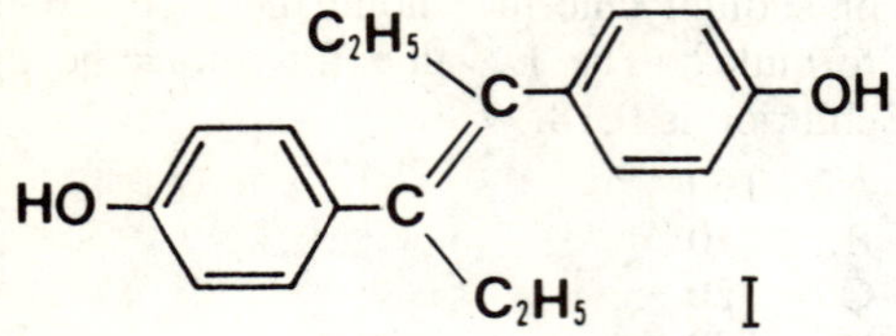

I

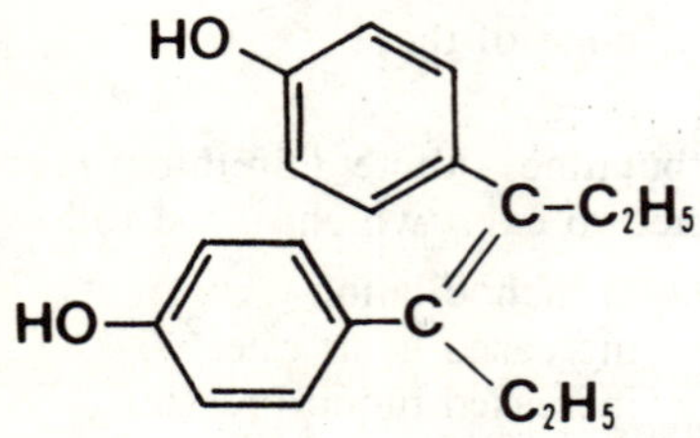

II

19. Which of the following is true of cholestyramine resin?
   A. it is not absorbed from the GI tract
   B. it is a cationic exchange resin
   C. it is used to increase the synthesis of cholesterol
   D. it is commercially available as a viscous syrup
   E. all of the above are true

20. The greatest drug concentration gradient between blood and tissues will occur when the drug is administered by
   A. the intradermal route
   B. the subcutaneous route
   C. intravenous push (bolus)
   D. the intramuscular route
   E. intravenous infusion (continuous)

21. The *National Formulary* specifies that a set of weights of what class should be used when performing the tests for evaluating prescription balances?
   A. A
   B. C
   C. P
   D. Q
   E. T

22. Penicillin-resistant organisms elaborate penicillinase, which inactivates the penicillin by
   A. oxidation to peroxypenicillin
   B. hydrolysis to penicilloic acid
   C. precipitation as the water-soluble penicillic acid
   D. chelation with heavy metals
   E. blocking the enzyme responsible for penicillin uptake by the organisms

23. Retinoic acid is used therapeutically
   A. by the oral route only
   B. to accelerate the production of epithelial cells in the skin
   C. to reverse the symptoms of psoriasis
   D. to promote healing of actinic keratoses
   E. for none of the purposes listed above

24. The structure shown below represents which category of surfactant?

$$C_{17}H_{35}\overset{\overset{\large O}{\|}}{C}-OCH_2\underset{\underset{\large OH}{|}}{C}HCH_2OH$$

   A. cationic
   B. amphoteric
   C. nonionic
   D. lipemic
   E. anionic

25. The recommended route of administration for diazoxide (Hyperstat®) when used in treating hypertensive crisis is
   A. deep IM
   B. IV push
   C. SC
   D. PO
   E. inhalation

26. Which of the following drugs is commonly used to treat drug-induced parkinsonism?
   A. dopamine (Intropin®)
   B. diazepam (Valium®)
   C. sodium valproate (Depakene®)
   D. methylphenidate (Ritalin®)
   E. benztropine (Cogentin®)

27. Convert the blood level of 0.2 mg/l to μg/dl.
   A. 0.0002 μg/dl
   B. 20 μg/dl
   C. 200 μg/dl
   D. 2000 μg/dl
   E. none of the above

28. Assume that drug A follows first-order kinetics and is eliminated entirely by renal excretion; how would the half-life of drug A be expected to change in a patient with impaired renal function? It will
   A. be increased only if liver impairment is also present
   B. be decreased only if liver impairment is also present
   C. be increased
   D. be decreased
   E. remain constant

29. Which of the following agents is indicated for use as an antipruritic agent because of its ability to antagonize the action of 5-hydroxytryptamine?

A. hydroxyzine (Atarax®)
B. chlorpheniramine maleate (Chlor-Trimeton®)
C. cyproheptadine (Periactin®)
D. promethazine (Phenergan®)
E. triamcinolone acetonide (Aristocort®)

30. The chemical reaction shown below is an example of

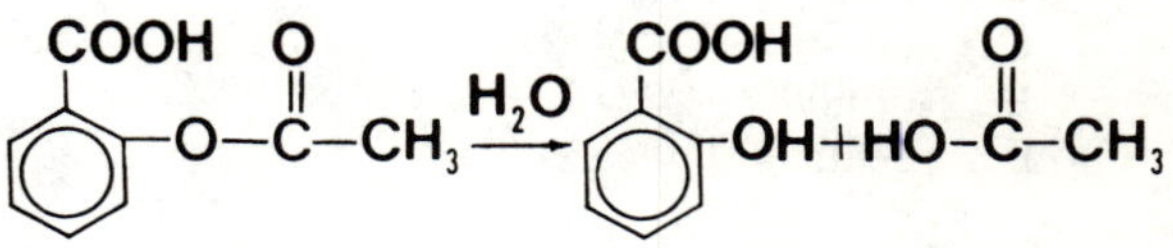

A. esterification
B. neutralization
C. hydrolysis
D. saponification
E. chelation

31. Acetylcysteine is usually administered by which of the following routes?

A. inhalation
B. IM
C. SC
D. orally
E. IV

32. A pharmacist wishes to prepare 120 g of 0.6% coal tar ointment. How much 1% coal tar ointment must be mixed with zinc oxide paste to obtain the desired strength?

A. 0.72 g
B. 7.2 g
C. 20 g
D. 48 g
E. none of the above

33. Colchicine is believed to relieve the pain of acute attacks of gout by

A. complexing uric acid in the urine
B. inhibiting the formation of sodium urate crystals
C. inhibiting the synthesis of uric acid
D. increasing the excretion of uric acid
E. blocking nerve transmission in the affected area

34. Although epinephrine is a useful drug for open-angle glaucoma, it is contraindicated in narrow-angle glaucoma because it

A. is a vasoconstrictor
B. is a mydriatic
C. is a carbonic anhydrase inhibitor
D. reduces the outflow of aqueous humor
E. stimulates the formation of aqueous humor

35. A pharmacy has 20 g of a 5% hydrocortisone cream. How many grams of a 1% hydrocortisone cream must be added to obtain a 2% strength cream?

A. 5 g
B. 20 g
C. 26.7 g
D. 60 g
E. none of the above

36. The process of reverse osmosis can be used to prepare

A. Alcohol USP
B. Isopropyl Alcohol USP
C. Milk of Magnesia USP
D. Purified Water USP
E. all of the above

37. Assuming that a fixed dose of a drug having a biological half-life of 24 hours is administered on a once-a-day basis, we would expect steady-state plasma levels to be attained after

A. 12 hours
B. one day
C. two days
D. five days
E. 10 days

38. The compound pictured below is

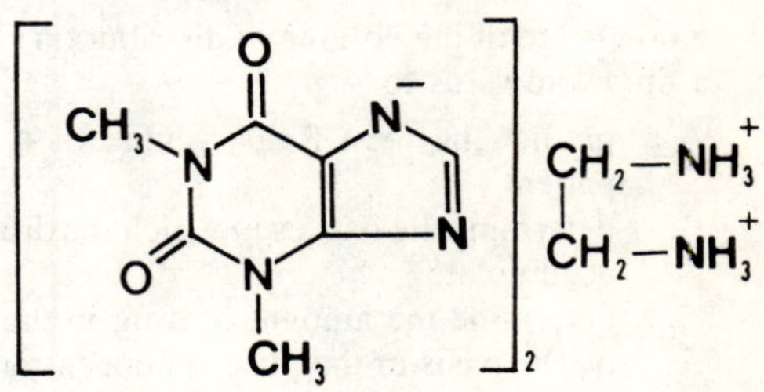

A. phenobarbital
B. aminophylline
C. uric acid
D. dimethyl xanthine
E. dixanthoethylenediamine

39. A patient who is on allopurinol (Zyloprim®) for gout is about to receive 6-mercaptopurine (Purinethol®) for acute lymphatic leukemia. Under these circumstances

A. some other uricosuric should be used
B. some other antineoplastic should be used
C. the dose of the allopurinol should be reduced

D. the dose of the 6-mercaptopurine should be reduced
E. a uricosuric drug will not be necessary because 6-mercaptopurine will also increase uric acid excretion

40. Clorox® contains 5.25% sodium hypochlorite. How many ml of Clorox® should be added to five gallons of water to obtain a final concentration of 1/500 sodium hypochlorite for a disinfecting solution?

A. 10
B. 38
C. 52.5
D. 76
E. 105

41. Disposable plastic syringes are molded from all of the following polymers *except*

A. nylon
B. polyethylene
C. polypropylene
D. styrene
E. all are used

42. Yellow wax is a/an

A. aliphatic fraction from petroleum
B. natural product from the honeycomb of the bee
C. mineral wax
D. purified wax from animal fat and bone
E. synthetic wax prepared from polymers

43. Knowledge of the volume of distribution (V_d) of a drug allows us to

A. predict the total fluid volume of a given patient
B. determine the tissues in which the drug will accumulate
C. determine the amount of drug in the body on the basis of the plasma concentration at any given time
D. calculate the half-life of the drug
E. determine the bioavailability of the drug

44. Sodium bisulfite is included in some pharmaceutical solutions as a/an

A. antimicrobial preservative
B. antioxidant
C. buffering agent
D. chelating agent
E. pH adjustor

45. The following structure is ____ aminobenzoic acid.

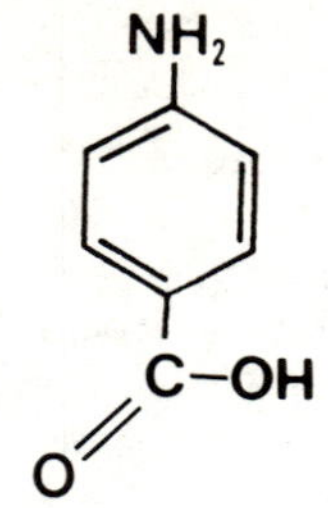

A. meta-
B. para-
C. duo-
D. ortho-
E. dextro-

46. A pharmacist adds 1 pint of 1:750 Zephiran® Chloride solution to 1 gallon of 0.9% Sodium Chloride Solution. What is the % W/V concentration of Zephiran® Chloride in the final dilution?

A. 0.015%
B. 0.017%
C. 0.13%
D. 0.9%
E. none of these

47. Polymyxin B and colistin are both members of the chemical group known as

A. polypeptides
B. macrolides
C. aminoglycosides
D. cephalosporins
E. sulfonylureas

48. Sixty-five mg of dextropropoxyphene HCl (Darvon®) is approximately equivalent to how much codeine?

A. 16.25 mg
B. 32.5 mg
C. 65.0 mg
D. 130 mg
E. 195 mg

49. A normal hematocrit for a healthy man would be

A. 0.5
B. 1.0
C. 10
D. 20
E. 45

50. The activity of topical nasal decongestants is mainly a

    A. direct counteraction to histamine
    B. drying effect on nasal fluids
    C. local vasoconstriction effect
    D. local vasodilation effect
    E. counter-irritation effect

Post-Test Answers

1. **B.** (Ph Calc:19)
2. **B.** (Pcol:109)
3. **D.** (Ph Chem:14)
4. **C.** (Pcol:64)
5. **D.** (Ph Calc:15)
6. **D.** (Pcol:28)
7. **D.** (Clin Pharm:182)
8. **C.** (Ph Calc:40)
9. **A.** (Pharm:36)
10. **D.** (Biopharm:1)
11. **C.** (Ph Chem:29)
12. **A.** (Pcol:37)
13. **C.** (Ph Calc:47)
14. **E.** (Pcol:21)
15. **C.** (Pcol:121)
16. **D.** (Ph Calc:26)
17. **B.** (Biopharm:48)
18. **B.** (Ph Chem:23)
19. **A.** (Pcol:13)
20. **C.** (Clin Pharm:89)
21. **C.** (Pharm:14)
22. **B.** (Ph Chem:42)
23. **B.** (Pcol:18)
24. **C.** (Ph Chem:176–79)
25. **B.** (Pcol:101)
26. **E.** (Clin Pharm:10)
27. **B.** (Ph Calc:2)
28. **C.** (Biopharm:58)
29. **C.** (Pcol:111)
30. **C.** (Ph Calc:164)
31. **A.** (Pcol:10)
32. **E.** (Ph Calc:50)
33. **B.** (Pcol:70)
34. **B.** (Clin Pharm:132)
35. **D.** (Ph Calc:14)
36. **D.** (Pharm:56)
37. **D.** (Biopharm:57)
38. **B.** (Ph Chem:6)
39. **D.** (Clin Pharm:184)
40. **B.** (Ph Calc:7)
41. **A.** (Pharm:44)
42. **B.** (Ph Chem:78)
43. **C.** (Biopharm:25)
44. **B.** (Pharm:22)
45. **B.** (Ph Chem:147, 154)
46. **A.** (Ph Calc:41)
47. **A.** (Pcol:38)
48. **B.** (Pcol:87)
49. **E.** (Clin Pharm:80)
50. **C.** (Pharm:138)